Nutrition and Disease Management for Veterinary Technicians and Nurses

Nutrition and Disease Management for Veterinary Technicians and Nurses

SECOND EDITION

By Ann Wortinger and Kara M. Burns

WILEY

This edition first published 2015 © 2015 by John Wiley & Sons, Inc.

First edition, 2007 © Blackwell Publishing

Editorial offices:

  1606 Golden Aspen Drive, Suites 103 and 104, Ames, Iowa 50014-8300, USA
  The Atrium, Southern Gate, Chichester, West Sussex, PO19 8SQ, UK
  9600 Garsington Road, Oxford, OX4 2DQ, UK

For details of our global editorial offices, for customer services and for information about how to apply for permission to reuse the copyright material in this book please see our website at www.wiley.com/wiley-blackwell.

Authorization to photocopy items for internal or personal use, or the internal or personal use of specific clients, is granted by Blackwell Publishing, provided that the base fee is paid directly to the Copyright Clearance Center, 222 Rosewood Drive, Danvers, MA 01923. For those organizations that have been granted a photocopy license by CCC, a separate system of payments has been arranged. The fee codes for users of the Transactional Reporting Service are ISBN-13: 978-1-1185-0927-2/2015.

Designations used by companies to distinguish their products are often claimed as trademarks. All brand names and product names used in this book are trade names, service marks, trademarks or registered trademarks of their respective owners. The publisher is not associated with any product or vendor mentioned in this book.

The contents of this work are intended to further general scientific research, understanding, and discussion only and are not intended and should not be relied upon as recommending or promoting a specific method, diagnosis, or treatment by health science practitioners for any particular patient. The publisher and the author make no representations or warranties with respect to the accuracy or completeness of the contents of this work and specifically disclaim all warranties, including without limitation any implied warranties of fitness for a particular purpose. In view of ongoing research, equipment modifications, changes in governmental regulations, and the constant flow of information relating to the use of medicines, equipment, and devices, the reader is urged to review and evaluate the information provided in the package insert or instructions for each medicine, equipment, or device for, among other things, any changes in the instructions or indication of usage and for added warnings and precautions. Readers should consult with a specialist where appropriate. The fact that an organization or Website is referred to in this work as a citation and/or a potential source of further information does not mean that the author or the publisher endorses the information the organization or Website may provide or recommendations it may make. Further, readers should be aware that Internet Websites listed in this work may have changed or disappeared between when this work was written and when it is read. No warranty may be created or extended by any promotional statements for this work. Neither the publisher nor the author shall be liable for any damages arising herefrom.

Library of Congress Data applied for

ISBN : 9781118509272

A catalogue record for this book is available from the British Library.

Wiley also publishes its books in a variety of electronic formats. Some content that appears in print may not be available in electronic books.

Typeset in 8.5/12pt MeridienLTStd by Laserwords Private Limited, Chennai, India

SKY10024405_012521

Contents

Preface

Nutrition is an area of veterinary medicine that is very easy for the technician to have an active role in. Many of the commercial food producers have even concentrated on educating technicians on nutrition. There are nutrition tracks at most national conferences, as well as on-line learning programs.

As with any other area of education, you still need to know the basics to understand what is being taught, and unfortunately this is often not addressed for technicians. While chemistry, microbiology and math are required at most schools, even these do not adequately address basic animal nutrition. We all are taught the basic nutrients in a diet: water, protein, fats and carbohydrates, but how do they work together, what happens to them inside the body and what changes occur with aging or disease?

So where does this leave a technician who wants to know more about nutrition, who wants to really understand what is going on inside the animal? Usually they start by going through the available veterinary nutrition books, if you aren't overwhelmed and terrified by the first chapter it's a miracle. These books are often more detailed than a technician needs or wants to know; you tend to get lost in these details and miss the basic points. If you go to human nutrition books, these do not address the unique nutritional needs of our most common species, dogs, cats, horses, birds and pocket pets, though they can often address basic nutrition in a less technical manner. Some people enroll in an online program, but the basics are still often missing from these and referencing these later on can be difficult. I love having reference books available whenever I have a question or need clarification on a point of interest, and I often have questions and need clarification. Many commercial food producers also provide technical helplines, but you still need to understand the basics before you can ask for clarification!

I have plowed through nutrition books from the very basic pet owner books to the extremely technical veterinary books; all of them have something to offer, but will you read long enough to understand it? I was very fortunate to have a number of veterinarians who were willing to explain the points I didn't understand, to correct me when I misunderstood a concept and to direct me to areas that I may find interesting. Without them, I would have had a much more difficult time understanding and utilizing nutrition in our day-to-day practice. After all, that is the ultimate goal of nutrition isn't it?

My goal in writing this book was to provide a book for a technician that was both relevant and technical but understandable and usable. This is not a dummied down version of a veterinary nutrition book, but one that focuses on the unique interests of technicians and how we use nutrition in practice and at home. For the second edition I have asked my good friend and partner in nutrition, Kara Burns to provide her spin on disease management and alternate species nutrition. I am very excited to have Kara helping to improve the second edition.

The book is organized into five sections. The first section addresses the basics of nutrition by looking at energy and nutrients, how the individual nutrients of water, carbohydrates, fats, proteins, vitamins and minerals are utilized by the body, digestions and absorption of these nutrients and finally energy balance. Section 2 covers nutritional requirements for cats and dogs by going through the history and regulation of pets food, understanding how to read pet food labels, understanding nutrient content and types of foods and how they differ, and evaluating raw food diets, preservatives and homemade diets. Section 3 covers different feeding regimens, body condition scoring both definition and use, and takes feeding from pregnancy and lactation through neonatal, growth and adult maintenance feeding and into geriatrics. Section 3 also covers feeding for performance animals, special feeding requirement for cats, nutrition myths, the use of nutritional support and assisted feeding techniques. Section 4 is new and covers nutritional management of disease, looking at GI disease, hepatic disease, weight management, FLUTD and others. The final section, also new, addresses the feeding management of other species, including horses, birds, and pocket pets. Each section will build on the information covered in previous sections, allowing for practical use of the information learned.

My cats and chickens are not thrilled when I start calculating caloric intake, nutrient distribution or metabolizable energy. I am sure that Kara's varied pet population feels much the same way, but they too will ultimately benefit from our knowledge, as have innumerable clients, patients, co-workers and students.

My hope is that through this book you to will come to appreciate the important role nutrition plays in veterinary medicine, both through prevention and therapeutic use. You will have a better understanding of basic digestion, nutrient use by the body and how food can affect our patients from the pre-natal period through their death (hopefully many years down the line). And lastly that you will bring nutrition into your practice and use it to improve the quality of care that is provided to your patients. Nutrition is an ever-evolving field in veterinary medicine, and I hope this book serves as a stepping stone for future learning. Kara and I love veterinary nutrition and we hope that you will come to love it too!

Ann Wortinger

Acknowledgments

Working on this second edition has been challenging on many fronts. I changed jobs half way through, continued with my speaking schedule, had a son get married and my youngest child graduated and moved out. Enough activities to distract the most hardy of writers.

By adding Kara Burns as cowriter, we have been able to expand the chapters and information provided, allowing both of us to further spread the nutrition word! As many of you know, Kara and I were on the organizing committee for the Veterinary Technician Specialty in Nutrition, and are now on the Executive committee for the VTS (Nutrition). A labor of love for both of us!

My feline editorial staff has changed since the last edition, Cheyenne-Abyssinian extraordinaire has been replaced by Dusty, our blind Detroit stray; we also lost Daisy much too soon and added Poppy a TNR rescue. Lily and Rose helped to train my new recruits in what is expected of a feline editorial staff at our house. You ladies had the unfailing ability to know exactly which book or article I was currently working out of, or would need next. You very kindly marked it with your furry bodies. Supervision was conducted from the back of my chair, when needed, and Dusty needed to be taught that crossing the keyboard was not the way to get across my desk. How does anyone work without a feline editorial staff?

Ann Wortinger

Writing *Nutrition and Disease Management for Veterinary Technicians and Nurses, Second Edition* with Ann Wortinger has been the realization of a dream. I do not believe there are two people with more passion for nutrition than Ann and myself. We both see the value of proper nutrition and the foundation for health that proper nutrition provides to veterinary patients. Thank you, Ann, for adding me as an author and for your friendship!

Thank you to the love of my life Ellen Lowery, DVM, PhD, MBA. You make my life complete and give me the courage to pursue all of my dreams. Thank you for your encouragement and support in this endeavor and for constantly supporting my desire to write this book!

My parents, Bernard "Red" and Marilyn Burns instilled in me a love of all animals. Additionally, I saw the power of nutrition first hand as my father dealt with Type 1 diabetes his entire life, eventually succumbing to complications of the disease. Veterinary nutrition fell naturally into place from these experiences.

I have an expansive editorial staff that has contributed their supervisory abilities along this writing journey. Felines Prancer, O'Malley, and Oreo have been consistently knocking all references off of my desk in an obvious attempt to keep me from sitting in one place for too long. Whenever I had a writing "block," I would sit back and watch our horses, Socks and Eddie, running through the pasture – what an awesome sight. All six of our birds would take turns providing beautiful sounds to help the writing process. And yes – Pudge and Fribble, the reigning "Best Dogs Ever" (Fribble has the additional title of "cutest dogever") were with me every step of the way. Thank you all for bringing such joy to my life.

Kara M. Burns

About the companion website

This book is accompanied by a companion website:

www.wiley.com/go/wortinger/nutrition

The website includes:

* Cases for self-study and review
* Review questions and answers
* The figures from the book in PowerPoint

SECTION 1
Basics of Nutrition

1 Nutrients and Energy

Introduction

Animals, unlike plants, are unable to generate their own energy, and require a balanced diet to grow normally, maintain health once they are mature, reproduce, and perform physical work.[1,2] Plants are able to convert solar energy from the sun into carbohydrates thorough a process called photosynthesis, but they too require water, vitamins and minerals for optimal growth and production. Animals in turn either eat plants or eat other animals that eat plants to obtain their energy.[1,2]

Nutrients

For animals, energy is provided in the diet through nutrients. Nutrients are components of the diet that have specific functions within the body and contribute to growth, tissue maintenance and optimal health.[1,2] Essential nutrients are those components that cannot be synthesized by the body at a rate adequate to meet the body's needs, so they must be included in the diet. These nutrients are used as structural components as with bone and muscle, enhancing or being involved in metabolism, transporting substances such as oxygen and electrolytes, maintaining normal body temperature and supplying energy.[1,2] Nonessential nutrients can be synthesized by the body and can be obtained either through production by the body or through the diet.[1,2] Nutrients are further divided into six major categories; water, carbohydrates, proteins, fats, vitamins and minerals.

Energy is not one of the major nutrients, but after water it is the most critical component of the diet with energy needs always being the first requirement to be met in an animal's diet.[1,2] After energy needs have been met, nutrients become available for other metabolic functions.[1,2] Approximately 50–80% of the dry matter of a dog's or cat's diet is used for energy.[1,2] The body obtains energy from nutrients by oxidation of the chemical bonds found in proteins, carbohydrates and fats.[2]

Oxidation is the process of a substance combining with oxygen resulting in the loss of electrons.[3] This oxidation occurs during digestion, absorption and transport of nutrients into the body's cells.[2] The most important energy-containing compound produced during this oxidative process is adenosine triphosphate (ATP), a common high-energy compound composed of a purine (adenosine), a sugar (ribose) and three phosphate groups.[2,3]

The biochemical reactions that occur within the body either use or release energy. Anabolic reactions require energy for completion, and catabolic reactions release energy upon completion.[2] ATP and other energy-trapping compounds pick up part of the energy released from one process and transfer it to the other processes.[2] This energy is used for pumping ions, molecular synthesis and to activate contractile proteins, these three processes essentially describe the total use of energy by the animal.[2] Without the energy supplied through the diet, these reactions would not occur and death would follow.[2]

ATP is the usable form of energy for the body, but not a good form of energy storage because it is used quickly after being produced.[2] Glycogen and triglycerides are longer-term storage forms of energy.[2] In fasting animals, when the body needs energy it uses stored glycogen first, stored fat second and finally as last resort amino acids from body protein.[2] The fatty acids found in triglycerides are not able to be converted into glucose; only the glycerol backbone can be utilized for this purpose. For proteins, they must undergo a process called gluconeogenesis to be converted into usable glucose, and not all proteins are able to undergo this process.[4]

Nutrition and Disease Management for Veterinary Technicians and Nurses, Second Edition. Ann Wortinger, Kara M. Burns
© 2015 John Wiley & Sons, Inc. Published 2015 by John Wiley & Sons, Inc.
Companion Website: www.wiley.com/go/wortinger/nutrition

Measures of Energy

Energy represents the capacity to do work. This is measured most commonly in the United States as a calorie. A calorie is the amount of heat that is required to increase the temperature of 1 kilogram of water from 14.5 °C to 15.5 °C (or 1 °C).[4] As this unit of measure is very small indeed, we commonly use the term kilocalorie (1000 calories). When we look at food labels, this is the unit that is being referenced, a kilocalorie, or kcal.

Although kcal is what is used in the United States, a joule is the SI unit measure of energy. 1 kcal = 4.184 joules. As with calories, a joule is a small unit of measure, and kilojoule (1,000,000 J) and megajoule (1000 J) are the units most commonly used in animal nutrition.[4]

Gross Energy

The total amount of potential energy contained within a diet is called gross energy (GE). GE in food is determined by burning the food in a bomb calorimeter and measuring the total amount of heat produced. Unfortunately, animals are not able to use 100% of the energy contained in a food; some of it is lost during digestion and assimilation of nutrients as well as in urine, feces, respiration and production of heat.[1,2]

Digestible Energy

Digestible energy (DE) refers to the energy available for absorption across the intestinal mucosa; the energy lost is that found in the feces. Metabolizable energy (ME) is the amount of energy actually available to the tissue for use; the energy lost is that found in the feces *and* urine. ME is the value most often used to express the energy content in pet foods.[1,2]

When GE values are readjusted for digestibility and urinary losses, ME values of 3.5 kilocalories/g are assigned to proteins and carbohydrates and 8.5 kilocalories/g to fats; these values are called Modified Atwater factors.[1,2] These were developed by AAFCO to produce an equation that would more accurately reflect the digestibility of commercial pet foods, which tend to have lower digestibility than typical human foods.[4]

The ME of a diet or food ingredient depends on both the nutrient composition of the food and the animal consuming it.[1,2] If a dog and horse are fed the same high-fiber diet, the horse will have a higher ME value due to its better ability at fiber digestion than would a dog. These same differences in digestion can be seen between dogs and cats though not to the same extent as seen with an herbivore.

Three possible methods can be used to determine the ME in a diet: direct determination using feeding trials and total collection methods, calculation from analyzed levels of protein, carbohydrates and fats in the diet, and extrapolation of data collected from other species.[1,2]

Feeding Trials

Feeding trials using the species of concern are the most accurate method of determining a food's ME content. However this can be very time-consuming and expensive and requires access to large numbers of test animals.[1,2] The American Association of Feed Control Officials (AAFCO), the government body that oversees pet food production, has certain requirements for feeding trials; in general they require a minimum of 8 animals for a maintenance diet, at least 1 year of age, being fed the food in question for a minimum of 26 weeks. The food consumption is measured and recorded daily, individual body weights should be recorded at the beginning, weekly and at the end, and a minimum data base of blood work is required at the beginning and end of the study. All animals are to be given a complete physical exam by a veterinarian at the beginning and end of the study; they should be evaluated for general health, body and hair condition with comments recorded. A number of animals, not to exceed 25% (2 animals), may be removed for nonnutrition related reasons only during the first two weeks of the study. A necropsy will be conducted on any animal that dies during the study. There are additional conditions for foods used during pregnancy, lactation or growth.[5] Manufactures of some of the premium pet foods routinely measure the ME of their formulated pet foods and ingredients through the use of controlled feeding trials.[1,2] Feeding trials are obviously a time-consuming and expensive way to test ME in pet foods, but are also the most accurate method and have the greatest potential to expose any deficiencies or excesses in a particular food.

Table 1.1 Examples of AAFCO certification claims

1 Animal feeding trials using AAFCO's procedures substantiate that … provides complete and balanced nutrition for maintenance.
2 This product is formulated to meet the nutritional levels established by the AAFCO dog food profile for adult dogs.
3 Animal feeding tests using AAFCO's procedures substantiate that … provides complete and balanced nutrition for all life stages of cats.
4 … is formulated to meet nutritional levels established by the AAFCO cat food nutrient profiles for growth and maintenance.[1,2]

Calculation Method

ME values can also be determined using the calculation method. This involves the use of mathematical formulas to estimate a food's ME from its analyzed protein, carbohydrate and fat content. The formulas used for dog and cat diets have constants that account for fecal and urinary losses of energy.[1,2] The method does not account for digestibility or quality of ingredients, therefore excesses or deficiencies may not be apparent. ME is calculated using standard values for each nutrient, when the actual energy provided by each nutrient may be different from the standard.

Actual GE for triglycerides range from 6.5–9.5 kcal/per gram, proteins range from 4.0 to 8.3 kcal/gram, and carbohydrates range from 3.7 to 4.3 kcal/gram. The standard values assigned to these nutrients are triglycerides 9.4 kcal/gram, proteins 5.65 kcal/gram and carbohydrates 4.15 kcal/gram.[4] These values reflect gross energy rather than the modified Atwater numbers typically assigned when doing pet food calculations. Gross energy does not account for fecal or urinary losses in a diet, or for the energy used during digestion.[4]

When direct data is not available for particular food ingredients in a particular species, data from other species can be used. This is especially common with cat food ingredients. The species most often used for comparison is the pig. Although this method of estimating ME is not as accurate as direct measurement, data collected from swine experiments have been reported to correlate well with values from other species with simple stomachs.[1,2]

The method used to attain AAFCO certification is required to be listed on the product label. Most companies that use feeding trials clearly state this; those that use calculation methods or extrapolation methods may be a little vague in how the certification is obtained (Table 1.1).

Energy Density

Energy density of a pet food refers to the number of kilocalories provided in a given weight or volume. In the United States, energy density is expressed as kilocalories (kcal) of ME per kg or pound of the food.[1,2] The energy density must be high enough for the animal to be able to consume enough food to meet its daily energy requirements. Energy density will be the primary factor that determines the amount of food eaten each day.[1,2] The ability to maintain a normal body weight and growth rate is the criteria used to determine the appropriate quantity of food to be fed.

Because energy intake determines total food intake, it is especially important that diets are properly balanced so that requirements for all other nutrients are met at the same time that energy requirements are met.[1,2] For this reason it is more appropriate to express levels of energy containing nutrients in a food in terms of ME rather than as a percentage of the food's weight (Table 1.2).[1,2]

Expressing nutrient content as units per 1000 kcal of ME is called nutrient density.[1,2] Remember, fats contain almost three times the energy of proteins or carbohydrates and may only be a small portion of the diet's weight, but supply a majority of the calories. If you look only at weight, a diet may look low fat, but in fact be just the opposite.

When evaluating different diets, it's important to look at the caloric distribution of a food as well as nutrient density, rather than the percentage of the food's weight, typically expressed as dry matter (DM). This will allow you to compare foods of differing moisture or energy contents. This method is somewhat limited when compared to the use of nutrient density because caloric distribution only considers the energy containing nutrients of the food. The AAFCO requires that the energy value of a pet food be expressed in kcal of ME (Table 1.3 and 1.4).[1,2]

Table 1.2 Example of nutrient density and nutrient distribution

Nutrient density:
Protein 21 gr/96.25 gr/100 kcal
Fat 23.8 gr/96.25 gr/100 kcal
Carbs 51.45 gr/96.25 gr/100 kcal

Nutrient distribution:
Protein 21 gr/96.25 gr/100 kcal = 22%
$\qquad$ (21÷96.25) × 100 = 22%
Fat 23.8 gr/96.25 gr/100 kcal = 25%
$\qquad$ (23.8÷96.25) × 100 = 25%
Carbs 51.45 gr/96.25 gr/100 kcal = 53%
$\qquad$ (51.45÷96.25) × 100 = 53%

Calorie calculation:
Protein 22% of 100 kcal = 22 kcals/ 96.25 grams of food
Fat 25% of 100 kcal = 25 kcal/96.25 grams of food
Carbs 53% of 100 kcal = 53 kcal/96.25 grams of food

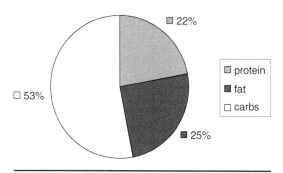

Table 1.3 Examples of nutrient density and caloric distribution

Dog food for growth, dry:
Calories (ME): 4491 kcal/kg, 485 kcal/cup
Caloric distribution:
$\quad$ Protein 29%
$\quad$ Fat 46%
$\quad$ Carbohydrate 25%

Dog food for maintenance, canned:
Calories (ME): 1108 kcal/kg, 409 kcal/can
Caloric distribution:
$\quad$ Protein 34%
$\quad$ Fat 58%
$\quad$ Carbohydrate 8%

Cat food for maintenance, dry:
Calories (ME): 4490 kcal/kg, 459 kcal/cup
Caloric distribution:
$\quad$ Protein 29%
$\quad$ Fat 47%
$\quad$ Carbohydrate 24%

Cat food, hairball formula, dry:
Calories (ME): 3692 kcal/kg, 280 kcal/cup
Caloric distribution:
$\quad$ Protein 30%
$\quad$ Fat 29%
$\quad$ Carbohydrate 41%

Therapeutic recovery diet, canned:
Calories (ME): 2000 kcal/kg, 340 kcal/can
$\quad$ 2.14 kcal/ml-canine
$\quad$ 2.11 kcal/ml-feline
Caloric distribution:
$\quad$ Protein 29%
$\quad$ Fat 66%
$\quad$ Carbohydrate 5%

Source: From P Roudebush DS Dzanis, J Debraekeleer, RG Brown (2000) Pet food labels. In MS Hand, CD Thatcher, RI Remillard, P Roudebush (eds), *Small Animal Clinical Nutrition* (4th edn), p. 155, Marceline, MO: Walsworth Publishing for Mark Morris Institute.

Excess energy intake is much more common in dogs and cats than is energy deficiency. The current estimates given by the American Veterinary Medical Association (AVMA) show that in excess of 40% of dogs and cats are overweight (10–15% above their desired body weight) and 25% of dogs are seen as obese (20–25% above their desired body weight).[6] Excessive energy intake has been shown to have several detrimental effects on dogs during growth, especially those of the large and giant breeds. Feeding growing puppies to attain maximal growth rate appears to be a significant contributing factor in the development of skeletal disorders such as osteochondrosis and hip dysplasia (Figure 1.1).[1,2]

Excessive energy intake during growth also affects the total number of fat cells the animal has, meaning that if the animal over-consumes during its growth phase, this can contribute to the development of obesity later in life. Once a fat cell has been formed, it will never go away,

and research has shown that the individual cells produce hormones that help it to retain its stored fat.[1,2,7] Obesity had been linked to the development of orthopedic problems later in life as well as increasing the incidence of diabetes, hyperlipidemia, pancreatitis and heart failure. A study conducted by Nestlé Purina demonstrated that by simply reducing the amount of food fed to a controlled group of Labradors by 25%, they on average lived

Table 1.4 Calculating nutrients as a percentage of metabolizable energy

Total calories in 100 grams of food
Protein = 3.5 kcal/gram × grams in food
Fat = 8.5 kcal/gram × grams in food
Carbohydrate = 3.5 kcal/gram × grams in food
Total calories/100 gram = protein calorie + fat calorie + carbohydrate calorie

Percentage of ME contributed by each nutrient (caloric distribution)
Protein = (protein calories/100 gram divided by total calories/100 gram) × 100 = % ME
Fat = (fat calories/100 gram divided by total calories/100 gram) × 100 = % ME
Carbohydrate = (carbohydrate calories/100 gram divided by total calories) × 100 = % ME

Source: From: LP Case, DP Carey, DA Hirakawa, *et al.* (2000) Energy and water. In Gross *et al.* (2nd edn), *Canine and Feline Nutrition*, pp. 3–14, St Louis, MO: Mosby; KL Gross, KL Wedekind, CS Cowell *et al.* (2000). Nutrients. In MS Hand, CD Thatcher, RL Remillard *et al.* (eds), *Small Animal Clinical Nutrition* (4th edn), pp. 21–36, Marceline, MO: Walsworth Publishing Mark Morris Institute

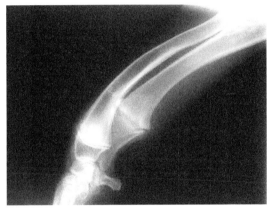

Figure 1.1 Radiograph of a Great Dane puppy with hypertrophic osteodystrophy due to overnutrition. This x-ray shows a line of lucency where destruction of the bone has occurred adjacent to the growth plates in the distal ulna. New bone production can also be seen outside of the bones. (Courtesy of Dr Dan Degner, with permission.)

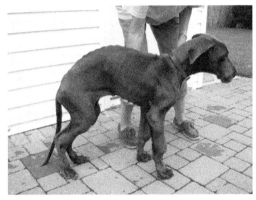

Figure 1.2 A Great Dane puppy showing the joint enlargement seen with hypertrophic osteodystrophy due to overnutrition. (Courtesy of Dr Dan Degner, with permission.)

1.5 years longer than their pair-mate, had less incidence of orthopedic problems, cancer and metabolic diseases (Figures 1.2 and 1.3).[8]

Inadequate energy intake results in reduced growth rate and compromised development of young dogs and cats and in weight loss and muscle wasting in adult animals. In healthy animals, this is most commonly seen in hard-working dogs, pregnant or lactating females that are being fed a diet that is too low in energy density.[1,2] This can also be seen in sick animals that are either unable or unwilling to eat, or those whose disease process cause energy loss or increased energy use.[9]

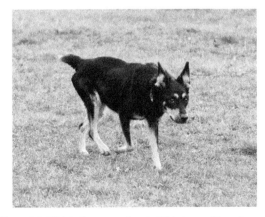

Figure 1.3 Weight loss secondary to Diabetes mellitus. A common complication of this disease is weight loss due to lack of glucose utilization by the cells, causing protein catabolism of the muscle to meet the body's energy requirements with the decreased energy availability.

References

1 Case LP, Carey DP, Hirakawa DA, Daristotle L (2000) Energy and water. In Gross *et al.* (eds), *Canine and Feline Nutrition* (2nd edn), pp. 3–14, St Louis, MO: Mosby.

2 Gross, KL, Wedekind KL, Cowell CS *et al.* (2000) Nutrients. In MS Hand, CD Thatcher, RL Remillard *et al.* (eds), *Small Animal Clinical Nutrition* (4th edn), pp. 21–36, Marceline, MO: Walsworth Publishing, Mark Morris Institute.

3 Whitney E, Rolfes SR (2008) Glossary. In *Understanding Nutrition* (11th edn), pp. 11–12, Belmont, CA: Thomson Wadsworth.

4 Delaney SJ, Fascetti AJ (2012) Basic nutrition overview. In AJ Fascetti, SJ Delaney (eds), *Applied Veterinary Clinical Nutrition*, pp. 9–21, Ames, IA: Wiley-Blackwell.

5 Hand MS, Thatcher CD, Remillard RL, Roudebush P (2000) AAFCO feeding protocols for dog and cat foods. In MS Hand, CD Thatcher, RL Remillard *et al.* (eds), *Small Animal Clinical Nutrition* (4th edn), p. 1056, Marceline, MO: Walsworth Publishing.

6 AVMA tips on preventing obesity in pets. http://www.avmamedia.org/display.asp?sid=396&NAME=Preventing_obesity_in_pets, accessed July 4, 2012.

7 Toll PW, Yamka RM, Schoenerr WD, Hand MS (2012) Obesity. In MS Hand, CD Thatcher, RL Remillard *et al.* (eds), *Small Animal Clinical Nutrition* (5th edn), p. 502, Marceline, MO: Walsworth Publishing, Mark Morris Institute.

8 Kealy RD, Lawler DF, Ballam JM *et al.* (2012) Effects of diet restriction on life span and age-related changes in dogs, *Journal of the American Veterinary Medical Association* **220**, 1315–20.

9 Donoghue S, Kronfeld DS, Case LP, *et al.* (1994) Feeding hospitalized dogs and cats. In JM Wills, KW Simpson (eds), *The Waltham Book of Clinical Nutrition of the Dog and Cat*, p. 29, Oxford: Butterworth-Heinemann.

2 Water

Introduction

Water is the single most important nutrient in terms of survivability. Animals can live for weeks without any food, using their own body fat and muscle for energy production, but a loss of only 10% of their body water can result in death.[1−3] It is also one of three nutrients that do not contribute any calories to the diet.

Within the body, water functions as a solvent that facilitates cellular functions and as a transport medium for nutrients and the end products of cellular metabolism. Water is able to absorb much of the heat that is generated during metabolic reactions with a minimal increase in temperature. Water also helps to transport heat away from the working organs through the blood.[1,2]

Water is an essential component in normal digestion because it is necessary for hydrolysis, the splitting of larger molecules into smaller ones through the addition of water.[1,2] Examples of hydrolysis would include lipase, an enzyme that hydrolyzes fats, amylase an enzyme that hydrolyzes amyloid, a complex carbohydrate and peptidase an enzyme that hydrolyzes peptides, complex groups of amino acids.[4] Elimination of waste products through the kidneys also requires a large amount of water, which acts as both a solvent for the toxic metabolites and as a carrier medium.[1,2]

Water is involved in regulating oncotic pressure that helps the body to maintain its shape; one manifestation of loss of oncotic pressure is seen with dehydration with loss of skin elasticity. Water is found in all the body fluids as well as helping to lubricate the joints and eyes, provides protective cushioning for the nervous system and aids in gas exchange in respiration by keeping the alveoli moist and expanded.[2]

Water accounts for the largest proportion of any of the nutrients in an animal's body, varying from 40% to 80% of the total amount. The percent of water varies with species, condition and age.[1,2] Generally, lean body mass contains 70–80% water and 20–25% protein, with adipose tissue containing 10–15% water and 75–80% fat. The younger and leaner the animal is, the more water it contains. The fatter the animal, the lower the animal's water content.[2]

Water Quality

Because of water's role as a solvent, the potential exists that other substances can enter the animal's body that hadn't been planned for. Salinity (water's salt content), nitrates, nitrites, inorganic chemicals and microbial contamination are examples of only a few contaminants that can be found in water supplies.[5] Routine measurement of water quality looks at these dissolved solids with a reading of total parts per million (ppm) and is reported as "total dissolved solids" (TDS). Water containing less than 5000 ppm TDS is generally considered acceptable for consumption. A level above 7000 ppm is considered unsuitable for livestock and poultry consumption.[5] Human recommendations are less than 500 ppm of TDS, and this is considered a better recommendation for companion animals.

For anyone with access to city water, TDS testing is done through the local public health department. For those persons using well water or other sources of water, having a commercial analytical laboratory screen the water for TDS, pesticide residues and other chemicals would be recommended.[2]

Water Loss

Water is lost in a number of ways. Obligatory loss from the kidneys is the minimum amount of water required by the body to rid itself of the daily load of urinary waste

Nutrition and Disease Management for Veterinary Technicians and Nurses, Second Edition. Ann Wortinger, Kara M. Burns
© 2015 John Wiley & Sons, Inc. Published 2015 by John Wiley & Sons, Inc.
Companion Website: www.wiley.com/go/wortinger/nutrition

products. Facultative loss is the remaining portion of the urine that is excreted in response to the normal water reabsorption rate of the kidneys and to mechanisms responsible for maintaining proper water balance in the body. Fecal water accounts for a much smaller portion of the water lost.[1] A third route of water loss is through evaporation from the lungs during respiration. Water can also be lost through perspiration, but this is only a very small portion of water loss for most companion animals. In dogs and cats evaporative and perspiration water loss are very important for the regulation of normal body temperature during hot weather.[1]

Water Gains

Daily water consumption must compensate for these continual losses. The total water intake daily comes from three possible sources: water present in the food, metabolic water and drinking water.[1]

The amount of water found in the diet depends on the type of food being fed; dry food can have a moisture content as low as 7%, with some canned foods being as high as 84%. Within limits, increasing the water content of a food increases the diets acceptability to the animal.[1]

Metabolic water is the water that is produced during oxidation of the energy-containing nutrients of the body. Oxygen combines with the hydrogen atoms removed from the carbohydrates, proteins, and fats in the food during digestion to produce water molecules.[1,6] The metabolism of fat produces the greatest amount of metabolic water on a weight basis, and protein catabolism produces the smallest amount.[1] Metabolic water accounts for a fairly insignificant portion of the water intake, being only 5–10% of the daily total intake.[1,5]

The most significant source of water intake is voluntary drinking. Numerous factors can affect an animal's voluntary oral intake including ambient temperature, type of diet being fed, level of exercise, physiologic state and health.[1,6] Water intake increases with an increase in ambient temperature and increasing exercise because of evaporative loss through the lungs due to panting to cool the body. The amount of food being fed can also affect water intake: as the calories increase so does the amount of waste products that the body needs to get rid of, increasing the amount of urine produced. If this increase in calories results in weight gain, there will also be an increased loss due to panting to help with thermoregulation.[1,6]

Voluntary Oral Intake

The type of diet being fed as well as the composition can dramatically affect voluntary oral intake of water. A study on dogs found that when the test animals were fed a diet containing 73% moisture, they obtained only 38% of their daily water needs from drinking water. When they were abruptly switched to a diet containing only 7% water, voluntary oral intake immediately increased to 95% or more of the total daily intake.[1] When cats are fed only canned food, their voluntary oral intake is likewise very low, in fact when cats are fed a food with very high water content; cats can maintain normal water balance with no additional drinking water.[6] This could be seen with liquid or gruel recovery diets as well as some commercial canned diets with a high amount of sauce.

Water requirements are related to maintaining appropriate water balance in the animal. Dogs and cats meet the majority of their water requirements through water included in food and voluntary oral intake. As a general guideline, the daily water requirement, expressed in ml/day for dogs and cats is roughly equivalent to the daily energy requirement (DER) in kcal/day. For dogs this is 1.6 × the resting energy requirement (RER), for cats 1.2 × RER.[2,5]

Domestic cats, descendents of desert animals, normally form more concentrated urine than do dogs. Actual water requirements for cats may be less than those for dogs. Water needs can best be met though access to clean, fresh water at all times.[2,5,6] Dogs will show thirst and drink voluntarily when body water decreases by 4% or less, cats do not voluntarily drink until they lose as much as 8% of their body water. In addition, cats that are fed dry food diets will typically consume less water per day than those fed canned food diets.[6]

If fresh, palatable, clean water is available and proper amounts of a balance diet are being fed, most dogs and cats are able to accurately self-regulate their water balance through voluntary oral intake.[1,2,6] Normally, thirst ensures that water intake meets or exceeds the body's requirements. Inadequate water intake can reduce appetite, reduces production on a number of levels including growth, lactation, reproduction and physical activity.[2]

References

1 Case LP, Carey DP, Hirakawa DA, Daristotle L (2000) Energy and water. In *Canine and Feline Nutrition* (2nd edn), pp. 3–14, St Louis, MO: Mosby.

2 Gross KL, Wedekind KL, Cowell CS *et al.* (2000) Nutrients. In MS Hand, CD Thatcher, RL Remillard *et al.* (eds), *Small Animal Clinical Nutrition* (4th edn), pp. 21–36, Marceline, MO: Walsworth Publishing for Mark Morris Institute.

3 Wills JM (1996) Basic principles of nutrition and feeding. In N Kelly, J Wills (eds), *Manual of Companion Animal Nutrition and Feeding*, pp. 14–15, Ames, IA: Iowa State Press.

4 Whitney E, Rolfes SR (2008) Digestion, absorption and transport. In *Understanding Nutrition* (11th edn), pp. 76–7, Belmont, CA: Thomson Wadsworth.

5 Gross KL, Jewell DE, Yamka RM *et al.* (2012) Macronutrients. In MS Hand, CD Thatcher, RL Remillard *et al.* (eds), *Small Animal Clinical Nutrition* (5th edn), pp. 51–3, Marceline, MO: Walsworth Publishing.

6 Case LP (2003) The cat as an obligate carnivore. In *The Cat: Its Behavior, Nutrition and Health*, pp. 295–7, Ames, IA, Iowa State Press.

3 Carbohydrates

Introduction

Carbohydrates are the major energy-containing part of plants, making up between 60% and 90% of their dry-matter weight.[1] This class of nutrients is made up of the elements carbon, hydrogen and oxygen, and is classified as monosaccharides, disaccharides, oligosaccharides or polysaccharides and have the generally formula of $(CH_2O)_n$.[1,2] The hydrogen and oxygen are usually present in the same ratio as that found in water (H_2O) giving rise to the name carbohydrate or hydrated carbon.[3]

Carbohydrates are not an essential nutrient, but rather provide energy for the essential systems to do their jobs. In those species where fiber is not easily digested, the nondigestible carbohydrates found in fiber can be important for normal gastrointestinal function and health.[4]

As a nutrient, carbohydrates act primarily as an energy source, allowing amino acids and fatty acids to be used for building and maintenance of the body. When more carbohydrates are consumed than are needed by the body for energy, it may be converted into body fat and stored, or serve as starting materials for the metabolism of other compounds.[3,4]

Monosaccharides

Monosaccharides are also called simple sugars, and are the simplest form of carbohydrates, being composed of sugar units containing between 3 and 7 carbon atoms.[1,2] The chief monosaccharides are glucose, fructose (fruit sugar), and galactose (milk sugar).[1,2] Monosaccharides can combine with one another to form polymers, and these can be enormous molecules containing many thousands of individual monosaccharide units.[3]

Glucose is a moderately sweet simple sugar found in commercially prepared corn syrup and sweet fruits such as grapes and berries. It is also the chief end product of starch digestion and glycogen hydrolysis in the body. Glucose is the form of carbohydrate found circulating in the blood stream and is the primary form of carbohydrate used by the body's cells for energy.[1] Glucose is a 6 carbon ring in the shape of a hexagon, onto which the hydrogen and oxygen compounds are attached. This 6 carbon configuration gives the monosaccharides their other name of hexoses. Glucose is also known as dextrose (Figure 3.1).[5]

Fructose, commonly called fruit sugar, is a very sweet sugar found in honey, ripe fruits and some vegetables. It is also formed from the digestion or hydrolysis of the disaccharide sucrose.[1] Fructose is also a 6 carbon sugar but the structure differs from glucose in that 2 of the carbons are outside of the ring structure giving the molecule a pentagon shape (Figure 3.2).[5]

Galactose is not found in a free form in foods. However, it makes up 50% of the disaccharide lactose, which is found in the milk of all mammals.[1] It has the same number and kinds of atoms as glucose, with only the position of 1 OH group being slightly different (Figure 3.3).[5]

Disaccharides

Disaccharides are made up of two monosaccharide units linked together. Lactose, the sugar found in mammalian milk, contains a molecule of glucose and a molecule of galactose. This is the only carbohydrate of animal origin.[1,2] Lactose intolerance, as seen in some adult animals, is caused by a deficiency of the enzyme beta-galactosidase. This deficiency prevents the glucose and galactose molecules from separating, making this a nondigestible carbohydrate.[3] Sucrose, commonly called table sugar, contains a molecule of glucose linked to a molecule of fructose. This is the most common sugar

Nutrition and Disease Management for Veterinary Technicians and Nurses, Second Edition. Ann Wortinger, Kara M. Burns
© 2015 John Wiley & Sons, Inc. Published 2015 by John Wiley & Sons, Inc.
Companion Website: www.wiley.com/go/wortinger/nutrition

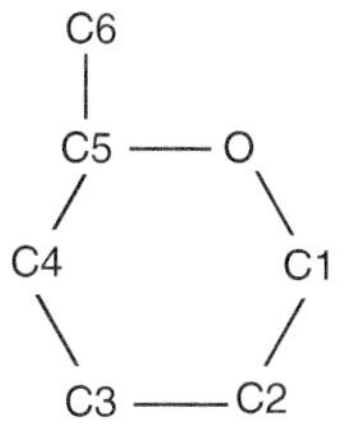

Figure 3.1 6 carbon hexagon glucose.

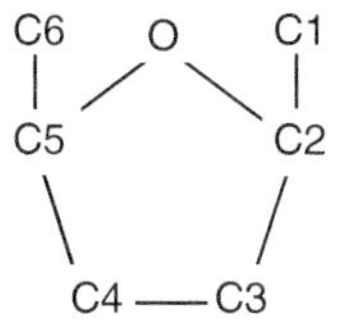

Figure 3.2 6 carbon pentagon fructose.

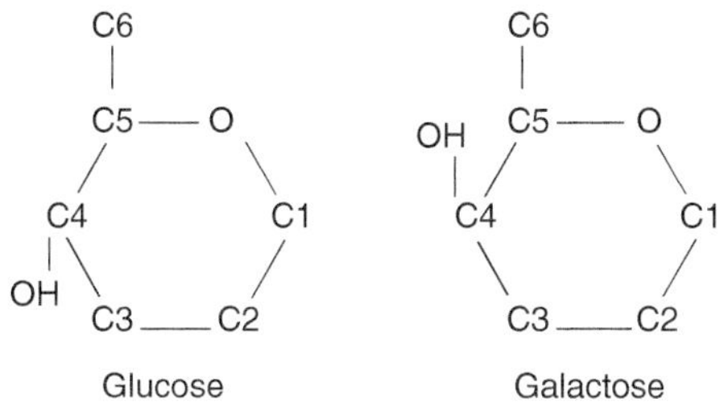

Figure 3.3 Glucose and galactose molecules.

found in plants.[1,2] Maltose is formed by linking two glucose molecules. This is produced whenever a starch molecule is broken down. This can be seen during digestion or during the fermentation process that yields alcohol. Maltose is a minor constitute of only a few foods.[5]

Oligosaccharides

Oligosaccharides are carbohydrates made up of 3–10 monosaccharide units making them polymers. These units may be the same or a mix of different monosaccharides. They are often difficult to digest and if found in quantity as with some plant materials, may be associated with gastrointestinal disturbances or flatulence.[2,3] Those that contain fructose are called fructooligosaccharides (FOS), but there are many other oligosaccharides found in plants.[2] FOS's in the diet improve intestinal flora,

increase nitrogen digestion and retention, improve stool quality and reduce fecal odors.[1]

This class of carbohydrates is used commonly for their prebiotic effects. A prebiotic is defined as "nondigestible food ingredients that selectively stimulate a limited number of bacteria in the colon to improve the host health."[6] This healthful effect is seen because these fibers are resistant to the breakdown by enzymes in the host intestines, but are able to be broken down by certain gut bacteria helping to support the limited growth of these bacteria. Prebiotic fibers are thought to reduce fecal odor by modifying fecal concentration of certain digestive by-products and improve immune function by influencing gut-associated immune cells.[6]

Polysaccharides

Polysaccharides consist of many thousands of monosaccharide units. They are found widely in plants being used for cell wall material (cellulose) and energy storage (starch in the form of amyloid and amylopectin for plants and glycogen for animals).[1,3] Cereal grains such as corn, wheat, sorghum, barley and rice are the major ingredients in pet foods that provide starch.[1] Complex carbohydrates of plant origin other than starch are referred to as dietary fiber, or nonstarch polysaccharides. These include cellulose, hemicellulose, pectin, and the plant gums and mucilages.[1,3] Plant fibers differ from starches and glycogen in that their monosaccharide units have a different bonding configuration (beta bonds instead of alpha bonds). These bonds resist digestion by the gastrointestinal enzymes of most monogastrics, making their energy unavailable for absorption in the small intestine (Figure 3.4).[1]

Certain microbes found in the large intestine of dogs and cats are able to break down fiber to varying degrees, even though the animal themselves are unable to break down the fiber.[1] This bacterial fermentation produces short-chain fatty acids (SCFAs) and other end products. The SCFAs that are produced in the greatest numbers are acetate, propionate and butyrate.[1] These SCFAs are a significant energy source for the enterocytes of the small intestine and colonocytes of the large intestine.[1] Fiber in the diet also functions as an aid in the proper functioning of the gastrointestinal tract and as a dietary diluent that decreases the total energy density of the diet.[1]

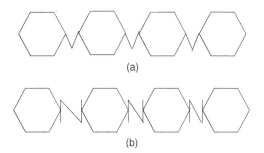

(a)

(b)

Figure 3.4 (a) Alpha enzymatic hydrolysis occurs at these sites. The enzymes must be able to fit like a key in a lock for the break to occur. (b) Cellulose with beta bonding. Alpha enzymes cannot break down these molecules as they don't "fit" into the lock properly.

Table 3.1 Dietary fiber fermentation in dogs

Fiber type	Solubility	Fermentability
Beet pulp	Low	Moderate
Cellulose	Low	Low
Rice bran	Low	Moderate
Gum arabic	High	Moderate
Pectin	Low	High
Carboxy mellthycellulose	High	Low
Methylcellulose	High	Low
Cabbage fiber	Low	High
Guar gum	High	High
Locust bean gum	High	Low
Xanthan gum	High	Moderate

Source: Reference 1.

Glycosaminoglycans are complex polysaccharides associated with proteins. They form integral parts of the interstitial fluid, cartilage, skin and tendons. The primary glycosaminoglycans are chondroitin sulfate and hyaluronic acid (Table 3.1).[2]

Carbohydrate Types

Polysaccharides that are able to be digested by the intestinal enzymes are designated as starches, while those that are resistant to digestion and instead undergo fermentation or bacterial digestion are designated as fibers.[6] For most starches, digestibility increases with the degree gelatinization.

Gelatinization is a process in which starch crystals are melted and hydrated (water added to the molecule) when heated or cooked. Extrusion cooking, a process used to produce dry pet foods, produces gelatinization through the application of heat as does the canning process.[6]

Carbohydrate Functions

Carbohydrates have several functions in the body. The monosaccharide glucose is an important energy source for many tissues. A constant supply of glucose is necessary for the proper functioning of the central nervous system (CNS), and glycogen, the storage form of glucose within the body, is present in the heart muscle as an important emergency energy source for the heart.[1] Glycogen stored in the liver and muscle can be hydrolyzed to supply additional energy to the cells when circulating glucose is low. The CNS and red blood cells are wholly dependent on glucose for energy, while other tissues within the body are able to utilize other substances to obtain energy.[6]

Carbohydrates also supply carbon skeletons for the formation of nonessential amino acids, and is needed for the synthesis of other essential body compounds such as glucuronic acid, heparin, chondroitin sulfate, the immunopolysaccharides, deoxyribonucleic acid (DNA) and ribonucleic acid (RNA).[1] When joined with proteins or lipids some carbohydrates also become important structural components in the body's tissues.[1] When metabolized for energy to carbon dioxide and water, they become a source of heat for the body.[2] Finally, simple carbohydrates and starches consumed in excess of the body's needs are stored as glycogen or converted to fat.[2]

Not only do carbohydrates provide energy for the body, digestible carbohydrates also have a protein sparing effect. By providing enough carbohydrates for the body to meet its energy needs, protein is spared from being used for energy and is available for use in tissue repair and growth.[1,2] Conversely, if insufficient carbohydrates are available in the diet, protein will be used to meet energy needs decreasing the amount available for tissue repair and growth.[1]

Cats and Carbohydrates

Cats have a unique metabolism among companion animals that limits their ability to efficiently use large amounts of absorbed carbohydrates.

- Low activities of the intestinal enzymes sucrose and lactase.
- Sugar transport system in the intestinal tract is not able to adapt to varying levels of dietary carbohydrates.
- Lack hepatic glucokinase activity, limiting their ability to assimilate simple sugars.
- Pancreatic amylase is only 5% of what dogs produce.
- No salivary amylase is produced.

These differences support the classification of cats as strict carnivores, but that does not mean that they cannot digest and utilize carbohydrates. If large amounts of carbohydrates are fed to cats (>40% dry matter), signs of maldigestion can be seen such as diarrhea, bloating and flatulence.[6] Differences can also be seen among the different carbohydrate sources and their effects on blood glucose. Normal cats can maintain a normal blood glucose level when fed diets that are low in carbohydrates and high in protein, by using a process called gluconeogenesis where protein is used for energy instead of carbohydrates.[6]

References

1 Case LP, Carey DP, Hirakawa DA, Daristotle L (2000) Carbohydates. In *Canine and Feline Nutrition* (2nd edn), pp. 15–18, St Louis, MO, Mosby.

2 Gross KL Wedekind KL, Cowell CS *et al.* (2000) Nutrients. In MS Hand, CD Thatcher, RL Remillard *et al.* (eds), *Small Animal Clinical Nutrition* (4th edn), pp. 36–48, Marceline, MO: Walsworth Publishing for Mark Morris Institute.

3 Price CJ, Bedford PCG, Sutton JB (1993) Nutrients and the requirements of dog and cats. In JW Simpson, RS Anderson, PJ Markwell (eds), *Clinical Nutrition of the Dog and Cat*, pp. 20–2, Cambridge, MA: Blackwell.

4 Delaney SJ, Fascetti AJ (2012) Basic nutrition overview. In AJ Fascetti, DJ Delaney (eds), *Applied Veterinary Clinical Nutrition*, p. 13, Ames, IA, Wiley-Blackwell.

5 Whitney E, Rolfes SR (2008) The carbohydrates, sugars, starches and fibers. In *Understanding Nutrition* (11th edn), pp. 101–8, Belmont, CA: Thomson Wadsworth.

6 Gross KL, Jewell DE, Yamka RM *et al.* (2012) Macronutrients. In MS Hand, CD Thatcher, RL Remillard *et al.* (eds), *Small Animal Clinical Nutrition* (5th edn), p. 77. Marceline, MO: Walsworth Publishing for Mark Morris Institute.

4 Fats

Introduction

Dietary fat is part of a group of compounds known as lipids that share the property of being insoluble in water (hydrophobic) but soluble in other organic solvents.[1,2] Lipids that are solid at room temperature are commonly called fats, and those that are liquid at room temperature are called oils.[2]

Lipids can be further categorized into simple lipids, compound lipids and derived lipids.[1] The simple lipids include triglycerides, which are the most common form of fat present in the diet, and waxes.[1] Triglycerides are made up of three fatty acids linked to one molecule of glycerol; the waxes contain a greater number of fatty acids linked to a long-chain alcohol molecule (Table 4.1).[1]

Compound lipids are composed of a lipid, such as a fatty acid, linked to a nonlipid compound. Lipoproteins, which carry fat in the blood stream, are a type of compound lipid. The derived lipids, products of both simple and compound fats, include sterol compounds, such as cholesterol and the fat soluble vitamins A, D, E and K.[1]

Triglycerides

Triglyceride is the most important fat in the diet, and can be differentiated in foods according to the types of fatty acids that each triglyceride molecule contains.[1] Fatty acids vary in carbon-chain length and may be saturated, monounsaturated or polyunsaturated.[1] Saturated fatty acids contain no double bonds between the carbon atoms and are therefore "saturated" with hydrogen atoms. Monounsaturated fatty acids have one double bond, and polyunsaturated fatty acids (PUFAs) contain two or more double bonds.[1] In general, the triglycerides in animal fats contain a higher percentage of saturated fatty acids than do those in vegetable

Table 4.1 Triglyceride molecule

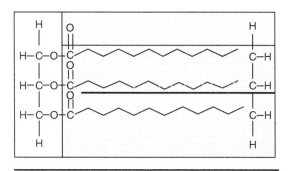

Source: Adapted from reference 5.
Yellow box highlights the glycerol molecule. Green boxes highlight the 3 fatty acid molecules. When combined they form a triglyceride molecule.

fats.[1] The more double bonds a fatty acid has, the less stable the molecule is and the more susceptible it is to oxidation resulting in rancidity.

Fats function in the body as a form of energy storage, major deposits of accumulated fat can be found under the skin (subcutaneous fat), around the vital organs and in the membranes surrounding the intestines (omental fat).[1,2] The deposits of fat also serve as insulators, protecting the body from heat loss, and as a protective layer around the vital organs to guard against physical injury.[1] Although animals have a limited capacity to store carbohydrates in the form of glycogen, they have an almost unlimited capacity to store surplus energy in the form of fat.[1] Fats also provide the body with essential fatty acids (EFAs) and provide a carrier for the fat soluble vitamins A, D, E and K.[1,2]

Fat also has numerous metabolic and structural functions. Fat provides insulation around myelinated nerve fibers and aids in the transmission of nerve impulses. Compound lipid molecules such as phospholipids and glycolipids, serve as structural components for cell

Nutrition and Disease Management for Veterinary Technicians and Nurses, Second Edition. Ann Wortinger, Kara M. Burns
© 2015 John Wiley & Sons, Inc. Published 2015 by John Wiley & Sons, Inc.
Companion Website: www.wiley.com/go/wortinger/nutrition

membranes and participate in the transport of nutrients and metabolites across these membranes.[1]

Lipoproteins

Lipoproteins provide for the transport of fats through the blood stream. Cholesterol is used by the body to form the bile salts necessary for proper fat digestion and absorption, and it is also a precursor for the steroid hormones.[1] Along with other lipids, cholesterol forms a protective layer in the skin that prevents excessive water loss and the invasion for foreign substances.[1]

Of any of the nutrients, fat provides the most concentrated form of energy almost 3 times that of carbohydrates and proteins. Each gram of fat provides 8.5 kcals, as oppose to the 3.5 kcals provided by proteins or carbohydrates. The digestibility of fat is usually higher than that of carbohydrates and proteins.[1] This is especially important when you need to increase caloric density of a food. By increasing the fat you can increase the available calories as well as the digestibility of the food (Table 4.2).

Essential Fatty Acids

Dietary fat provides a source of the essential fatty acids (EFAs). The EFAs are generally recognized as linoleic acid, alpha-linolenic acid and arachidonic acid. These are either omega 3 EFAs (alpha-linolenic acid) or omega 6 EFAs (linoleic acid and arachidonic acid).[1,2] The omega 3 and omega 6 fatty acids are essential because the body is unable to synthesize them. The omega 9 fatty acids and saturated fatty acids are able to be synthesized by the body and are seen as nonessential fatty acids.[2] All of the EFAs are polyunsaturated fatty acids (PUFAs), with the position of the first double bond being denoted by the omega term, when counting from the terminal (methyl) end of the chain.[1,2]

In most animals, gamma-linolenic acid and arachidonic acid can by synthesized from linoleic acid. If adequate linoleic acid is provided in the diet, there would be no dietary requirement for gamma-linolenic acid or arachidonic acid. The exception to this would be with the cat that requires a dietary source of arachidonic acid irregardless of the amount of linoleic acid found in

Table 4.2 Lipoprotein classes[5]

Lipoprotein	Acronym	Protein: lipid ratio	■ Triglycerides Cholesterol
Chylomicron	CM	1:99	
Very low-density lipoprotein	VLDL	10:90	
Low-density lipoprotein	LDL	25:75	
High-density lipoprotein	HDL	50:50	

Table 4.3 Fatty acid structure[1,2]

Saturated-lauric acid (12:0)

$CH_3-CH_2-CH_2-CH_2-CH_2-CH_2-CH_2-CH_2-CH_2-CH_2-CH_2-COOH$

Monounsaturated-palmitoleic acid (16:1n-7)

$CH_3-CH_2-CH_2-CH_2-CH_2-CH_2-CH=CH-CH_2-CH_2-CH_2-CH_2-CH_2-CH_2-CH_2-COOH$

Polyunsaturated linoleic acid (18:2n-6)

$CH_3-CH_2-CH_2-CH_2-CH_2-CH=CH-CH_2-CH=CH-CH_2-CH_2-CH_2-CH_2-CH_2-CH_2-CH2-COOH$

Alpha-linolenic acid (18:3n-3)

$CH_3-CH_2-CH=CH-CH_2-CH=CH-CH_2-CH=CH-CH_2-CH_2-CH_2-CH_2-CH_2-CH_2-CH_2-COOH$

Arachidonic acid (20:4n-6)

$CH_3-CH_2-CH_2-CH_2-CH_2-CH=CH-CH_2-CH=CH-CH_2-CH=CH-CH_2-CH=CH-CH_2-CH_2-CH_2-COOH$

---

the diet. Cats lack the metabolic pathway necessary to perform the conversion of linoleic acid to arachidonic acid.[1,3] Research has also shown that dogs cannot effectively convert alpha-linoleic acid to docosahexaenoic acid (DHA), so oils derived from fish oils rather than seed oils are a better source if long-chain omega-3 fatty acids are desired.[4]

Unlike many other nutrients, instead of being broken down for digestion and use by the body, fats undergo elongation and desaturation (losing hydrogen atoms) for use in the body. Unsaturated fatty acids cannot be converted between families such as the omega 3 or omega 6 families, and monounsaturated and saturated fatty acids can not be converted to EFAs (Table 4.3).[2]

The first number is the number of carbon atoms, the n designation indicates the number of double bonds and the last number is the location of that double bond from the terminal methyl (CH_3) end.

The best sources for linoleic acid (omega 6 family) are vegetable oils such as corn, soybean and safflower oils. Pork fat and poultry fat also contain appreciable amounts of linoleic acid, but beef fat and butter fat contain very little.[1] Arachidonic acid (omega 3 family) can be found only in animal fats; this is especially important in cat diets. Because of the essential requirement for arachidonic acid, cats can not be fed a balanced vegetarian diet as the only source of arachidonic acid is in animal fats.[3] Some fish oils are rich in arachidonic acid as well as being found in small amounts in poultry and pork fat.[1]

The EFAs have multiple functions within the body, including synthesis of prostaglandins and leukotrins.[4] Omega 6 fatty acids have functionally distinct effects compared with those of the omega 3 family.[2] Eicosanoids (a product of any of the omega EFAs families) that are produced from the omega 3 family are less immunologically stimulating than those from the omega 6 or 9 families. This means that they have less potential to produce an inflammatory reaction in the body.[2]

This is important in situations where decreasing the inflammatory response is desired, such as before and after surgery, after trauma, burns, injury or some types of cancer or assisting in the control of dermatitis, arthritis, inflammatory bowel disease and colitis.[2] Adjusting the omega 3 to omega 6 fatty acid ratio in therapeutic diets can assist in decreasing these responses.

The skin contains a large store of arachidonic acid, but is unable to convert linoleic acid to arachidonic acid at this site.[4] Adding arachidonic acid to food where it was previously absent increases food efficiency and enhances skin condition by reducing water loss through the skin.[2] This causes a shinier, glossier coat with less skin flaking.

Lipids are also essential for the absorption of the fat-soluble vitamins A, D, E and K. The type of fat that is required for this absorption is not specific.[2]

Fatty acid deficiencies in the diet impair wound healing, cause a dry lusterless coat, scaly skin, and change the lipid film on the skin, which can predispose the animal to skin infections. With an inadequate amount of fats, the fat soluble vitamins are also not properly absorbed and deficiencies in these can be seen.[2]

Most importantly to our animals, fats improve the palatability and texture of the diets being fed.[1,2] The problem with this would be as the fat content of the diet increases, so does the caloric density and palatability:

this can easily lead to over consumption of the diet, in turn leading to obesity.

References

1 Case LP, Carey DP, Hirakawa DA, Daristotle L (2000) Fats. In Gross *et al.* (eds), *Canine and Feline Nutrition* (2nd edn), pp. 19–22, St Louis, MO: Mosby.

2 Gross, KL, Wedekind KL, Cowell CS *et al.* (2000) Nutrients. In MS Hand, CD Thatcher, RL Remillard *et al.* (eds), *Small Animal Clinical Nutrition* (4th edn), pp. 59–66, Marceline, MO: Walsworth Publishing, Mark Morris Institute.

3 Case LP (2003) The cat as an obligate carnivore. In *The Cat: Its Behavior, Nutrition and Health*, pp. 300–2, Ames, IA: Iowa State Press.

4 Outerbridge CA (2012) Nutritional management of skin diseases. In AJ Fascetti, SJ Delaney (eds), *Applied Veterinary Clinical Nutrition*, p. 158, Ames, IA: Wiley-Blackwell.

5 Whitney E, Rolfes SR (2008) The lipids: triglycerides, phospholipids, and sterols. In *Understanding Nutrition* (11th edn), pp. 138–55, Belmont, CA: Thomson Wadsworth.

5 Protein and Amino Acids

Introduction

Proteins are large, complex molecules composed of hundreds to thousands of amino acids. These amino acids are composed of carbon, hydrogen, oxygen, nitrogen and sometimes sulfur and phosphorus atoms.[1−3] Although hundreds of amino acids exist in nature, only 20 are commonly found as protein components.[2] Proteins are linear polymers of amino acids in which the amino group of one amino acid and the carboxyl group of another amino acid are joined together through a peptide bond. Amino acids joined together are called peptides; two bonded together are a dipeptide, three a tripeptide and more than three a polypeptide.[2] Once hydrolysis begins in the body, simple proteins yield only amino acids or their derivatives.[1] Proteins can also become bonded to other molecules; this yields a useful basis for simple classification.[4]

Simple proteins give rise to their basic amino acids units only. Examples would include:

- Albumins are globular proteins found in egg white, blood plasma and milk.
- Collagens are fibrous proteins present in connective tissue and are converted to gelatin on prolonged boiling.
- Elastins are fibrous elastic proteins found in arterial walls and skin.[4]

Conjugated proteins give rise to other distinctive substances in addition to amino acids.

- Glycoproteins contain carbohydrates as seen with mucus.
- Lipoproteins contain lipid and function to carry fat throughout the bloodstream as seen with LDL (low density lipoproteins), HDL (high density lipoproteins) and VLDL (very low density lipoproteins).
- Phosphoproteins contain a phosphorus group such as casein in milk.

- Chromoproteins contain a pigment group such as heme in hemoglobin.
- Nucleoproteins combine proteins and nucleic acids, as with DNA and RNA.[1,2,4]

Protein is required in the diet to provide a source of amino acids to build, repair and replace body proteins. They also supply nitrogen for the synthesis of the nonessential amino acids and other nitrogen containing compounds.[3] Amino acids are divided into two groups, nonessential and essential.[1] The distinction between these two groups is that the essential amino acids must be included in the diet, while the nonessential amino acids can be synthesized by the body from other precursors at a rate sufficient to meet physiologic needs (Table 5.1).[1]

Some proteins are conditionally essential, in that they are required in amounts exceeding the body's ability to produce them at times, usually during certain

Table 5.1 Essential and nonessential amino acids for dogs and cats

Essential amino acids	Nonessential amino acids
Arginine	Alanine
Histidine	Asparagine
Isoleucine	Aspartate
Leucine	Cysteine
Lysine	Glutamate
Methionine	Glutamine
Phenylalanine	Glycine
Taurine (cats only)	Hydroxylysine
Tryptophan	Hydrosyproline
Threonine	Proline
Valine	Serine
	Tyrosine

Source: Reference 1.

Nutrition and Disease Management for Veterinary Technicians and Nurses, Second Edition. Ann Wortinger, Kara M. Burns
© 2015 John Wiley & Sons, Inc. Published 2015 by John Wiley & Sons, Inc.
Companion Website: www.wiley.com/go/wortinger/nutrition

physiologic or disease conditions.[2] Nitrogen, found in the side amine group on the protein, is essential for the synthesis of the nonessential amino acids, and is also required for synthesis of other nitrogen-containing molecules including nucleic acids, purines, pyrimidines and certain neurotransmitter substances.[5]

Functions of Proteins

Proteins in the body have numerous functions. They are the major structural components of hair, feathers, skin, nails, tendons, ligaments and cartilage.[1] Contractile proteins such as myosin and actin are involved in regulating muscle action. All of the enzymes that catalyze the body's essential metabolic reactions and are essential for nutrient digestion and assimilation are also protein molecules.[1] Many hormones that control the homeostatic mechanisms of various body systems are composed of protein such as insulin and glucagon, both of which are involved in control of normal blood sugar levels. Proteins found in the blood act as important carrier substances, including hemoglobin to carry oxygen between the lungs and the cells, lipoproteins which help transport fats throughout the body and transferrin which carries iron through the blood.[1] Plasma proteins are also involved in maintenance of the acid-base balance acting as the largest source of buffers in the blood. Finally, proteins are involved in the body's immune system in the form of immunoglobulins to make the antibodies that provide resistance to disease.[1]

The cat has the highest overall protein requirement when compared to any other mammal, including the dog.[3] This is not due to a higher requirement for essential amino acids, but rather because of some nitrogen catabolic enzymes in the liver of the cat that are permanently set to handle a high level of dietary protein; their activity is not modified or down-regulated even when the cat is receiving a low protein diet.[4] Cats also lack the ability to conserve nitrogen from the body's general nitrogen pool. This inflexibility of liver enzyme activity and fixed high rate of catabolic activity basically obligates cats to consume a high-protein diet.[3]

All proteins in the body are in a constant state of renewal and degradation. Though tissues vary in their rate of turnover, all protein molecules in the body are eventually catabolized and replaced.[1-4] During periods of growth or reproduction, additional protein is needed for the creation of new tissue. A regular supply of protein and nitrogen is necessary to maintain normal metabolic processes and provide for tissue maintenance and growth. The body does have the ability to synthesize new proteins from amino acids, provided that all of the necessary amino acids required for that protein synthesis are available to the tissue cells.[1] A high rate of protein synthesis occurs in the production of red and white blood cells, epithelial cells of the skin and those lining the GI tract and the pancreas.[2] Muscle protein composes nearly 50% of the total body protein, but only accounts for 30% of the new protein synthesized. Visceral and organ proteins consist of a smaller portion of the total body protein but account for 50% of the new proteins synthesized.[2] Rates of protein synthesis and degradation for any particular protein can change under different physiologic conditions.[2]

Protein consumed over what the animal requires is viewed as surplus. As amino acids are not able to be stored in the body above the small amount found in each cell in the amino acid pool, surplus amino acids are either used directly for energy production or converted to glycogen and stored in the muscle or liver or fat and stored in adipose tissue.[5]

Dietary Protein

The body does not care where the amino acids come from for its use, whether they are synthesized by the body, supplied in the diet as single amino acids or as intact proteins. Because of this, it can accurately be said that the body does not have a "protein requirement," but rather an amino acid requirement.[1] Absorbed amino acids and small di- and tripeptides are reassembled into "new" proteins by the liver and other tissues in the body.[2] After absorption, the amino acids go toward tissue synthesis, especially muscles and liver, synthesis of enzymes, albumin, hormones and other nitrogen-containing compounds and deamination (removal of the amine group) and use of the remaining carbon skeletons for energy.[2]

Proteins in the diet serve several functions. They provide the essential amino acids (which in turn are used for synthesis of protein in the growth and repair of tissue) and they are the body's primary source of nitrogen.[1] Nitrogen is essential for the synthesis of the nonessential amino acids and other nitrogen-containing compounds such as nucleic acids and certain neurotransmitter substances. Amino acids in the diet can also be metabolized for energy.[1] The gross energy of amino acids, once fecal and urinary losses are accounted for, are approximately the same as carbohydrates, 3.5 kcal/g.[1] A secondary function of proteins in dog and cat diets is to provide a source of flavor. Different flavors can be created when proteins in the diet are cooked in the presence of carbohydrates and fats. As the protein content in the diet increases, the food generally becomes more palatable and acceptability by the animal increases.[5]

Structural proteins in all tissues, especially in muscle, liver and serum albumin, can be considered as amino acid stores. These stores are not the same as the fat and carbohydrate stores, as they represent active, functional tissue. Use of these stores by the body for amino acids will decrease the function and ability of the animal.[2] Muscle stores represent the largest reserve from which amino acids can be drawn from in times of need, though too much loss of body protein can impair muscle function, including decreased cardiac and respiratory function.[2]

The degree to which a dog or cat is able to use the protein in the diet as a source of amino acids and nitrogen is affected by both the digestibility and the quality of the protein.[1] Proteins that are highly digestible and contain all of the essential amino acids in their proper proportions relative to the animal's needs are considered high-quality proteins. Those that are either low in digestibility or limiting in one or more of the essential amino acids are of lower quality.[1] The higher the quality of the protein in the diet, the less quantity will be needed by the animal to meet all of its essential amino acid needs.[1]

Protein Quality

The chemical score is an index that involves comparing the amino acid profile of a given protein with the amino acid profile of a reference of very high quality. Egg protein is typically used as the reference protein, and is given a chemical score of 100. The essential amino acid that is in greatest deficit in the test protein is called the limiting amino acid because it will limit the body's ability to use that protein.[1] The percentage of that amino acid present in the protein relative to the corresponding value in the reference protein determines the chemical score of the test protein.[1] The three amino acids in food proteins that are most often limiting are methionine, tryptophan and lysine. Having a chemical score can be helpful information concerning the amino acid deficits of a protein source, but its value is based entirely on the level of the most limiting amino acid in the food and does not take into account the proportions of all of the remaining amino acids.[1]

Biologic value is defined as the percentage of absorbed protein that is retained by the body. It is a measure of the ability of the body to convert absorbed amino acids into body tissue.[1] One problem with using biologic value as a measurement of protein quality is that is does not account for protein digestibility. In theory, if a small portion of a very indigestible protein that is absorbed is used efficiently by the body, it could still have a very high biologic value.[1] Protein quality can only be determined through the use of feeding trials, and digestibility is not usually listed on the product label (Table 5.2).[5]

Multiple protein sources are often combined together in pet foods to improve the overall quality and amino acid profile when foods are formulated. By combining

Table 5.2 Protein quality of common pet food ingredients

Ingredient	Percent protein	Chemical score	Biologic value
Egg (dried)	45–49%	100	94
Casein	80%	58	80
Beef, pork, lamb, chicken	29%	69	74
Soybean meal	48%	47	73
Whole corn	8%	41	59
White rice	7%	43	65
Wheat	14%	43	65
Collagen	88%	0	0

Source: Reference 2.

proteins based on their relative amino acid excesses and deficiencies, a food can be formulated with a higher-quality protein profile. This method of improving protein quality is called protein complementation.[2] Amino acid fortification is another method for improving the protein quality in foods. In this method one or more amino acids are added to a food when the main source of protein may be limiting. This is seen most commonly with methionine and lysine.[2]

Taurine

Taurine is an essential amino acid in cats, which in most mammals can be synthesized from methionine and cysteine. It belongs to a separate group of amino acids, called amino-sulphonic acids, and does not form part of the polypeptide chains like the other amino acids.[3,4] Cats have a very limited ability to synthesize taurine from other sulfur-containing amino acids, and therefore have an increased dietary requirement for it.[3,4] Taurine is necessary for bile acid conjugation to aid in digestion of fats and is necessary for normal retinal function and myocardial function.[3] Taurine is present only in animal tissues. Consumption of a diet containing high levels of plant products and cereal grains may not provide sufficient taurine, even if meat-based products are included in the diet.[3]

Taurine requirements for cats consuming canned foods are substantially higher than that for cats consuming dry foods.[3,4] The heat used to process the canned foods can damage the protein in the diet and lead to the production of indigestible protein by-products. These products are less digestible than untreated protein and travel to the large intestine where they are fermented by intestinal microbes. These bacterial populations responsible for the fermentation also degrade taurine.[3] This ultimately increases the fecal loss of taurine for the cats fed canned food diets. As a substantial proportion of the taurine requirements of adult cats are to replace the taurine lost in the feces through bile loss, anything that increases this loss also increases their requirements.[3]

References

1 Case LP, Carey DP, Hirakawa DA, Daristotle L (2000) Protein and amino acids. In Gross *et al.* (eds), *Canine and Feline Nutrition* (2nd edn), pp. 23–8, St Louis, MO: Mosby.
2 Gross, KL, Wedekind KL, Cowell CS *et al.* (2000) Nutrients. In MS Hand, CD Thatcher, RL Remillard *et al.* (eds), *Small Animal Clinical Nutrition* (4th edn), pp. 48–59, Marceline, MO: Walsworth Publishing.
3 Case LP (2003) The cat as an obligate carnivore. In *The Cat: Its Behavior, Nutrition and Health*, pp. 303–8, Ames, IA: Iowa State Press.
4 Simpson JW, Anderson RS, Markwell PJ (1993) Nutrients and the requirements of dog and cats. In CJ Price, PCG Bedford, JB Sutton (eds), *Clinical Nutrition of the Dog and Cat*, pp. 23–7, Cambridge, MA: Blackwell.
5 Case LP, Daristotle L, Hayek M, Raasch MF (2011) Protein and amino acids. In *Canine and Feline Nutrition* (3rd edn), pp. 21–5, St Louis, MO: Mosby.

6 Vitamins

Introduction

Vitamins are defined by their physical and physiologic characteristics. In order for a substance to be classified as a vitamin it must have five basic characteristics: (1) it must be an organic compound different from fat, protein and carbohydrate, (2) it must be a component of the diet, (3) it must be essential in minute amounts for normal physiologic function, (4) its absence must cause a deficiency syndrome, and (5) it must not be synthesized in quantities sufficient to support normal physiologic function.[1] These definitions are important, because not every vitamin is essential for every species.

Vitamins are needed in minute quantities to function as essential enzymes, enzyme precursors or coenzymes in many of the body's metabolic processes.[1,2] A general classification scheme for vitamins divides them into two groups: the fat soluble vitamins – A, D, E and K, and the water soluble vitamins – Vitamin C and the B-complex vitamin group.[2] Unlike carbohydrates, proteins or fats, vitamins do not supply any energy for the animal. However, they are essential in assisting the enzymes in releasing energy from these nutrients.[3]

For dogs and cats, the only essential water-soluble vitamins are the B-complex vitamins. Dogs and cats are able to synthesize vitamin C from glucose, unlike humans and guinea pigs for which vitamin C is an essential vitamin.[4] The fat-soluble vitamins A, D, and E are seen as essential, while vitamin K can typically be manufactured in adequate amounts by the intestinal microflora.[4]

Because of the differences in water solubility and chemical structure in vitamins, they are absorbed into the body through a variety of means.[1] Fat-soluble vitamins require bile salts and fat to form micelles for absorption: they are then passively absorbed through the lacteals (usually in the duodenum and ileum) and transported with chylomicrons to the liver via the lymphatic system.[1] Water soluble vitamins are absorbed by way of active transport, some vitamins requiring a carrier protein as with B12 (cobalamin) and the protein, intrinsic factor, where others require a sodium dependent, carrier-mediated absorption pump.[1]

Fat soluble vitamins can be stored in the body's lipid deposits, making them more resistant to deficiency, but are also more likely to result in toxicity.[1,2] Water soluble vitamins are depleted at a faster rate because of limited storage, and are less likely to cause toxicity, but more likely to become deficient.[1,2]

Vitamin requirements differ based on the lifestage of the animal. Growing and reproducing animals are making new tissues and therefore require higher levels of vitamins, minerals, protein and energy for optimal performance.[1] As animals age, metabolic and physiologic changes may also increase the requirements for vitamins.[1] Various disease conditions may also affect vitamin status. Prolonged starvation deprives animals of vitamins and other nutrients, and depletes the vitamin stores. Polyuric diseases such as diabetes mellitus and chronic renal failure may increase the excretion of water-soluble vitamins. Additionally, certain drugs, mainly antibiotics, may decrease the intestinal microflora responsible for vitamin K synthesis, and diuretic drug therapy may increase the excretion of water-soluble vitamins.[1] Since vitamins are organic compounds, they can be destroyed by a variety of means rendering them unable to perform their duties.[3]

Synthetic and naturally made vitamins are used by the body in the same way, though they may have different availabilities.[1] All commercial pet foods contain vitamin supplementation. It is very difficult to formulate a diet that meets all the vitamin requirements entirely from ingredient sources. Because of these vitamin additions, it is usually unnecessary and perhaps unwise to supplement commercial foods with

Nutrition and Disease Management for Veterinary Technicians and Nurses, Second Edition. Ann Wortinger, Kara M. Burns
© 2015 John Wiley & Sons, Inc. Published 2015 by John Wiley & Sons, Inc.
Companion Website: www.wiley.com/go/wortinger/nutrition

additional vitamin supplements.[1] Supplementation may be necessary in light of certain diseases, but should be part of a monitored long-term treatment plan directed by the veterinary team.[1]

Fat Soluble Vitamins

Vitamin A

Plants do not contain vitamin A per se, but instead contain provitamins in the form of carotenes and carotenoids. Beta-carotene has the greatest vitamin A activity as compared to the other carotenoids, but has only half the potency of pure vitamin A.[1] The carotenoids are the dark red pigments in plants that provide the deep yellow/orange color of many plants.[2] Vitamin A can also be found in some animal tissues, with highest concentrations found in the liver and fish liver oils, as well as milk and egg yolks.[1,2]

Vitamin A is absorbed almost exclusively as retinol into the lymphatic system with low-density lipoproteins (LDL) and transported to the liver, where it is deposited mainly in the hepatocytes and parenchymal cells.[1] A special transport protein called retinol-binding protein is responsible for picking up vitamin A from the liver and transporting it throughout the body.[5]

Vitamin A is necessary for normal functioning in vision, bone growth, reproduction, tooth development and maintenance of epithelial tissue including the mucous membranes lining the respiratory and gastrointestinal tracts.[1]

With vitamin A deficiencies, differentiation of new epithelial cells fails to occur, and normal epithelial cells are replaced with dysfunctional cells. Epithelial cells that do not function properly lead to lesions in the epithelium and increased susceptibility to infection.[1] Normal spermatogenesis in males and normal estrous cycles in females are also dependent on vitamin A.[2] Without vitamin A, the rods in the eyes become increasingly sensitive to light changes, which eventually leads to night blindness.[2]

Vitamin A toxicities can results in skeletal malformation, spontaneous fractures and internal hemorrhage.[1] Other signs may include anorexia, slow growth, weight loss, skin thickening, increased blood clotting time, enteritis, congenital abnormalities, conjunctivitis, fatty infiltration of the liver and reduced function of the liver and kidneys.[1]

Unlike dogs and most other animals, cats require preformed vitamin A or retinol. They lack the intestinal enzyme necessary to convert beta-carotene to active vitamin A.[1,2,4,6] Preformed vitamin A can only be found in animal tissues further supporting the evidence that cats are obligate carnivores.[1,2,6]

Vitamin D

Vitamin D consists of a group of compounds that regulate calcium and phosphorus metabolism in the body. The two most important of these compounds are vitamin D2 – ergocalciferol and vitamin D3 – cholecalciferol. Vitamin D2 is found primarily in harvested or injured plants, but not in living plant tissue. Because of this it is only of importance to herbivores.[2] Vitamin D3 is synthesized in the skin of animals when its precursor 7-dehydrocholesterol is exposed to ultraviolet light from the sun.[2] The 7-dehydrocholesterol is made in the liver from the fatty acid, cholesterol.[5] This form of vitamin D can be obtained either through synthesis in the skin or from consumption of animal products that contain cholecalciferol.[2] Cholecalciferol is most often associated with animal sourced products, while ergocalciferol is associated with plant sourced products.[5]

Both ingested and endogenous vitamin D3 is stored in the liver, muscle and fat tissue. Cholecalciferol is an inactive storage form of vitamin D. To become active it must first be transported from the skin or intestines to the liver where it is hydroxylated (an OH compound is added) to 25-hydroxycholecalciferol. This compound is then transported to the kidneys, where it is further converted by the addition of another OH group to one of several metabolites, the most active form being called calcitriol.[1,2,5] Although inactive vitamin D is considered a vitamin, calcitriol (1,25-dihydroxy vitamin D3) is often classified as a hormone because it is produced by the body and because of its mechanism of action.[2,5]

The primary function of vitamin D is to enhance intestinal absorption, mobilization, retention and bone deposition of calcium and phosphorus.[1] In the intestines vitamin D stimulates the synthesis of calcium binding protein, which enhances absorption of dietary calcium and phosphorus.[2] Vitamin D also affects normal bone growth and calcification by acting with parathyroid hormone (PTH) to mobilize calcium from the bone, and by causing an increase in phosphate reabsorption in the kidneys. The net effect of vitamin D's actions in the intestines, bones and kidneys is an increase in plasma calcium and phosphorus to the level that is necessary to allow for normal mineralization and remodeling of the bone.[2] Other target cells for vitamin D outside of the bones include cells of the immune system, brain and nervous systems, pancreas, skin, muscles and cartilage and reproductive organs.[5]

Signs of vitamin D deficiency are frequently seen with simultaneous deficiencies or imbalances of calcium and phosphorus. Clinical signs generally include rickets in young animals, enlarged costochondral junctions, osteomalacia and osteoporosis in adult animals and decreased plasma calcium and inorganic phosphorus concentrations.[1]

Vitamin D toxicity is usually associated with increases in vitamin D3 rather than vitamin D2. Excessive intake can result in hypercalcemia, soft tissue calcification and ultimately death.[2] Of the fat soluble vitamins, this one is most likely to have toxic effects when consumed in excessive amounts.[5]

Marine fish and fish oils are the richest natural sources of vitamin D in foods, but may pose a risk for toxicity. Researchers have found that moist foods generally contain higher levels of vitamin D than do dry foods and some moist foods exceeded the AAFCO maximal allowances.[1] Other dietary sources include fresh water fish and egg yolks. Beef, liver and dairy products contain smaller amount of vitamin D. The most common synthetic source of vitamin D in pet foods includes deactivated animal sterol in the form of sheep lanolin (cholecalciferol), vitamin D3 supplementation, deactivated plant sterol (ergocalciferol) and vitamin D2 supplementation.[1,4]

For most animals, exposure to direct sunlight for UV production of vitamin D is poor due to their living situations (primarily house pets), darkly pigmented skin or thick hair coats.[2] It has been suggested that if the skin of dogs and cats were exposed to sunlight, rather than shaded by their hair, they would be able to synthesize adequate amounts of vitamin D. However, research done by Drs Hazewinkel and Morris has not supported this theory.[4]

Vitamin E

Vitamin E is made up of a group of chemically related compounds called the tocopherols and tocotrienols.[1,2] Alpha tocopherol is the most active form of vitamin E in the body, and is the compound most commonly found in pet foods. Unfortunately, this form is also the least

potent in the form of an antioxidant in food stuffs. Delta tocopherol is the most potent antioxidant for foods, but is also the least biologically active form.[1] Because of this mix of activities, vitamin analyses of food stuffs are not a reliable means of determining vitamin activity.[1] Most foods add mixed tocopherols to cover all the bases; biologic activity and antioxidant activity.

Within the body, vitamin E is found in at least small amounts in almost all the tissues, with the liver able to store the largest amounts.[2] Vitamin E is absorbed from the small intestine by nonsaturable, passive diffusion into the intestinal lacteals and is transported via the lymphatics to the general circulation.[1] Absorption of vitamin E is enhanced by the simultaneous digestion and absorption of dietary fats. There is a very high correlation between tocopherol levels and the total lipid or cholesterol concentration in the plasma.[1] The vitamin is found in highest concentrations in membrane-rich cell fractions such as the mitochondria and microsomes.[1]

The need for vitamin E in the diet is markedly influenced by dietary composition, with increased need seen with increased levels of polyunsaturated fatty acids (PUFAs) in the diet, oxidizing agents, vitamin A, carotenoids and trace minerals. Decreased need is seen in increased levels of fat-soluble antioxidants, sulfur-containing amino acids and selenium.[1]

The chief function of vitamin E in the diet is as a potent antioxidant functioning to prevent the chain reaction of free radicals producing more free radicals.[5] PUFAs that are present in the foods and in the lipid membranes of the body's cells are very vulnerable to oxidative damage. Vitamin E interrupts the oxidation of these fats by donating electrons to the free radicals that induce lipid peroxidation.[2] Vitamin E also protects vitamin A and sulfur-containing amino acids from oxidative damage.[2]

Vitamin E has a close relationship with the trace mineral selenium. Selenium is a cofactor for the enzyme glutathione peroxidase, which functions to reduce the peroxides that are formed during the process of fatty acid oxidation. The inactivation of these peroxides by glutathione peroxidase protects the cell membrane from further oxidative damage.[1,2,5] By preventing the oxidation of cell-membrane fatty acids and the formation of peroxides, vitamin E spares selenium, while selenium creates a similar effect and is able to reduce the animal's vitamin E requirement.[1,2,5]

Deficiencies in vitamin E are seen primarily in the neuromuscular, vascular and reproductive systems with most signs being attributed to membrane dysfunction as a result of oxidative damage and disruption of critical cellular processes.[1] Clinical signs in dogs include degenerative skeletal muscle disease associated with muscle weakness, degeneration of testicular germinal epithelium and impaired spermatogenesis and failure of gestation. In cats, deficiency signs include steatitis, focal interstitial myocarditis, and focal myositis of skeletal muscle and periportal mononuclear infiltration of the liver.[1]

Vitamin E is one of the least toxic vitamins; animals can apparently tolerate very high doses without adverse effects. However, at extremely high doses, antagonism with other fat-soluble vitamins may occur, resulting in impaired bone mineralization, reduced hepatic storage of vitamin A and coagulopathies as a result of decreasing absorption of vitamins D, A and K.[1]

Vitamin E is synthesized only by plants, the richest sources being vegetable oils and to a lesser extent seeds and cereal grains. Tocopherol concentrations are highest in green leaves. Animal tissues tend to be low in vitamin E, with the highest levels being found in fatty tissues.[1]

Vitamin K

Vitamin K comprises a group of compounds called the quinones. Vitamin K1 (phylloquinone) occurs naturally in green leafy plants, and vitamin K2 (menoquinone) is synthesized by bacteria in the large intestine.[1,2,5] Vitamin K3 (menadione) is the most common form of synthetic vitamin K and has a vitamin activity two to three times higher than that of natural vitamin K1.

Vitamin K is required for normal blood clotting, as it is needed for the production of normal prothrombin (factor II) and for the synthesis of clotting factors VII, IX and X in the liver.[1,2,5] Vitamin K is also involved in the synthesis of osteocalcin, a protein that regulates the incorporation of calcium phosphates in growing bone.[1]

Vitamin K is found in green leafy vegetables such as spinach, kale, cabbage and cauliflower. Generally, animal sources contain lower amounts of vitamin K, though liver, egg, alfalfa meal, oilseed meal and certain fish meals are fairly good sources.[1,2] The synthesis of vitamin K by intestinal bacteria of dogs and cats can contribute at least a portion, if not all of the daily requirements for these species.[2] Coprophagy increases vitamin K absorption in dogs.[1]

Deficiency can occur with intestinal malabsorption diseases, ingestion of anticoagulants (mouse or rat poisons), destruction of the gut microflora by antibiotic therapy, and congenital defects.[1] Vitamin K3 has lower lipid solubility and is the most effective form of vitamin K for cases of malabsorption, while vitamin K1 is the only form of vitamin K effective in anticoagulant poisonings.[1] Deficiency can also be seen in cats being fed certain commercial foods containing high levels of salmon or tuna.[1]

Toxicity has only been reported once, and occurred secondary to warfarin (rodenticide) ingestion when vitamin K1 was given intravenously instead of subcutaneously or orally, as recommended.[1]

Water Soluble Vitamins

B-Complex Vitamins

The B-complex vitamins are all water soluble vitamins that were originally grouped together because of similar metabolic functions and occurrence in foods.[2] These nine vitamins act as coenzymes for specific cellular enzymes that are involved in energy metabolism and tissue synthesis.[2] Coenzymes are small organic molecules that must be present with an enzyme for a specific reaction to occur, similar to a key being required for a lock to engage.[2] The vitamins thiamin (B1), riboflavin (B2), niacin, pyridoxine (B6), pantothenic acid, and biotin are all involved in the conversion of food to energy. Folic acid, cobalamin (B12) and choline are important for cell maintenance and growth and/or blood cell synthesis.[1,2]

Sources for the B-complex vitamins include organ meats, as well as the germinal parts of grains and yeasts. Vitamin B12 is the exception, as it can only be obtained from animal sources.[4]

Thiamin

Thiamin, also called vitamin B1, is a component of the coenzyme thiamine pyrophosphate, which plays an important role in carbohydrate metabolism.[1-3,6] The thiamin requirement of an animal would be directly related to the carbohydrate content of the diet being fed.[2,6]

Thiamin is hydrolyzed to free thiamin by intestinal phosphatases before absorption by intestinal cells. Absorption takes place primarily in the jejunum by an active, carrier mediated transport system. The absorbed thiamin is transported in red blood cells and plasma with tissues then taking up the thiamin. The heart, liver and kidneys have the highest concentrations of thiamin in the body.[1]

A deficiency of thiamin results in an impairment of carbohydrate metabolism with accumulation of pyruvic and lactic acids within the body. This causes clinical signs related to the central nervous system because of the dependence of this system on a constant source of carbohydrate, in the form of glucose for energy.[2,6]

Thiamin deficiencies can be seen with inadequate dietary intake, or with high intake of foods containing thiamine antagonists. Thiaminases are found in high concentrations in raw fish, shellfish, bacteria, yeast and fungi. Thiaminases are destroyed by cooking.[1]

Thiamine can be readily found in many foods, with good sources being brewer's yeast, whole grain cereals, organ meats and egg yolk. Thiamine is heat labile, and is progressively destroyed by cooking.[1,2,6]

Riboflavin

Riboflavin, vitamin B2, is the precursor to a group of enzymatic cofactors called flavins. Flavins when linked to proteins are called flavoproteins.[1] It is named for its yellow color (flavin) and because it contains the simple sugar D-ribose (ribo).[2] It is relatively stable with heat-processing, but is easily destroyed by exposure to light and irradiation.[2]

Riboflavin functions in the body as a component of two different coenzymes, flavin mononucleotide and flavin adenine dinucleotide.[2] Both of these coenzymes are required in oxidative enzyme systems that function to release energy from carbohydrates, fats and proteins as well as in several biosynthetic pathways.[2]

After absorption in the intestinal tract, about 50% of the riboflavin in the blood is bound to albumin and the other half to globulins.[1] Additionally, microbial synthesis of riboflavin occurs in the large intestine of most species.[2] The amount synthesized is dependent on the carbohydrate content of the diet.[1,3]

Deficiency in dogs and cats is uncommon, but signs of dermatitis, erythema, weight loss, cataracts, impaired reproduction, neurologic changes and anorexia can be seen. Toxicity has not been reported in the dog or cat.[1,3]

Because there appears to be little storage of riboflavin in the body, daily intake of this vitamin is critical.[1] Good sources of riboflavin include dairy products, organ meats, muscle meats, eggs, green plants and yeast. Cereal grains are poor sources of riboflavin.[1]

Niacin

The term niacin encompasses both nicotinic acid and nicotinamide (also known as niacinamide) and is closely associated with riboflavin in cellular oxidation-reduction enzyme systems.[2,5,6] After absorption in the intestines, niacin is rapidly converted by the body into nicotinamide, the metabolically active form of the vitamin.[2] Nicotinamide is then incorporated into two different coenzymes, nicotinamide adenine dinucleotide (NAD) and nicotinamide adenine dinucleotide phosphate (NADP).[2,5,6] These coenzymes function as hydrogen-transfer agents in several enzymatic pathways involved in the use of fat, carbohydrate and protein.[2,6] Most animals can also synthesize niacin as an end-product of the metabolism of the essential amino acid tryptophan.[1,2]

Niacin is a fairly stable vitamin and processing conditions may actually release some bound niacin, which increases availability.[1] Niacin deficiency may occur when foods low in niacin and tryptophan are eaten such as corn and other grains. This deficiency results in a condition called pellagra, or black tongue. Signs seen are dermatitis, diarrhea, dementia and death. Clinical deficiencies in dogs in not common, as most commercial foods are adequately supplemented. However cats, because they are not able to synthesize substantial amounts of niacin from tryptophan and require preformed niacin, can develop deficiencies when fed high cereal diets.[1]

Niacin can be found in a wide variety of foods, the greatest levels being found in yeast, animal and fish by-products, cereals, legumes and oilseeds. Unfortunately, a large portion of the niacin found in many plant sources is in a bound form and unavailable for absorption. The niacin found in animal sources is primarily in the unbound, available form.[1,2] Niacin is less vulnerable to destruction during food processing and storage than are the other water-soluble vitamins.[3]

Pyridoxine

Vitamin B6 comprises three different compounds: pyridoxine, pyridoxal and pyridoxamine. All three are convertible in the dog and cat to the coenzyme pyridoxal 5'-phosphate which is the biologically active form of the vitamin.[1,2,6] Pyridoxine is involved in a wide range of enzyme systems, particularly associated with amino acid metabolism and to a lesser extent in the metabolism of glucose and fatty acids.[1,2,6] Pyridoxal 5'-phosphate is also required for the synthesis of hemoglobin and the conversion of tryptophan to niacin.[2] The pyridoxine requirements in the diet vary based on the protein levels in the diet.[2]

All three forms of B6 are freely absorbed via passive diffusion in the small intestine.[1] The predominate form found in the blood is pyridoxal phosphate, which is tightly bound to proteins.[1] Only small amounts of vitamin B6 are stored in the body, with any excesses and products of metabolism being excreted in the urine.[1]

Reduced growth, muscle weakness, neurologic signs, mild microcytic anemia, irreversible kidney lesions, decreased steroid hormone activity and anorexia are all signs of pyridoxine deficiency.[6] Oxalate crystalluria is also a notable sign of pyridoxine deficiency in cats. Naturally occurring deficiencies in dogs and cats have not been reported. Deficiencies have only been seen in specially formulated, deficient diets or owner made deficient diets.[1]

The incidence of toxicity is apparently very low; earliest detectable signs include ataxia and loss of small motor control.[6]

Vitamin B6 is widely distributed in foods, occurring in the greatest concentrations in meats, whole grain products, vegetables and nuts.[1] Plant tissues contain mostly pyridoxine, where animal tissues contain mostly pyridoxal and pyridoxamine.[1] Pyridoxine is far more stable than either of the other two forms, thus processing loss is greatest in foods containing high amounts of animal tissue.[1]

Pantothenic Acid

Pantothenic acid is derived from the Greek word "pantos" meaning "found everywhere or all" because this vitamin occurs in all body tissues and in all forms of living tissue.[1,2] Once absorbed, pantothenic acid is phosphorylated by adenosine triphosphate (ATP) to form coenzyme A.[1,2,6] This is one of the most important coenzymes and is involved in the metabolism of carbohydrates, fats and some amino acids within the citric acid cycle.[1,2,6]

Coenzyme A and acyl carrier protein are the primary forms of pantothenic acid found in foods. Both forms are degraded to pantothenic acid in the small intestine in a series of steps. Absorption occurs via a sodium-dependent energy-requiring process. At high concentrations, simple diffusion occurs throughout the small intestine. Pantothenic acid is transported in the free acid form in plasma. Red blood cells, which carry most of the vitamin, contain primarily acetyl-coenzyme A.[1]

Dogs with pantothenic acid deficiency have erratic appetites, depressed growth, fatty livers, decreased antibody response, hypocholesterolemia and can progress to coma in later stages.[1] Cats with pantothenic acid deficiencies can develop fatty livers and become emaciated. Pantothenic acid is generally regarded as nontoxic. No adverse reactions or clinical signs are seen other than gastric upset in animals consuming large quantities.[1]

Pantothenic acid is found in virtually all foodstuffs, so a naturally occurring deficiency is unlikely.[2,6] The most important sources are meats, especially liver and heart, egg yolk, dairy products and legumes.[1,2] Losses during food processing can be substantial because pantothenic acid is readily destroyed by freezing, canning and refining processes.[6]

Folic Acid

Folic acid is also known as vitamins B10 and B11 as well as pteroylglutamic acid.[1,6] This is a family name for a group of vitamins with related biologic activity. Other common names include folate, folates and folacin.[1] Folic acid requires enzymatic changes to form the active compound tetrahydrofolic acid; from this molecule the folate coenzymes used in the body are made.[6]

Folic acid acts as a one carbon methyl donor and acceptor molecule in intermediary metabolism.[1,2] An important role of folic acid is its involvement in the synthesis of thymidine, a component of deoxyribonucleic acid (DNA).[2] Vitamin B12 is also closely paired with folic acid in the production of methionine from homocysteine.[1]

Natural sources of folic acid undergo hydrolysis by intestinal enzymes and absorbed by enterocytes. Folic acid must be in the reduced form (i.e. dihydro, tetrahydro) to participate in the one-carbon metabolic reactions.[1] It is found most commonly in the "bound" form combined with a string of amino acids (glutamate) forming a compound known as polyglutamate.[3] Intestinal enzymes hydrolyze the polyglutamate to monoglutamates and several other glutamates. These are further reduced enzymatically to the active forms.[3]

Folic acid is synthesized by bacteria in the intestine and this largely meets the daily requirement of dogs and cats under normal circumstances.[6] It is required daily in the diet, as no reserves are kept in the body.[1] Naturally occurring deficiencies would be uncommon, but could be seen with deficient diets and with intestinal disease.[6] Clinical signs of folate deficiency are poor weight gain, anemia, anorexia, leukocytopenia (low white blood cell count), glossitis and decreased immune function. There have been no reported cases of folate toxicity as excess folate is sent to the liver and added to bile and disposed of through the intestines.[1,3]

Folic acid is found in green, leafy vegetables, organ meats and egg yolks. The vitamin is destroyed by heating, prolonged freezing and during storage in water.[1,2]

Biotin

Biotin was originally known as the "bios" factor. It is a sulfur-containing vitamin that functions as a coenzyme in several carboxylation reactions.[1,2,6] It acts as a carbon dioxide carrier in reactions in which carbon chains are lengthened, specifically in certain steps of fatty acid, nonessential amino acid and purine synthesis. In its active form it is always found covalently bound to a protein (apoprotein).[1]

After ingestion, biotin must be hydrolysed from protein by the enzyme biotinidase to be absorbed by the intestine. After hydrolysis, free biotin is absorbed through the intestine and transported through the blood to the tissues. Bacteria in the intestines are also able to synthesize biotin for use by the body.[6]

Naturally occurring biotin deficiencies are very rare in dogs and cats. Feeding raw egg whites and oral antibiotic use are probably the two most common causes.[1] Egg white contains a compound called avidin, which binds to biotin and makes it unavailable for absorption by the body.[1,2] Cooking destroys avidin, and allows the biotin in the egg to be used. Avidin can also prevent absorption of endogenously produced biotin by the intestinal bacteria.[6] Clinical signs of biotin deficiency include poor growth, dermatitis, lethargy, and neurologic abnormalities.[1] Biotin toxicity has not been reported in dogs and cats.[1]

The biotin requirement is thought to be met by two sources, diet and intestinal microbes since mammalian tissue is unable to synthesize it.[1] Biotin is widely found in many foods, but bioavailability varies greatly. Oilseeds, egg yolks, alfalfa meal, liver, and yeast are good sources of biotin. Marked losses of biotin can occur as a result of oxidation, canning, heat and solvent extraction of foodstuffs.[1,2]

Cobalamin

Vitamin B12 is the only vitamin that contains a trace element, cobalt. Cobalamin is the largest and most complex of the B vitamins.[1] When isolated from natural sources it is usually found in the form of cyanocobalamin, when transformed to a metabolically active coenzyme the cyano group is replaced by another chemical group attached to the cobalt group.[6]

Cobalamin and its metabolites are important in one-carbon metabolism during various biochemical reactions, and are involved in fat and carbohydrate metabolism as well as myelin synthesis.[1,2] The function of vitamin B12 is closely linked to that of folate.[1,2,6]

Cobalamin absorption depends on dietary intake and adequate gastrointestinal tract function. In most animals, absorption of cobalamin from the diet is facilitated by a group of glycoproteins called intrinsic factors, which are produced by the pancreas and gastric mucosa.[1,2] The absence of these factors can lead to vitamin B12 deficiency.[1,2] Most B12 deficiencies are not due to poor intake, but rather poor absorption. Inadequate absorption typically occurs either due to lack of hydrochloric acid in the stomach or lack of intrinsic factor.[3]

Vitamin B12 deficiency is very rare, but may result in poor growth and neuropathies. Because vitamin B12 is only made by microbes and found in animal tissues, a vegetarian diet may lead to deficiencies.[1] Microwave heating inactivates vitamin B12.[3] Toxicities have not been found in dogs and cats other than those given excessive amounts parenterally.[1]

Good sources of cobalamin include organ meats, fish and dairy products. This vitamin is unique in that once it is absorbed from the diet; excess amounts can be stored by the body. The primary place of storage is the liver, though muscle, bone and skin can also contain small amounts.[2] The body is so efficient at storing and recycling B12 that deficiencies may take years to develop.[3]

Choline

Choline is classified as one of the B-complex of vitamins, even though it does not entirely satisfy the strict definition of a vitamin.[1] Choline, unlike the other B-vitamins, can be synthesized in the liver from the amino acid serine. In this reaction, methionine acts as a methyl donor, with folic acid and cobalamin also being needed. It is required in much larger quantities by the body than the other B vitamins.[1,2] Because of this, even though it is an essential nutrient, not all animals require it as a dietary supplement making it a conditionally essential nutrient.[1,3] Choline also does not function as a coenzyme or cofactor as do most other vitamins, but is an integral part of cellular membranes.[1]

Choline functions as an integral part of cellular membranes as the phopholipid lecithin, promotes lipid transport as phosphatidylcholine, as a neurotransmitter as acetylcholine and as a source of methyl groups for transmethylation reactions.[1,2,5,6]

Choline is released from lecithin in the diet by digestive enzymes in the intestinal tract, and absorbed from the jejunum and ileum mainly by a carrier-mediated process. Once absorbed, choline is transported through the lymphatic system in the form of phosphatidylcholine bound to chylomicrons.[1]

Because on its synthesis in the liver, its presence in many foods and the ability of methionine to spare choline, dietary deficiencies of choline have not been reported in cats and dogs.[2]

Dietary sources include egg yolks, organ meats, legumes, dairy products and whole grains.[2]

Vitamin C

Ascorbic acid can be synthesized from glucose by plants and most animals including dogs and cats. Chemically its structure is closely related to that of the monosaccharide sugars.[1,2] Vitamin C functions in the body as an antioxidant and free radical scavenger.[1] Ascorbic acid is best know for its role in collagen synthesis though it is also involved in drug, steroid, and tyrosine metabolism, as well as electron transport in cells.[1] It is necessary for synthesis of carnitine to act as a carrier for the acyl groups across mitochondrial membranes.[1] Larger doses may play an important role in immune function and protecting against carcinogens.[1] Ascorbic acid acts as a nitrate scavenger, thereby reducing nitrosamine-induced carcinogenesis.

Dogs and cats are able to synthesize adequate amounts of ascorbic acid; therefore dietary amounts are absorbed by passive diffusion in the intestinal tract. Ascorbic acid is produced in the liver from either glucose or galactose through the glucuronate pathway.[1] Absorption efficiency in the intestines is unusually high ~80–90%.[1] Vitamin C is transported in the plasma in association with albumin. It is found widely distributed in all body tissues, with the pituitary and adrenal glands having the highest concentrations.[1] During periods of stress, the adrenal glands release vitamin C, together with hormones into the blood.[3]

Deficiency is unlikely due to dogs and cats being able to synthesize most if not all of their requirements.[2] Toxicity has not been seen in dogs and cats.[1]

Sources of vitamin C include fruits, vegetables and organ meats. Vitamin C content of most foods decreases dramatically during storage and processing as it is easily destroyed by oxidative processes. Exposure to heat, light, alkalis, oxidative enzymes and the minerals copper and iron can all increase losses of vitamin C activity.[2]

Vitamin-like Substances

Carnitine

L-carnitine is a natural compound found in all animal cells.[1] Its primary function is to transport long-chain fatty acids across the inner mitochondrial membrane into the mitochondrial matrix for oxidation.[1,3] It is synthesized primarily in the liver, and stored in the skeletal and cardiac muscles.[1,2]

Lysine, methionine, ascorbic acid, ferrous ions, vitamin B6 and niacin are all important in L-carnitine metabolism; these nutrients are required substrates and cofactors for enzymes involved in biosynthesis.[1]

Clinical signs of L-carnitine deficiency include chronic muscle weakness, fasting hypoglycemia, cardiomyopathy and hepatomegaly.[1] In many cases of deficiency, no clinical signs are seen.[1]

Carotenoids

This is a group of pigments that exhibit vitamin-like activities. More than 600 different compounds are classified as carotenoids, but fewer than 10% can be metabolized into vitamin A.[1] The carotenoids found in greatest numbers in a variety of foods include beta-carotene, alpha-carotene, lutein, lycopene, beta-cryptoxanin, zeaxanthin, canxanthin and astaxanthin.[1]

Carotenoids are digested and absorbed into the body using bile salts. Carotenoids are incorporated into micelles where they are absorbed by the small intestinal lacteals by way of passive diffusion.[1] After transportation in chylomicrons in the lymphatic system, they are bound to lipoproteins and transported into the bloodstream.[1]

Carotenoids have biologic activity beyond their vitamin A role. Carotenoids with nine or more double bonds function as antioxidants, and they also protect cell membranes by stabilizing the oxygen radicals produced.[1]

Carotenoids are found abundantly in orange and green vegetables, highly pigmented fruits and some species of fish.[1]

Bioflavonoids

The bioflavonoids are another group of red, blue and yellow pigments consisting of over 4000 different compounds, but are not classified as carotenoids. Like the carotenoids, they also have vitamin-like activities.[1]

Flavonoids are usually found naturally as glycosides linked to sugars. Mammalian enzymatic systems are unable to hydrolyze flavonoids, but the necessary enzymes are present in the gut microflora.[1] After hydrolysis and absorption in the small intestines, flavonoids are bound in the liver.

The flavonoids have a sparing effect on vitamin C; they also have the ability to perform similarly to vitamin C. Flavonoid reactions are involved in the antioxidant system for lipid and water environments.

Bioflavonoids are found most abundantly in the skins and peels of colored fruits and vegetable.[1]

References

1 Gross KL, Wedekind KL, Cowell CS *et al.* (2000) Nutrients. In MS Hand, CD Thatcher, RL Remillard *et al.* (eds), *Small Animal Clinical Nutrition* (4th edn), pp. 80–95, Marceline, MO: Walsworth Publishing.

2 Case LP, Carey DP, Hirakawa DA, Daristotle L (2000). Vitamins. In *Canine and Feline Nutrition* (2nd edn), pp. 29–40, St Louis, MO: Mosby.

3 Whitney E, Rolfes SR (2008) The water soluble vitamins: B vitamins and vitamin C. In *Understanding Nutrition* (11th edn), pp. 323–57, Belmont, CA: Thomson Wadsworth.

4 Delaney SJ, Fascetti AJ (2012) Basic nutrition overview. In AJ Fascetti, SJ Delaney (eds), *Applied Veterinary Clinical Nutrition*, pp. 13–14, Chichester, West Sussex, UK: Wiley-Blackwell.

5 Whitney E, Rolfes, SR (2008) The fat soluble vitamins: A, D, E, and K. In *Understanding Nutrition* (11th edn), pp. 369–86, Belmont, CA: Thomson Wadsworth.

6 Simpson JW, Anderson RS, Markwell PJ (1993) Nutrients and the requirements of dog and cats. In CJ Price, PCG Bedford, JB Sutton (eds), *Clinical Nutrition of the Dog and Cat*, pp. 30–7, Cambridge, MA: Blackwell.

7 Minerals

Introduction

Minerals are the inorganic portion of the diet. Some are required in large quantities because they form a major part of the body's structural components while others are only required in small quantities for the chemical processes of metabolism.[1]

As with most other nutrients, problems with minerals in the diet are usually related more to excesses or imbalances with other nutrients rather than a result of actual deficiencies in the diet.[2] Because of this, in a diet that is known to be nutritionally complete in its mineral content, further supplementation is at best wasteful, and at worst dangerous to the health of the animal.[1]

More than 18 minerals are believed to be essential for mammals. By definition, macrominerals are required by the animal in the diet in percentage amounts, where microminerals are required at a part per million (ppm) level.[3] Unlike vitamins, minerals are inorganic compounds that always retain their original chemical structure. Once they enter the body, they will remain there until excreted. Minerals can also not be destroyed by heat, air, acid or mixing.[4]

Minerals are used by the body for structural components as seen with calcium, phosphorus and magnesium in bones and teeth, as portions of body fluids and tissues as with the electrolytes sodium, potassium, phosphorus, chloride, calcium and magnesium, and as catalysts/cofactors in enzyme and hormone systems as seen with iodine and selenium and in the oxygen delivery system as seen with iron in hemoglobin.[3]

Availability of minerals from the diet, as well as how effectively the mineral can be used by the individual animal, can be affected by a number of things. These include the chemical form of the mineral which effects solubility, the amounts and proportions of other dietary components that the mineral interacts with metabolically, the age, gender and species of the animal, the intake of the mineral, the body's need (amount found in the body's stores), and environmental factors.[3]

Meat-derived foods are considered a more available source of certain minerals that plant derived foods. The organic forms of minerals found in meats are often more available or as available as those from inorganic mineral supplements, while those found in plants are often less available.[3] Meats, unlike plants do not contain anti-nutritional factors, such as phytate, oxalate, goitrogens and fibers. These all have the potential to reduce mineral availability in the diet.[3] Also different forms of minerals differ in availability based on what they are combined with; generally sulfur and chloride forms have the best availability, followed by carbonates, with oxides being the most poorly available.[3]

Macrominerals

Calcium

Calcium has two important functions within the body. It is necessary for the formation and maintenance of the skeleton and teeth, and it acts as an intracellular messenger that allows cells to respond to stimuli such as hormones and neurotransmitters.[3]

Calcium serves two physiologic functions in bones, as structural material and as a storage site for calcium.[3] The amount of calcium absorbed from the diet can range from 25% to 90%, depending on the calcium status, the form of the calcium and intake in the diet.[3] The calcium found in blood, lymph, and other body fluids accounts for only ~1% of the total calcium in the body; the remaining 99% is found in the bones and teeth.[3]

Calcium absorption by the body can be actively regulated by vitamin D, facilitated or passively absorbed. Irregardless of how the calcium is absorbed, vitamin D is the most important regulator of calcium absorption.[3] Vitamin D helps to make the calcium-binding protein needed for absorption of calcium.[4] Absorption of

Nutrition and Disease Management for Veterinary Technicians and Nurses, Second Edition. Ann Wortinger, Kara M. Burns
© 2015 John Wiley & Sons, Inc. Published 2015 by John Wiley & Sons, Inc.
Companion Website: www.wiley.com/go/wortinger/nutrition

calcium is most efficient during times of inadequate intake, and decrease as calcium needs are met. Blood calcium levels change only in response to abnormal regulatory control, not due to levels found in the diet.[4]

Deficiencies are uncommon today in well-formulated pet foods. Though calcium imbalances can occur as a result of poor feeding practices. Calcium deficiencies are most commonly seen when dogs and cats are fed "table scrap" diets or all meat diets consisting primarily of muscle and organ meats.[2,3] This type of diet is very low in calcium, and high in phosphorus that can develop into nutritional secondary hyperparathyroidism. The low dietary levels of dietary calcium stimulates the release of parathyroid hormone (PTH), the PTH increases the resorption of calcium from the bone in an attempt to increase the plasma calcium levels. Eventually this can lead to significant bone loss with resultant pathologic fractures.[2,3] Calcium excesses are most commonly due to dietary supplementation, especially of large breed, fast growing puppies. By over-supplementing the diet with calcium, deficiencies can be produced in other nutrients as well as the potential for causing increased incidence of osteochondritis dessecans (OCD), hypertrophic osteodystrophy (HOD), and Wobbler's syndrome to name only a few.[2,3]

A relative calcium deficiency can also be seen with eclampsia, though this is more of a problem of calcium homeostasis in the body.[2] Eclampsia is seen most often in small breed dogs, and less frequently in cats.[2] This is usually seen 2–3 weeks after parturition and is caused by a failure of the mother's calcium regulatory system to maintain plasma calcium levels when there is loss of calcium in the milk.[2] With subnormal calcium plasma levels, seizures and tetany can be seen. Prognosis is good if treatment is started at an early stage.[2] Excess calcium supplementation to try to prevent this problem can actually exacerbate it. When calcium intake is high, the PTH level is low. As milk production increases, calcium is lost in the milk. Normally PTH would be stimulated to release calcium from the bone to maintain plasma levels. The PTH is unable to respond quickly enough to prevent dangerously low plasma levels from occurring in the mother.[2] The best course of preventative action is to feed a high-quality commercial diet that has been formulated for growing animals and gestation from the time of pregnancy though parturition and lactation.[2]

Calcium can be found in meat meals because of their bone content, soybean meal and flaxseed meal. Grains and meats without bones are poor sources of calcium. The most common supplements used in pet foods include calcium carbonate (limestone), calcium sulfate, calcium chloride, calcium phosphate and bone meal.[3]

Phosphorus

After calcium, phosphorus is the largest constituent found in bones and teeth. Phosphorus is a structural component of RNA and DNA as well as energy generating compounds such as ATP, as part of the phospholipids found in cell membranes, and combined with structural proteins as with phosoproteins.[3,4] Phosphorus salts in the form of phosphates are found in the bones and teeth, but also in all the cells in the body, and as a part of the major buffer system regulating the acid-base balance in the body.[4] These functions make it essential for cell growth and differentiation, energy use, transfer and metabolism, fatty acid transport and amino acid and protein formation.[3,4] Generally, phosphorus is more available from animal-based ingredients than from plant-based ingredients.[3] Phosphorus found in meats is primarily in the organic form, while that found in plants is in the form of phytic acid which is only about 30% available to monogastric animals.[3] Phytic acid is a phosphorus containing compound that can bind other minerals, including calcium, and make them unavailable for absorption.[2]

Regulation of phosphorus within the body involves the coordinated efforts of both the intestines and the kidneys. When dietary intake is low, intestinal absorption is highly efficient and the kidneys decrease urinary losses. When dietary intake is high, intestinal absorption decreases and urinary losses increase.[3]

High levels of phosphorus can be found in meats, eggs and milk products. The primary supplements used in pet foods include calcium phosphate, sodium phosphate and phosphoric acid.[3]

Magnesium

Magnesium in the third largest mineral constituent found in the body after calcium and phosphorus.[3] It is involved in the metabolism of carbohydrates and lipids as well as acting as a catalyst for a wide variety of enzymes. As a cation (a positively charged particle) in the intracellular fluid, magnesium is essential for the cellular metabolism of both carbohydrates and proteins. Protein synthesis also requires the presence of ionized magnesium.[2] Magnesium can be found in soft tissue and bone as well as the intracellular and extracelluar fluids.[2] Over half of the magnesium found in the body is located in the bones.[4] A number of dietary and physiologic factors can negatively impact magnesium absorption, including high levels of phosphorus, calcium, potassium, fat and protein in the diet.[3]

Magnesium homeostasis within the body is controlled primarily through the kidneys; because of this certain drugs can cause increased renal excretion of magnesium. These would include diuretics, aminoglycosides, cisplatin, cyclosporine, amphotericin and methotrexate.[3]

A deficiency of magnesium in the diet results in signs of weakness, ataxia with eventual progression to seizures. Naturally occurring magnesium deficiency is usually not seen in healthy dogs and cats.[2] Avoiding excess magnesium is recommended to prevent the formation of struvite crystals and stones in the urine.[3] In sick animals, magnesium deficiencies can be seen with gastrointestinal and kidney diseases.[3]

Sources of magnesium in the diet include ingredients containing bone (bone meals), oilseeds (flaxseed and soybean meal), and unrefined grains and fiber sources (wheat bran, oat bran, beet pulp). Common supplements found in pet foods are magnesium oxide and magnesium sulfate.[3]

Sodium and Chloride

Sodium and chloride are the major electrolytes of the extracellular fluids, and are important for maintaining osmotic pressure, regulating acid-base balance and transmitting nerve impulses and muscle contractions.[2,3] Sodium ions must also be present in the intestinal lumen for absorption of sugars and amino acids.[3] Calcium absorption and mobilization is affected by the presence of sodium, and the absorption of several vitamins such as riboflavin, thiamin and ascorbic acid is sodium dependent.[3]

Sodium and chloride are readily absorbed from the small intestine, with excretion primarily in the urine though small amounts can be in the feces and perspiration.[3] In very low sodium diets, the body has a remarkable ability to conserve sodium by excreting very low amounts in the urine.[3]

Concentrations of sodium in the body are regulated by various hormones acting to maintain a constant sodium/potassium ratio in the extracellular fluid.[3]

Sodium requirements are influenced by reproductive status, lactation, rapid growth and heat stress.

When consuming a diet with high levels of sodium, a secondary increase in water intake is seen as well as an increase in urination with high salt excretion by the kidneys.[2] Studies have indicated that dogs and cats are resistant to salt retention and hypertension when fed diets high in sodium when compare to humans.[2]

Fish, eggs, dried whey (milk protein), poultry by-product meal and soy isolate are all high in sodium and chloride.[3] Typical dietary supplements added to pet foods include salt, sodium phosphates, calcium chloride, choline chloride, potassium chloride and sodium acetate.[3]

Microminerals

Iron

Iron is present in several enzymes and other proteins responsible for oxygen activation, for electron transport and for oxygen transport. Iron found in food exists primarily as heme iron present in hemoglobin and myoglobin and as nonheme iron found in grains and other plants.[3] The amount of iron absorbed from food is dependent on the iron status of the body, the availability of dietary iron, and the amounts of heme and nonheme iron found in the food.[3]

Ferrous iron has lost 2 electrons and has a net positive charge of +2. When iron has been oxidized, it loses another electron for a net loss of 3 electrons, giving it a positive charge of +3 resulting in ferric iron.[4] Ferrous iron can be oxidized to ferric iron, and ferric iron can be reduced to ferrous iron.[4] These different forms of iron allow it to participate in the electron transport chain that transfers hydrogen and electrons to oxygen forming water, and in the process makes ATP for energy use.[4]

Iron is transported by plasma to the bone marrow where it is used for hemoglobin synthesis in red blood cells.[3] It is stored primarily as ferritin and hemosiderin in the liver, bone marrow and spleen.[3] Excretion of iron is limited, with only small amounts being found in the urine. The iron appearing in the feces is primarily unabsorbed iron, though it is continually lost in sweat, hair and nails.[3]

Excesses of iron in the diet should be avoided because of potential antagonism with other minerals primarily copper and zinc.[3] Chronic blood loss will eventually deplete iron stores and cause a microcytic, hypochromic anemia. This is seen most commonly with parasitic infections, both intestinal in the form of hookworms and external with fleas and ticks.[3] Young animals are especially at risk due to their low iron stores and the low iron content in milk.[3]

Some dietary factors in foods can bind with nonheme iron inhibiting absorption from the gastrointestinal tract. These include phytate (phytic acid) found in legumes, whole grains and rice; vegetable proteins in soybeans, other legumes and nuts; calcium found in milk and polyphenols in grain products.[4]

High levels of iron are found in most meats, especially organ meats, other sources include beet pulp, soymill run and peanut hulls.[3] Typical iron additives used in pet foods include ferrous sulfate, ferric chloride, ferrous fumarate, ferrous carbonate, and iron oxide.[3] Iron oxide is not biologically available to dogs and cats but is added to foods to give it a "meaty red" color.[3]

Zinc

Second only to iron, zinc is the most abundant micromineral found in the body. It is important for carbohydrate, lipid, protein and nucleic acid metabolism. It is necessary for the maintenance of normal skin integrity, taste and immunologic functioning.[2,3] Zinc also helps with growth and development as well as synthesis, storage and release of the hormone insulin from the pancreas.[4]

Homeostasis is controlled through absorption and excretion. Absorption occurs primarily in the small intestine. This absorption is markedly affected by other dietary components.[3] Phytate, found in many plants decreases zinc absorption while certain materials such as citrate, picolinate, EDTA and amino acids such as histidine and glutamate increase zinc absorption.[3] The liver is the primary organ involved with zinc metabolism. Storage of zinc is limited except in the bone. Stores only increase slightly when dietary levels increase.[3]

Zinc can be recycled in the body from the pancreas to the intestines and back to the pancreas in a process called enteropancreatic circulation of zinc.[4] Once outside of the intestines, zinc is transported in the plasma bound to albumin and transferrin.[4]

Signs of zinc deficiency can be seen in animals being fed high cereal diets due to the phytate found in them. This, in combination with calcium, combines to form an insoluble complex of phytate, calcium and zinc.[3] Deficiency can be seen even when zinc levels in the diet are lower recommended levels.[3] The only reported cases of toxicity have been due to dietary indiscretion as seen with the eating of pennies, die-case nuts from animal carriers and baby lotions containing zinc.[3] Excesses in the diet can interfere with absorption of other minerals primarily iron and copper.[3]

Zinc can be found in most meats, fiber sources and dicalcium phosphate. Zinc supplements used most often include zinc oxide, zinc sulfate, zinc chloride and zinc carbonate.[3]

Copper

Copper is used by the body for iron absorption and transport and hemoglobin formation. Most of the copper found in the body is bound to the plasma protein ceruloplasmin. This protein functions as a carrier of copper and in the oxidation of plasma iron. Copper is also required for the conversion of the amino acid tyrosine to the pigment melanin and for the synthesis of connective tissues collagen and elastin as well as for production of ATP.[2] Copper is needed for normal osteoblast activity during skeletal growth.[2] Like iron, copper is needed in many of the metabolic reactions related to the release of energy.[4]

Absorption of copper occurs throughout the intestinal tract, with the major portion being in the small intestine.[3] The liver is the primary site of copper metabolism, with hepatic concentrations reflecting an animals' intake and copper status.[3] Excess copper is excreted in the bile.[2]

Copper deficiency results in a hypochromic, microcytic anemia similar to that seen with iron deficiency. Other signs of deficiency can include depigmentation of colored hair coats, and impaired skeletal development in young animals.[2] Excessive copper can result in interference with zinc and iron metabolism.[3]

The richest sources of copper include legumes, whole grains, nuts, shellfish and seeds, most organ meats are also rich in copper.[4] Typical dietary supplements include cupric sulfate, cupric carbonate and cupric chloride.[3]

Selenium

Selenium shares some of the chemical characteristics of the mineral sulfur, allowing it to substitute for sulfur in the amino acids methionine, cysteine and cysteine.[4] Selenium is an essential component of the enzyme glutathione peroxidase, which helps to protect cellular and subcellular membranes from oxidative damage.[2,3] Glutathione peroxidase deactivates lipid peroxides that are formed during oxidation of cell-membrane lipids.[2] Vitamin E protects the polyunsaturated fatty acids (PUFAs) in cell membranes from oxidative damage, preventing the release of lipid peroxides. By reducing the number of peroxides that are formed, vitamin E spares the cellular use of selenium.[2] Selenium also helps to spare vitamin E by preserving the pancreas, allowing for normal fat digestion and thus normal vitamin E absorption, and by reducing the amount of vitamin E required to maintain lipid membrane integrity through the availability of glutathione peroxidase.[3]

Selenium deficiencies or toxicities have not been reported in dogs and cats.[3] Selenium availability in food is highly influenced by whether the selenium is from foods or found as a supplement.[3] Selenium availability averages ~30% in ingredients of animal origin, and ~50% in ingredients of plant origin.[3]

Sources of selenium include fish, eggs and liver. Common supplements found in pet foods include sodium selenite and sodium selenate.[3]

Iodine

Iodine is required by the body for the synthesis of the hormones thyroxine and triiodothyronine by the thyroid gland.[2] Thyroxine stimulates cellular oxidative processes and regulates the basal metabolic rate.[2] This affects thermoregulation, reproduction, growth and development, circulation and muscle function.[3]

The thyroid gland effectively traps iodine daily to ensure adequate supplies for production of the thyroid hormones.[3] This trapping mechanism regulates a more or less constant iodine supply to the thyroid glands over a wide range of plasma levels.[3] Iodine requirements are influenced by physiologic state and diet.[3] Lactating animals require more dietary iodine because of loss through the milk.[3] The hypothalamus regulates thyroid hormone production by controlling the release of the pituitary's thyroid-stimulating hormone (TSH).[4]

The principle sign of iodine deficiency is goiter, an enlargement of the thyroid gland.[2] Naturally occurring dietary deficiency does not usually occur, but diets containing "goitrogenic compounds" can lead to this. Certain compounds found in peas, peanuts, soybeans and flaxseed can bind iodine making it unavailable for use.[3]

Fish, eggs, iodized salt and poultry by-product meal are good sources of iodine. Common supplements found in pet foods include calcium iodate, potassium iodide and cuprous iodide.[3]

Chromium

Chromium participates in the carbohydrate and lipid metabolism. Like iron, it also has different charges, with the Cr+++ ion being the most stable.[4] Chromium helps to maintain glucose homeostasis by enhancing the activity of the hormone insulin. Research has not shown that chromium supplements effectively improve glucose or insulin response in diabetics though.[4]

Chromium can be found in a variety of foods such as liver, brewer's yeast and whole grains.[4]

References

1 Simpson JW, Anderson RS, Markwell PJ (1993) Nutrients and the requirements of dog and cats. In CJ Price, PCG Bedford, JB Sutton (eds), *Clinical Nutrition of the Dog and Cat*, pp. 27–30, Cambridge, MA: Blackwell.

2 Case LP; Carey DP, Hirakawa DA, Daristotle L (2000) Vitamins and minerals. In *Canine and Feline Nutrition* (2nd edn), pp. 123–8, St Louis, MO: Mosby.

3 Gross KL, Wedekind KL, Cowell CS *et al.* (2000) Nutrients. In MS Hand, CD Thatcher, RL Remillard *et al.* (eds), *Small Animal Clinical Nutrition* (4th edn), pp. 66–80, Marceline, MO: Walsworth Publishing.

4 Whitney E, Rolfes SR (2008) Water and the major minerals. In *Understanding Nutrition* (11th edn), pp. 408–24, Belmont, CA: Thomson Wadsworth.

8 Digestion and Absorption

Introduction

The role of digestion is to break up the large complex molecules found in many nutrients into their simplest, most soluble forms so that absorption and use by the body can take place.[1] The two basic types of action involved in this process are mechanical digestion as seen with chewing and peristaltic action in the stomach and intestines, and chemical or enzymatic digestion as seen with the splitting of chemical bonds of the complex nutrients.[1]

The three major types of foods requiring digestion are fats, carbohydrates and proteins. Before fats can be absorbed they need to be hydrolyzed to glycerol, free fatty acids and some mono and diglycerides. Complex carbohydrates are broken down to the simple sugars of glucose, fructose and galactose for use by the body. Proteins are hydrolyzed to their simple amino acids units and some dipeptides.[1,2] The process of digestion begins when food first enters the mouth, and continues until the excretion of waste products and the undigested portion of the foods in the feces.[1]

Digestive Tract

The digestive tract can be described as a hollow tube which starts at the mouth and continues all the way to the anus.[3] Within this tube, various changes take place to allow ingested nutrients to be processed and utilized.[3]

In all species, the mouth functions to bring food into the body and start the initial breaking down of the food by chewing and mixing the food with saliva.[1] Saliva is produced in response to the sight and smell of food. It acts as a lubricant to make both chewing and swallowing easier and serves to liquefy the parts of the food that stimulate the taste buds and impart flavor to the food.[1,2] Saliva is composed of water, salts, mucus and for dogs,

amylase to initiate digestion of carbohydrates.[4] Cats lack salivary amylase, which in other animals starts carbohydrate digestion in the mouth.[5]

The tongue serves to help move the food bolus around the mouth and when the food bolus begins to liquefy, allows the animal to taste the food it has consumed.[4] Unlike many herbivores that thoroughly chew their food, dogs and cats often swallow large bites of food with little or no chewing.[1−3] The teeth of dogs and cats have few flat chewing surfaces as would be seen with an herbivore. An additional distinction can be seen with cats, which have fewer premolars and molars than do dogs. The additional teeth provide dogs with an increased capacity to chew and crush their food.[1,2] The dental pattern seen with dogs is suggestive of a more omnivorous diet, while that of cats is typical of the pattern seen with most other obligate carnivores.[1]

From the mouth the food passes into the esophagus. When empty the esophagus is a collapsed tube with longitudinal folds.[3] The lining of the esophagus contains many goblet cells which secrete a large amount of mucus to further assist in the lubrication of food during swallowing.[1,3] At the end of the esophagus is the cardia or cardiac sphincter, a muscular ring that allows food to pass into the stomach, but constricts back down to prevent reflux of stomach contents back into the lower esophagus.[1−3]

Swallowing involves a series of three steps; the first is under voluntary control, the remaining two are involuntary.[3] Swallowing is initiated by the formation of a bolus of food within the mouth; this is then pushed against the hard palate by the tongue and projected back into the pharynx.[3] Sensory receptors in the pharynx start the second step of swallowing by detecting the food bolus and closing the nasopharynx by upward movement of the soft palate. The pharyngeal muscles contract forcing the bolus of food into the esophagus, the last phase of swallowing involves detection of the

Nutrition and Disease Management for Veterinary Technicians and Nurses, Second Edition. Ann Wortinger, Kara M. Burns
© 2015 John Wiley & Sons, Inc. Published 2015 by John Wiley & Sons, Inc.
Companion Website: www.wiley.com/go/wortinger/nutrition

food bolus within the cranial esophagus. This detection produces a peristaltic wave moving the food bolus down the esophagus into the stomach. A second peristaltic wave will often follow, ensuring that the food has been completely emptied into the stomach.[3]

The stomach acts as a reservoir for ingested food, and initiates the digestion process.[3] By acting as a reservoir, the stomach allows for ingestion of a few large meals throughout the day rather than multiple smaller meals.[1] The stomach in cats is smaller than that found in dogs. Cats consume several smaller meals throughout the day (usually 10–20 meals); therefore they did not need to have a large capacity stomach.[2,5]

Chemical digestion of protein starts in the stomach, as well as mixing of the food with the gastric secretions. The stomach also controls entry of food into the small intestine.[1] The gastric secretions are composed of mucus to protect the stomach lining and further lubricate the food, hydrochloric acid to provide the proper pH for the necessary enzymatic reactions to occur, and pepsinogen a proteolytic enzyme.[1] Hydrochloric acid converts the pepsinogen into the active enzyme pepsin. This initiates the hydrolysis of protein molecules to smaller polypeptide units.[1] The acidic environment of the stomach serves to protect the animal from bacterial growth and kills most bacteria entering the body through the mouth.[4] The sight, smell and taste of food, together with the presence of food in the stomach, stimulate the secretion of hydrochloric acid and pepsinogen.

The stomach has a built in pacemaker which produces five slow waves per minute, some of which initiate muscular contractions.[3] These peristaltic movements slowly mix the ingested food with the gastric secretions, preparing it for entry into the small intestine.[1] Thorough mixing of the ingested food results in the production of a semifluid mass of food called chyme. Chyme must pass through the pyloric sphincter of the stomach to enter the small intestine for further digestion. The pyloric sphincter acts to control the rate of passage of chyme into the small intestine. The rate of emptying can be affected by osmotic pressure, particle size and viscosity of the chyme.[1] Generally, larger meals have a slower rate of emptying than do small meals, liquids leave the stomach faster than do solids, and very high fat meals may cause a decrease in stomach emptying rate. Diets that contain soluble fiber such as pectin, guar gum or fructooligosaccharides can cause a decreased rate of emptying when compared to diets that contain insoluble dietary fibers such as cellulose, peanut hulls and hemicelluloses.[1] At this stage of digestion, even though the food is now semisolid chyme, the carbohydrates and fats are almost unchanged in composition, but the proteins have been partially hydrolyzed into smaller polypeptide units.[2] The majority of digestion up to this point has been primarily mechanical in nature, which is all about to change.[1]

The small intestine starts at the pylorus and ends at the ileocecocolic junction. It is divided into three parts, the duodenum, jejunum and ileum. The duodenum is the first and shortest portion of the small intestine and is the site where the pancreatic and bile ducts enter the intestine.[3] The jejunum and ileum form the main portion of the small intestine, there is no clear divisions between the different parts of the small intestine.[3]

Further mechanical digestion can also occur in the small intestine through the contraction of the muscle layers.[1] These contractions continue to mix the food with intestinal secretions, increasing the exposure of digested food particles to the surface of the intestine and slowly propel the food mass through the intestinal tract.[1]

Both the pancreas and glands located in the duodenal mucosa secrete enzymes into the intestinal lumen that begin the chemical digestion of fat, carbohydrate and protein. These enzymes include intestinal lipase, amino peptidase, dipeptidase, nucleotidase, nucleosidase and enterokinase.[1] Intestinal lipase converts fat to monoglycerides, diglycerides, glycerol and free fatty acids. Amino peptidase breaks the peptide bond located at the terminal end of the protein molecule, slowly releasing single amino acid units from the protein chain.[1] Dipeptidase breaks the peptide bond of dipeptides to release two single amino acid units. Both nucleotidase and nucleosidase hydrolyze nucleoproteins to their constituent bases and pentose sugars.[1] Enterokinase converts inactive trypsinogen secreted by the pancreas into its active form of trypsin, once activated, trypsin is able to activate more of itself as well as the other protease enzymes.[3] The cells of the brush border that lines the intestines completes the final digestion of carbohydrates through the secretion of the enzymes maltase, lactase and sucrase- the brush border enzymes. These convert the disaccharides maltose, lactose and sucrose into the base monosaccharides of glucose, fructose and galactose.[1]

The pancreas is responsible for secreting the enzymes trypsin, chymotrypsin, carypeptidase and nuclease.[1] Most of these are secreted in the inactive form and are activated by other components in the small intestine after release.[1] The pancreas also produces lipase and amylase which are responsible for hydrolysis of fats and starches into smaller units. The acidic chyme produced in the stomach is neutralized by bicarbonate salts produced in the pancreas, this helps to adjust the intestinal pH to provide an optimal environment for the digestive enzymes to work.[1,4]

Bile Salts

Bile salts are essential for the production of a lipid/water interface to permit lipase digestion of the triglycerides.[3] They are produced in the liver from cholesterol and concentrated and stored in the gall bladder. Bile's primary function in the small intestine is the emulsification of dietary fat and the activation of certain lipases.[1,4] The intestinal contractions ensure thorough mixing of the fat, lipase and bile salts. This produces an emulsion of small fat droplets called micelles.[3]

Hormones in Digestion

Hormonal control of digestion in the small intestine involves several parts. Secretin is produced by the duodenal mucosa in response to the entry of chyme from the stomach.[1] Secretin stimulates the release of bicarbonate from the pancreas and controls the rate of bile release from the gall bladder. Cholecystokinin is also released from this portion of the duodenal mucosa in response to the presence of fat in the chyme. This hormone stimulates the contraction of the gall bladder, causing the release of bile into the intestinal lumen.[1] Cholecystokinin is also called pancreozymin, and stimulates the release of the pancreatic enzymes.[1]

In dogs and cats the chemical digestion of food is completed in the small intestine. Absorption involves the transfer by the body of digested nutrients from the intestinal lumen into the blood or lymphatic system for delivery to tissues throughout the body.[1] Like digestion, the primary site of absorption also occurs in the small intestine.[1]

Digestion after the Intestines

Amino acids units are absorbed into the enterocytes lining the small intestine by specific carriers using an energy-dependent active process. Different carriers are used for different classes of amino acids.[3] Once absorbed, the amino acids are sent to the liver by way of the portal vein.[3]

After the brush border enzymes have broken down the carbohydrates into their smallest particles they are absorbed by the enterocytes using specific carriers in an active energy-requiring process. When the monosaccharides are in the enterocytes, they are rapidly released into the capillaries and transported to the liver.[3]

The micelles produced in the intestines are absorbed through a passive process into the enterocytes along with absorption of the fat soluble vitamins.[3] Within the enterocyte the fatty acids reform into triglyceride and attach to lipoproteins to form chylomicrons. These chylomicrons are released into the lacteal, the part of the intestinal lymphatics that absorbs fats, for transportation to the liver and other tissues.[3] The bile remains within the intestinal lumen, and eventually travels down to the jejunum to be reabsorbed and circulated back to the liver for reuse.[1]

Water and electrolytes both flow across the intestinal mucosa in response to osmotic pressure.[1] Most of the minerals are absorbed by the body in the ionized form, meaning they carry an electrical charge. The water soluble vitamins are absorbed by passive diffusion, though some may be absorbed by active processes when dietary levels are especially low.[1]

The liver further processes the absorbed monosaccharides and amino acids that arrive through the portal vein.[1] Some of the monosaccharides are converted to glycogen for storage, and some are secreted directly into the circulation. Some amino acids are released directly into the bloodstream where they are available to the tissues for absorption into the cells. Excess amino acids are either converted to other nonessential amino acids or metabolized by the liver and converted to fat for storage.[1] Once these amino acids are converted to fats, they can no longer be used for protein production.

Large Intestine Digestion

The large intestine begins at the ileocecocolic valve and continues as the cecum, ascending, transverse and descending colon, rectum and anus.[3] These divisions are clearly demarcated based on their location within the abdomen.[3]

The contents of the small intestine enter the colon through the ileocecolic valve.[1,3] The cecum is small in dogs and cats and consists of an intestinal pocket next to the junction of the colon and small intestine, and serves no known function in these animals.[3] In nonruminant herbivores such as the rabbit and horse, the cecum is quite large and has highly enhanced digestive capacities.[1]

The colon has three primary functions, the absorption of water and electrolytes, and the fermentation of food residues by the resident bacterial population and storage of feces in the rectum.[3]

Unlike the small intestine, the large intestine has no villi and therefore has limited capacity for absorption of nutrients. It can absorb water and electrolytes quite well, though it has no mechanisms for active transport.[1] The absorption of water by the large intestine is very important in ensuring passage of formed feces and preventing dehydration.[3] Normally, water is passively absorbed from the colon following the active energy-dependent absorption of sodium chloride.

The bacterial colonies of the large intestine are able to digest some of the insoluble fiber and other nutrients in the diet that have escaped digestion in the small intestine. These bacteria are able to produce certain short chain fatty acids (SCFAs), the most important being butyrate which is used by the colonocytes for energy rather than using glucose or amino acids.[1] The microflora in the colon not only produces SCFAs but also the vitamins biotin and vitamin K, carbon dioxide and methane.[6]

When amino acids reach the colon undigested, the bacteria produce the amines indole and skatole. In addition hydrogen sulfide gas is produced from the sulfur-containing amino acids.[1] Hydrogen sulfide gas, indole and skatole impart strong odors to the feces and are responsible for flatulence.[1] Certain types of carbohydrates found in legumes such as soybeans are resistant to digestion by the enzymes of the small intestine. When these carbohydrates reach the colon and the resident bacteria, there is a resultant production of intestinal gas (flatulence). The degree to which flatulence and strong fecal odors occur in dogs and cats that are fed poorly digestible materials varies with the amounts and types of materials fed as well as the resident bacteria that are present in the individual animals.[1,2]

Any material that survives the digestive process in the stomach, small and large intestines is viewed as nondigestible and is termed waste material.[5] By the time feces have been excreted, the body has extracted all the usable energy, vitamins, minerals and fiber found in the food.

References

1 Case LP, Carey DP, Hirakawa DA, Daristotle L (2000) Digestion and Absorption. In *Canine and Feline Nutrition* (2nd edn), pp. 53–60, St Louis, MO: Mosby.

2 Case LP (2003) The cat as an obligate carnivore. In *The Cat: Its Behavior, Nutrition and Health*, pp. 303–8, Ames, IA, Iowa State Press.

3 Simpson JW, Anderson RS, Markwell PJ (1993) Anatomy and physiology of the digestive tract. In CJ Price, PCG Bedford, JB Sutton (eds), *Clinical Nutrition of the Dog and Cat*, pp. 1–18, Cambridge, MA: Blackwell.

4 Whitney E, Rolfes SR (2008) Digestion, absorption and transport. In *Understanding Nutrition* (11th edn), pp. 71–89, Belmont, CA: Thomson Wadsworth.

5 Kirk CA, Debraekeller J, Armstrong PJ (2000) Normal cats. In MS Hand, CD Thatcher, RL Remillard *et al.* (eds), *Small Animal Clinical Nutrition* (4th edn), pp. 291–337, Marceline, MO: Walsworth Publishing.

6 Gross KL, Jewell DE, Yamka RM *et al.* (2010) Macronutrients. In MS Hand, CD Thatcher, RL Remillard *et al.* (eds), *Small Animal Clinical Nutrition* (5th edn), pp. 74–5, Marceline, MO: Walsworth Publishing, Mark Morris Institute.

9 Energy Balance

Introduction

Energy in food is different from nutrients in that intake must be kept close to requirements. Energy balance is when an animal's intake is sufficient to meet its needs, and minimal changes in the energy stored by the body occur.[1,2] Positive energy balance happens when caloric intake exceeds energy expenditure and weight gain can occur.[2] In growing and pregnant animals, excess energy is converted primarily to lean body tissue; in adult animals excess energy is stored primarily as fat, with only some increase in lean body tissue.[1,2] A negative energy balance occurs when caloric intake is insufficient to meet energy expenditures. When this is the case, weight loss and decreases in both fat and lean body stores can occur.[1,2] A very specific amount of energy is required by animals to maintain a given body weight. Slight variations in this requirement can result in increases and decreases in body weight.[3]

Units of Measure

Energy is the capacity of the body to do work. To measure the energy used we typically use the calorie. A calorie is defined as the amount of heat required to raise the temperature of 1 ml of water 1°C.[3] Because this amount of energy is actually very small, what we use in nutrition to express energy content is actually a kilocalorie, or 1000 calories. You may see this expressed as "kcal," "kilocal," "big calorie" or "Calorie" (note the uppercase "C"). In large animal nutrition, a megacalorie (Mcal) may be used, which is equivalent to 1,000,000 calories or 1000 kcals.

While we think of calories as being a metric expression, the actual metric unit used to designate measurement of energy is the joule.[3] To convert from calories to joules you multiple calories by 4.184 to obtain joules. As with calories, joules are a very small unit of measure and are more commonly expressed as kilojoule (1000 joules) and megajoule (1,000,000 joules).[3]

Energy content of food is expressed as the amount of energy (kcals) per unit of weight or volume. The weight of a given volume of food will vary based on the density of food, which can vary greatly.[3]

Daily Energy Requirements

The daily energy requirement (DER) for dogs and cats depends on the amount of energy that the body expends on a daily basis.[2] Energy balance though is achieved by matching input and output over a long period of time.[1] Even a small imbalance maintained over a long period of time can cause weight gain or weight loss dependent on the direction of the imbalance.[1]

The principal mechanism for control of energy balance is thought to be through regulation of intake, though some variation in output can be important.[1] The energy requirement of the animal and the energy density of the food will determine the quantity of food eaten on a daily basis.[1] But a highly palatable food can lead to excess intake over energy expenditure and a poorly palatable food can lead to an insufficient intake to meet energy requirements. Regulation of intake is considered to be a negative feedback system, meaning that as weight increases, intake will decrease, and when weight decreases, intake will increase.

Energy expenditure can be divided into four major areas, resting energy requirement (RER), voluntary muscular activity expenditure, body heat production, and meal induced thermogenesis.[2]

Nutrition and Disease Management for Veterinary Technicians and Nurses, Second Edition. Ann Wortinger, Kara M. Burns
© 2015 John Wiley & Sons, Inc. Published 2015 by John Wiley & Sons, Inc.
Companion Website: www.wiley.com/go/wortinger/nutrition

Resting Energy Requirements

Resting energy requirement (RER), also called resting metabolic rate, accounts for the largest portion of an animal's energy expenditure representing ~60–75% of the total daily intake.[2] RER is the amount of energy used while resting quietly in a thermo neutral environment in a nonfasted animal.[1,2,4] This represents the energy required to maintain homeostasis in all of the integrated systems of the body during rest.[2] Factors influencing RER include sex and reproductive status, thyroid and autonomic nervous system function, body composition, body surface area and nutritional status.[2] As an animal's lean body mass increases, or body surface area increase, RER also increases.[2]

Common Measurements of Energy

Basal energy requirement (BER)
The energy requirement for a normal animal in a thermo neutral environment, awake but resting in a fasting state. Also known as basal metabolic rate (BMR) or basal energy expenditure (BEE). As it is difficult to have an animal cooperate with the activity restrictions required to measure BER, the term resting energy expenditure (REE) is more commonly used in veterinary medicine.[3]

Resting energy requirement (RER)
The energy requirement for a normal animal at rest in a thermo neutral environment, awake but not fasted. RER accounts for energy used for digestion, absorption and metabolism of nutrients and recovery from physical activity. Also known as resting metabolic rate (RMR) or resting energy expenditure (REE).

Maintenance energy requirement (MER)
The energy requirement for a moderately active adult animal in a thermo neutral environment. MER accounts for energy used for obtaining, digesting and absorbing nutrients in an amount to maintain body weight, as well as energy used for spontaneous activity. MER is the amount of energy required to maintain an animal at its current weight and body composition. It is also known as metabolic energy expenditure (MEE).

Daily energy requirement (DER)
The energy required for average daily activity of any animal, dependent on lifestyle and activity. DER includes energy necessary for work, gestation, lactation and growth, as well as energy needed to maintain normal body temperature.

Gross energy (GE)
The total amount of heat produced by burning a specific amount of food in a bomb calorimeter. Neither water nor minerals, in the form of ash, are combustible. Therefore they contribute no calories or energy to the GE of a diet.

Digestible energy (DE)
The energy in a food that is left over after digestion. The energy remaining in feces is subtracted from GE to obtain this amount.

Metabolizable energy (ME)
The energy in a food available to the animal after losses from feces, urine and combustible gasses are subtracted from GE.

Kilocalorie (kcal)
The energy needed to raise the temperature of 1 gram of water from 14.5 to 15.5 °Celsius. 1 kcal = 1000 calories.

3500 kcal
The amount of energy change required to lose or gain 1 pound. To lose or gain 1 kilogram we would multiply 3500 by 2.2 to obtain 7700 kcals.[3–5]

Energy Expenditure

Voluntary muscular activity, or exercise, is the most variable area of energy expenditure. Muscular activity accounts for ~30% of the total energy expenditures.[2] The amount of energy expended is directly affected by the duration and intensity of the activity, though the amount of energy used can also increase as weight increases.[2]

RER can be affected by body composition, age, caloric intake and hormonal status.[2] RER also naturally decreases as an animal ages and losses lean body tissue.[2] Changes in RER can also occur secondary to energy restriction. When caloric intake is decreased, hormones will cause an initial decrease in energy requirements to conserve body tissue.[2,5] If caloric restriction continues, RER will be readjusted and won't be corrected until levels of lean body tissue return to normal.[2] Persistent overeating, or positive energy balance, can lead to an increase in energy expenditure in part due to the increase in lean body mass with weight gain, but also due to increased meal-induced thermogenesis. Accumulated fat in adipose tissue does not increase the energy requirements for the animal, except through increased energy used to move.[2,5]

Reproductive status affects energy requirements with neutered animals having significantly lower estimated RER than to intact animals. The decrease in energy requirements occurring immediately after neutering is estimated to be ~25%. This is due to both a change in body composition (less lean body tissue) but also a decrease in activity levels, and hormones.[2] Intact animals tend to be more active both during breeding season but also in territorial disputes that are usually not as much of a concern for a neutered animal. The loss of the androgenic hormones decrease lean body mass for the neutered animal.

Body Heat Production

Body heat is also known as heat increment. This is the energy associated with ingestion, digestion, absorption and metabolism of food. Heat increment accounts for ~10–15% of the total daily energy expenditure in dogs and cats.[3] The degree of heat produced during digestion can vary based on meal size and the nutrient composition of the meal. A high protein diet will produce the greatest amount of heat, while a high fat diet will produce the least amount of heat.[3]

The ingestion of nutrients causes heat production through the process of digestion and absorption.[2] The use of digestive enzymes by the body allows these chemical reactions to occur at the relatively low temperatures found within the body. To achieve the same results in an industrial process would require much more extreme conditions of temperature, pH or highly reactive ingredients.[5] The final amount of calories used is ultimately dependent on the composition of the diet as well as the nutritional status of the animal.[2]

Facultative Thermogenesis

Facultative thermogenesis refers to the amount of energy required to maintain body temperature when an animal is outside of its thermoneutral zone. For adult dogs, the thermoneutral zone is considered to be between 20–25 °C and 30–35 °C (68–77 °F and 86–95 °F). For cats, the thermoneutral zone is not entirely known, but is estimated to be between 30 °C and 38 °C (68 °F and 100 °F).[3]

Adaptive thermogenesis is the change in the RER secondary to environmental stresses. These stresses include changes in ambient temperature both heat and cold, alterations in food intake and emotional stress.[2] This process allows the body to maintain the energy balance despite changes in caloric intake by being less efficient in energy use.[2]

For animals living outdoors, facultative thermogenesis can be a major source of energy expenditure if they experience temperatures well outside of their thermoneutral zones.[3]

Voluntary Oral Intake

Voluntary food intake is regulated by both internal physiologic controls and external cues.[2] The animal also receives cues from the body in the form of physical signs such as stomach contractions when empty stimulating eating or stomach distention when full inhibiting eating.[5] There are also numerous neural and hormonal mechanisms that provide direct stimulation or inhibition to eating. Glucagon and insulin would be examples of two such hormones.[5] Glucagon is a peptide produced in the intestines that causes a decrease in food intake. Insulin on the other hand is produced by the pancreas and stimulates hunger and increased food intake.[2] The administration of exogenous steroids can have the same effect as insulin on hunger and food intake. The exogenous steroids do not increase the energy requirement for the body but do increase appetite. This can commonly be seen with administration of corticosteroids.

External controls of food intake include stimuli such as diet palatability, food composition, food texture and the timing and environment of meals.[2] Feeding a highly palatable diet is considered a primary environmental factor contributing to the over consumption of food which in turn leads to obesity.[2] This can be seen with high-fat diets, calorically dense diets and foods that offer a variety of palatable flavors.[2]

Both dogs and cats have definite taste and texture preferences. The majority of dogs prefer canned and semi-moist foods over dry food, with beef being the preferred flavor and cooked meat preferred over raw.[2] Dogs also have a strong preference for sucrose, while cats have been shown to lack the taste receptors in their tongues to even detect sugars.[2,6] Dogs and cats can detect several specific amino acids that are only weakly bitter to people. These amino acids and peptides help to give foods their meaty and savory aromas and tastes. They also respond to selected nucleotides and fatty acids that appear to increase the meaty taste perception in foods. A nucleotide that accumulates in decomposing meat is distasteful to cats, but not to dogs. This may help explain dog's fascination with dead animals.[6] Both dogs and cats prefer warm food over cold food, with increasing palatability seen with increased fat levels in the diet.[2]

The timing of meals as well as the environment that they are offered in can affect eating behavior.[2] Dogs and cats rapidly become conditioned to receiving their meals at a specific time of day; this can be seen with both behavioral and physical signs.[2] Activity will generally increase at anticipated mealtimes, and gastric secretions and motility increase in anticipation of eating.[2]

The number of animals being fed can also increase the amount of food consumed with each meal, in dogs this is a phenomenon called social facilitation. This causes a moderate increase in interest in food and an increased rate of eating. The degree that this affects individual dogs can vary greatly.[2] Social hierarchies between dogs can also affect the amount of food eaten; with subordinate dogs eating less in the presence of dominate dogs during mealtimes.[2]

For cats, the smell of food is the primary determinant for food acceptance. When they are unable to smell, they will continue to refuse all attempts to feed them.[7] Cats do not appear to participate in social facilitation in eating, and do not appear to be affected by the presence of another cat when they are eating.[7]

The frequency of meals can affect both food intake and metabolic efficiency. With increased meal frequency, there is actually an increase in energy loss through increased thermogenesis. With smaller, more frequent meals the body uses more energy to digest, absorb and metabolize the food than when one or two larger meals are fed.[2]

Nutrient Composition

The nutrient composition of the food can affect both the nutrient metabolism and the amount of food voluntarily eaten by the animal.[2] Most animals will decrease their intake of a high-fat diet to compensate for energy needs, though the greater caloric density of the diet with increased palatability can still cause increased energy intake in some animals.[2] The body is also metabolically more efficient at converting dietary fat to body fat for storage than it is at converting dietary carbohydrate or protein to body fat. Because of this, if an animal is eating calories in excess of its requirements of a high fat diet, they will gain more weight than if they were consuming the same number of calories in a high protein or high carbohydrate diet.[2]

The addition of treats and table scraps to the diet can also over-ride the satiety cues the body gives. These treats tend to be highly desirable and appealing, and even if full the animals will not turn them down.[2] This leads to an increase in energy intake and obesity because owners seldom will decrease the amount of "regular food" offered to the pet when also giving treats. Feeding a variety of new food types can also cause the same affect by introducing novelty.[2]

Estimated Energy Requirements

Many formulas have been used to calculate the estimated energy requirements for animals. Dogs represent a unique challenge in that their sizes have one of the widest ranges in the animal kingdom, from the 4 lb Chihuahua to the 200 lb Great Dane. Cats tend to have a smaller range of sizes, usually between 4 and 20 lb. Some of these use algometric formulas, some linear equations and still some use body surface area (BSA). All of these formulas are helpful, but all still are only estimates of actual caloric needs. Numerous charts have also been devised that allow quick access to estimate energy needs (Table 9.1).

Obviously, if you're using a calculator that does not have an exponential key, you'll have to use one of the linear formulas. All of these formulas have been

Table 9.1 Formula(s) for calculating MER in adult maintenance in kcals/day, using body weight (BW) in kilograms

Canine	Feline
Inactive $99 \times BW^{0.67}$ (Ref. 2)	Inactive $60 \times BW$ (Refs 11, 12)
Active $132 \times BW^{0.67}$ (Ref, 2)	Moderately active $70 \times BW$ (Ref. 12)
Very active $160 \times BW^{0.67}$ (Ref. 2)	Highly active $80 \times BW$ (Ref. 12)
Endurance/performance $300 \times BW^{0.67}$ (Ref. 8)	Kitten 0–3 month $250 \times BW$ (Ref. 12)
<2 kg [BER $70 \times BW^{0.75}$] $\times 1.3$–2.0 (Ref. 9)	Kitten 3–5 month $130 \times BW$ (Ref. 12)
>2 kg [BER $(30 \times BW) + 70$] $\times 1.3$–2.0 (Ref. 9)	<2 kg [BER $70 \times BW^{0.75}$] $\times 1.3$–2.0 (Ref. 9)
$1500 \times BSA$ (Ref. 10)	>2 kg [BER $(30 \times BW) + 70$] $\times 1.3$–2.0 (Ref. 9)

Table 9.2 Example of calculating amount of food to be fed to individual animal

Using the linear formula
10 lb dog = 4.5 kg
RER = (wt in kg) $\times$ 30) + 70
MER = RER $\times$ 1.3
MER = [(30 $\times$ 4.5 kg) + 70] $\times$ 1.3
MER = 136.36 $\times$ 1.3
MER= 177.27 kcal/day
Diet A = 326 kcal/cup
Feeding amount = 177.27/326
Feeding amount = .54 cup/day
This is based on a standard 8 oz measuring cup

Table 9.3 Life stages and increased energy needs

Life stage – canine	Energy requirement
Post weaning	2 $\times$ adult MER
40% adult weight	1.6 $\times$ adult MER
80% adult weight	1.2 $\times$ adult MER
Late gestation	1.25-1.5 $\times$ adult MER
Lactation	3 $\times$ adult MER
Prolonged physical work	2- 4 $\times$ adult MER
Decreased environmental temperature	1.2- 1.8 $\times$ adult MER

Life stage – feline	Energy requirement
Post weaned	250 kcal/kg BW
20 weeks	130 kcal/kg BW
Late gestation	1.25 $\times$ adult MER
Lactation	3-4 $\times$ adult MER

compared, and when calculated out the results are within a reasonable distance of each other. You can also use charts that have the MER calculated out and work from these numbers. Ultimately all energy estimates will need to be adjusted based on the desired response from the animal; weight gain, weight maintenance or weight loss. Variability between individual animals, sexual status and environmental living conditions can result in a difference up or down of up to 25% of the calculated energy need.[2]

Using these equations and the energy density of the food, the amount of food to be fed to the individual animal can be calculated (Table 9.2).[2]

Certain life stages can result in increased energy needs. These would include growth, gestation, lactation, periods of strenuous physical work and exposure to extreme environmental conditions (Table 9.3).[2]

Water requirements can be expressed in one of two ways, either 2–3 $\times$ the dry matter (DM) intake of the food, expressed in grams or using the MER kcal/day estimates to also calculate water requirements.[2] The best recommendation is to have plenty of clean, fresh water available at all times, regardless of the animal's physiologic state, caloric intake or dry matter intake.[2]

References

1 Will JM (1996) Basic principles of nutrition and feeding. In N Kelly, J Wills (eds), *Manual of Companion Animal Nutrition and Feeding*, pp. 19–21, Ames, IA: Iowa State Press.

2 Case LP, Carey DP, Hirakawa DA, Daristotle L (2000) Energy balance. In *Canine and Feline Nutrition* (2nd edn), pp. 75–88, St Louis, MO: Mosby.

3 Delaney SJ, Fascetti AJ (2012) Determining energy requirements. In AJ Fascetti, SJ Delaney (eds). *Applied Veterinary Clinical Nutrition*, pp. 23–42, Ames, IA: Wiley-Blackwell.

4 Gross KL, Wedekind KL, Cowell CS *et al.* (2000) Nutrients. In MS Hand, CD Thatcher, RL Remillard *et al.* (eds), *Small Animal Clinical Nutrition* (4th edn), pp. 31–3, Marceline, MO: Walsworth Publishing.

5 Burger IH (1993) A basic guide to nutrient requirements. In JM Wills, KW Simpson (eds), *The Waltham Book of Companion Animal Nutrition*. pp. 6–10, Tarrytown, NY: Pergamon.

6 Crane SW, Griffin RW, Messent PR (2000) Introduction to commercial pet foods. In MS Hand, CD Thatcher, RL Remillard, P Roudebush (eds), *Small Animal Clinical Nutrition* (4th edn), p. 123, Marceline, MO, Walsworth Publishing.

7 Horwitz D, Soulard Y, Junien-Castagna A (2008) The feeding behavior of the cat. In P Pibot, V Biourge, D Elliott (eds), *Encyclopedia of Feline Clinical Nutrition*, p. 445. Aimargues, France, Aniwa SAS.

Further Reading

Gross KL, Jewell DE, Yamka RM, *et al.* (2010) Macronutrients. In *Small Animal Clinical Nutrition* (5th edn). MS Hand, CD Thatcher, RI Remillard, *et al.* (eds), p. 55. Marceline, MO: Walsworth Publishing.

Xia L, Weihua L, Hong W, *et al.* (2005) Pseudogenization of a sweet-receptor gene accounts for cats indifference toward sugar. *PLoS Genet* **1**(**1**): 27–35.

Case LP (1999) Nutrient requirements. In *The Dog: Its Behavior, Nutrition and Health*, p. 279, Ames, IO: Iowa State Press.

Simpson JW, Anderson RS, Markwell PJ (1993) Anorexia, enteral and parenteral feeding. In *Clinical Nutrition of the Dog and Cat*, p. 107, Cambridge, MA: Blackwell.

Appendix D (2000) In MS Hand, CD Thatcher, RL Remillard *et al.* (eds), *Small Animal Clinical Nutrition* (4th edn), p. 1010, Marceline, MO: Walsworth Publishing.

Donoghue S (1996) The underweight patient. In N Kelly, J Wills (eds), *Manual of Companion Animal Nutrition and Feeding*, p. 103, Ames, IA: Iowa State Press.

Case LP (2003) The cat as an obligate carnivore. In *The Cat: Its Behavior, Nutrition and Health*, p. 293, Ames, IO: Iowa State Press.

10 Nutrition Calculations

Introduction

Math is a part of our everyday world; we find it everywhere from balancing your checkbook to calculating calories for Mrs Smith's overweight Bassett. The more comfortable we are with doing these calculations, the more accurate our results will be. While not as potentially devastating as a drug dosage error, miscalculating calories, energy or food intake can have an equally bad outcomes for our patients.

Ideally, the veterinarian will tell you what diet requirements they want, and you can take everything from there. Determining caloric requirements, figuring feeding volumes and even percent of weight loss desired. The better your skills, the more challenged and less bored you will be in your work every day, and the more you can help your patients.

Units of Measure

In the United States, we commonly use the US customary units: these are the pounds, ounces, inches and feet that we are all familiar with. As we all know, there is no consistency between weight, volume and length, and you just have to memorize the conversions. Weight is measured in ounces, pounds and tons, length is measured in inches, feet, yards and miles, and volume is measured in ounces, cups, pints, quarts and gallons. Conversions between the various units are tedious and often confusing. We learn early on that:

1 cup (c) = 8 ounces (oz)
16 ounces (oz) = 1 pound (lb or #)
2 pints (pt) = 1 quart (qt)
4 quarts (qt) = 1 gallon (gal)
12 inches (in or ") = 1 foot (ft or ')
3 feet (ft) = 1 yard (yd)
5280 feet (ft) = 1 mile (m)
2000 pounds (lb or #) = 1 ton (t)

There is no rhyme or reason for the units; we just need to know them.

The metric system was developed after the French Revolution in 1795 as a means of making measuring more consistent and removing regional differences. The biggest advantage of this unit of measure is that it is divided in equal parts throughout the entire system. By simply moving decimal points you can go from one unit of measure to another. Also conversions between weight, length and volume are easier to figure out than with the US Customary units.

For metric units, weight is measured in grams, volume is measured in liters and length is measured in meters. By moving your decimal point to the right or to the left you can divide or multiple the unit being measured and easily convert from, for example, milligrams to kilograms. Everything is determined by units of 10, maintaining consistency throughout the entire system. We know that:

1 millimeter (mL) = 1 centimeter (cc)
1000 mL = 1 liter (L)
1000 grams (g) = 1 kilogram (kg)
1 kilogram (kg) = 1 liter (L)
10 centimeters (cm) = 1 decimeter (dm)
    = 0.10 meter (m)

Each space to the left of the decimal point increases the value by a power of 10. Conversely, each space to the right of the decimal point decreases the value by a power of 10. The most common units seen in medicine include:

Deci- 10^{-1} (d)
Centi- 10^{-2} (c)
Milli- 10^{-3} (m)
Micro 10^{-6} (μ)
Deca- 10^{1} (d)
Hecto- 10^{2} (h)
Kilo- 10^{3} (k)

Nutrition and Disease Management for Veterinary Technicians and Nurses, Second Edition. Ann Wortinger, Kara M. Burns
© 2015 John Wiley & Sons, Inc. Published 2015 by John Wiley & Sons, Inc.
Companion Website: www.wiley.com/go/wortinger/nutrition

To convert from one unit to the other you simply determine the number of spaces to move your decimal point right or left. This provides much more consistency and easier math than does the US Customary units.

Converting Units

The biggest problem we have with the two most common units of measure, the US Customary units and the metric units, is that they have very little in common. If you're like most technicians, you weigh your patients in pounds on the scale and then have to convert this to kilograms to calculate drug dosages or fluid rates. This is an extra step that we've given ourselves by not using metric in our everyday lives. If we send medications or foods home with clients, we have to reconvert these amounts back to a value that they can utilize and recognize, resulting in even more conversions for us!

Like the US Customary units, we just have to know the conversions to do these calculations accurately.

1 kg = 2.2 lb
1 lb = 0.45 kg
1 teaspoon (tsp) = 5 ml
1 tablespoon (Tbl) = 15 mL
1 oz = 30 mL
1 cup = 240 mL
1 centimeter = 2.54 inches

The hardest part is remembering what needs to be done where and using what conversion. The most common nutrition calculation we deal with is converting between pounds and kilograms.

Example:
1 lb = 2.2 kg
1 kg = 0.45 lb
A 10 lb cat would weigh 4.5 kg
10 lb/2.2 = 4.5
A 25 lb dog would weigh 11.4 kg
25 lb/ 2.2 = 11.4.

To convert from kilograms to pounds you would multiply rather than divide by 2.2

Example:
A 5 kg cat would weigh 11 lb
$$5 \text{ kg} \times 2.2 = 11 \text{ lb}$$

A 25 kg dog would weigh 55 lb
$$25 \text{ kg} \times 2.2 = 55 \text{ lb}.$$

If these conversions are done incorrectly, the result would be an over 2 fold increase or decrease in the desired value. This is a pretty big amount. When converting from pounds to kilograms, your final number should be smaller. When converting from kilograms to pounds your final number should be bigger.

Calculating Resting Energy Requirements (RER)

This is our base calculation when figuring out daily calorie requirements. You can use either a linear formula such as:

$$(\text{wt in kg} \times 30) + 70 = \text{RER}$$

Or a logarithmic formula such as:

$$70 \times \text{kg body weight}^{0.75}$$

Using the linear formula is easier mathematically, but is not seen as being as accurate over a wide range of body weights (<2 kg and >30 kg) as the logarithmic formula.

Example:
Body weight 28 lb
Convert to kg = 28/2.2 = 12.7 kg
RER = (BW kg × 30) + 70 = (12.7 × 30) + 70 = 452 kcals/day.

The logarithmic formula is more difficult, especially when using a four-function calculator, but can be done.

Example:
Body weight 28 lb
Convert to kg = 28/2.2 = 12.7 kg
RER = 70 × BW in kg$^{0.75}$ = (kg × kg × kg, $\sqrt{}$, $\sqrt{}$) × 70
(12.7 × 12.7 × 12.7 $\sqrt{}$, $\sqrt{}$) = 6.7 × 70 = 471 kcals/day.

As both of these formulas are estimates of the animal's actual energy requirements, any adjustments of intake should be determined by the animal. If they are hungry or losing weight, then increase the volume being fed. If they are gaining weight or are vomiting, then decrease the volume being fed.

Calculating Daily Energy Requirements (DER)

Daily energy requirements are calculated from the RER, but utilize the animal's activity level to supply any extra calories required for daily maintenance.

$$DER = RER \times 1.0 - 1.6$$

(dependent on energy expenditure)

Example:

Body weight 28 lb or 12.7 kg
RER = 452–471 kcal/day
DER = 452–471 × 1.0–1.6.

Our dog is moderately active and goes on (2) 60 minute walks/day. We will select 1.4 as our DER correction factor.

DER = 452–471 × 1.4 = 633–659 kcal/day

As with RER if the animal is gaining weight on the amount of food fed, cut back. If they are hungry or losing weight, increase the amount fed.

Calculating Feeding Amounts

The feeding amounts are determined by the caloric density of the food selected, and the kcal requirements for that animal. If you choose to follow the package direction on feeding volume, the animal will most likely not lose weight, and may very well gain weight as calories are not a "one size fits all" equation.

Take the kcals required and divide that by the caloric density of the food selected.

Example:

Calories needed/day = 633–659 kcals
Calorie density of the food:
259 kcal/cup (standard 8 oz measuring cup)
417 kcal/can
633–659/259 kcal/cup = 2.44–2.54 cups
633–659/417 kcal/can = 1.5–1.58 cans.

As we want to make this as user-friendly as possible for the owner, we need to select a unit of measure they can achieve. It is unlikely that a client will know how to

get 0.44 parts of a cup, but could easily do 0.5. The same is true for the canned volume. We can tell the client to feed 0.58 parts of a can – what is the likelihood that they will be able to comply with this request? They can easily figure out 0.5 parts of a can though.

For this animal, I would recommend either 2.5 cups of dry food/day or 1.5 cans of canned food/day. Many clients like to feed a combination of canned and dry foods, how will that affect your feeding volumes?

Take the kcals/day and determine either how much canned you want to feed/day or how much dry you want to feed/day and then determine the remaining amount.

Example:

BW 28 lb/12.7 kg
DER = 633–659 kcals/day
259 kcal/cup (standard 8 oz measuring cup)
417 kcal/can.

The owner wants to feed 1 can of food divided into 2 feedings, with the remaining calories supplied by the dry food.

DER = 633 – 659–417 (1 can of food) = 216–242 calories remaining that can be supplied by dry food

216–242/259 kcals/cup = 0.83 – 0.93 cups/day.

I would likely recommend a "scant" 1 cup of dry food. This is taking the measuring cup and not quite filling it up. Make sure that clients understand what is meant by 1 cup. A level cup not a heaping cup. And a standard 8 oz measuring cup is what is used in the kitchen, not a 7/11 Big Gulp cup!!

Converting Guaranteed Analysis to Energy Density

Energy density is the percent in the diet of a nutrient x the modified Atwater factor for that nutrient = kcal/100 gm of food. Energy density differs from metabolizable energy (ME) in that nondigestible energy lost through feces and urine is not accounted for. Energy lost through "dietary thermogenesis" is also not accounted for: this is the energy required for digestion and assimilation of nutrients in the body. Also remember that when working with the Guaranteed Analysis, the numbers are represented as minimums (protein and fat) and maximums (crude fiber and moisture) and not the actual values found in that food. As long as the food meets these numbers, the actual values can vary significantly.

Modified Atwater factors for protein and carbohydrates are 3.5 kcal/gram, for fats they are 8.5 kcal/gram. This is the number of calories for that nutrient found in 1 gram of food.

Example:

Dog Kibble Guaranteed

P 6.0% × 3.5 = 21 kcal/gm protein
F 2.8% × 8.5 = 23.8 kcal/gm fat
CHO 14.7% × 3.5 = 51.45 kcal/gm CHO
96.25 kcal/gm/100 kcal

Note: carbohydrates are not usually listed on the Guaranteed Analysis, and must be extrapolated from the nitrogen free extract or the manufacturer can be contacted for the actual digestible carbohydrate content.

Energy Density equals

Energy density is useful to determine the actual percentage a particular nutrient contributes to the caloric content. Take the calculated kcal/grams; divide that by the total kcals/grams for all nutrients. Multiply by 100 to find the percentage.

Example:

P 21/96.25 × 100 = 22%
F 23.8/96.25 × 100 = 25%
CHO 51.45/96.25 × 100 = 53%

When looking at the Guaranteed Analysis you would assume that only 2.8% of the calories come from fat. By calculating the energy density you can see that in fact 25% of the calories come from fat.

Calculating Nutrients as a Percent Metabolizable Energy (ME) Total Calories in 100 Grams of Food

Protein = 3.5 kcal/gram × grams in food

Fat = 8.5 kcal/gram × grams in food

Carbohydrate = 3.5 kcal/gram × grams in food

Total calories/100 gram = protein calorie + fat calorie

+ carbohydrate calorie

Percentage of ME Contributed by Each Nutrient (Caloric Distribution)

Protein = (protein calories/100 gram divided by

total calories/100 gram) × 100 = % ME

Fat = (fat calories/100 gram divided by total calories

/100 gram) × 100 = % ME

Carbohydrate = (carbohydrate calories/100 gram

divided by total calories)

× 100 = % ME

Example:

Dry Dog Food (as Fed)

Moisture 8%
P 21.4% × 3.5 = 74.9 kcal/100 grams of food
F 10.1% × 8.5 = 85.85 kcal/100 grams of food
CHO 52.3% × 3.5 = 183.05 kcal/100 grams of food
Total calories per 100 gm = 344 kcals
ME estimate
P = (74.9/344) × 100 = 22%
F = (85.85/344) × 100 = 25%
CHO = (183.05/344) × 100 = 53%

Calculating Meals per Can/cup/bag

Many times when we send food home, the client wants to know how long the food will last. With canned food this is an easier calculation, but with dry foods this can be more of a mental math challenge to come up with. The main reason for this challenge is that we're feeding the food in cups, but the manufacturer is selling it in pounds.

We can figure out how many ounces are in each cup of food by weighing it on the baby or small animal scale, and then seeing how many "meals" are in the bag.

Example:

We want to feed 2.5 cups of dry food/day to our patient. We sell the client a 20 lb bag of food. How long will this bag be expected to last the client?
1 cup of food = 5.5 ounces (if this was water 1 cup = 8 ounces, but food is usually less dense)
20 lb bag of food = _____ ounces (oz)

Remember 1 lb = 16 oz

20 lb × 16 = 320 oz

Take the 320 oz/5.5 oz/cup = 58 cups of food

Each meal is 2.5 cups

58 cups/2.5 cups/day = 23 days worth of food

Cost of Feeding

Many clients assume that the better the brand of food, the more expensive it will be to feed. By calculating the cost/meal we can demonstrate that the actual cost is not that much higher or may be even lower between different brands of foods.

We just covered how to figure out the number of meals in a bag of food. By taking that amount and dividing the actual cost of the food you can determine the cost/meal. Again this is easier to do with canned food, but make sure that when comparing, you compare dry food to dry food, and canned food to canned food. With the substantial differences in moisture content, canned food is inherently higher in price than would be dry food.

When using a therapeutic diet, it is many times helpful to equate feeding the food to allowing less medication to be administered, thus decreasing the overall cost of medication and ease of administration. Therapeutic diets are more expensive than over the counter (OTC) foods, but they provide benefits that cannot be achieved with OTC foods. Many times there is not an equivalent food available OTC because you need to have a veterinarian managing the disease processes not the client.

Example:

Canned food:

Your patient requires 1.25 cans of food twice daily. The cost/can is $0.89/can

(1.25 × 2) × 0.89 = $2.23/day × 30 = $66.75/month

Dry food:

Therapeutic dog diet

20 lb bag = $43.00

20 lb × 16 = 320 oz

Take the 320 oz/5.5 oz/cup = 58 cups of food

Each meal is 2.5 cups

58 cups/2.5 cups/day = 23 days worth of food

On a per meal basis $43.00/23 days = $1.87/day to feed

If we look at a "less expensive" brand of OTC food that is cheaper, but lacks the therapeutic value of the veterinary diet, but is also less digestible, we'll see that the OTC food may actually be more expensive or similar in cost to feed.

Low-cost dog food

20 lb = $32.00

1 cup of food = 5.5 ounces (if this was water 1 cup = 8 ounces, but food is usually less dense)

20 lb bag of food = _____ ounces (oz)

Remember 1 lb = 16 oz

20 lb × 16 = 320 oz

Take the 320 oz/5.5 oz/cup = 58 cups of food

Each meal is 3.5 cups (less caloric density than therapeutic diet)

58 cups/3.5 cups/day = 16 days worth of food

On a per meal basis $32.00/16 days = $2.00/day to feed

This calculation shows that because you have to feed more of the less expensive food, you get less feeding days/bag, and the overall cost/meal is more expensive.

Conclusion

By knowing how to do these common calculations, we can offer better nutrition to our patents and clients. Go forth and use your calculator with confidence and astound those around you!

Further Reading

Bill R (2000) *Medical Mathematics and Dosage Calculations for Veterinary Professionals*, Ames, IA: Blackwell Publishing.

Ramsey JJ (2012) Determining energy requirements. In S Delaney, A Fascetti (eds), *Applied Veterinary Clinical Nutrition*, pp. 23–45, Ames, IA: Wiley-Blackwell.

SECTION 2
Nutritional Requirements of Dogs and Cats

11 History and Regulation of Pet Foods

Introduction

Until the mid-1800s, dogs and cats were fed primarily table scraps with supplemental scavenging.[1] Some owners may have fed homemade food formulas made from human foods but no commercial pet foods were available until 1860.[1,2]

The first commercially prepared dog food was produced by James Spratt, an American living in London in 1860.[1,2] On his trip across the Atlantic to England, he was not impressed with the dry biscuits fed to his dog aboard the ship. Once in London he developed a dry kibble or "dog cake" that he sold to the English huntsman for their dogs.[1] Following his success with this food in England he expanded his sales to include the United States, where production was continued until the late 1950s when it was purchased by General Mills.[1,2]

In the early 1900s several other people saw the success that Mr Spratt was having with his dry "dog cakes" and began to develop and sell their own formulas. In 1907 F.H. Bennett, an Englishman, developed and produced Milk-Bone dog biscuits in New York City.[1,2] At that time, Milk-Bones were marketed as a complete dog food.[1]

Until the early 1920s, Messrs Spratt and Bennett were the two primary producers of commercial pet food. In the early 1920s the Chappel brothers of Rockford, Illinois produced the first batches of canned commercial food. They began by canning horse meat for dogs under the Ken-L-Ration brand name, following this with a dry food in the 1930s.[1,2] By the mid-1920s Samuel and Clarence Gaines of the Gaines Food Company from Sherburne, New York began selling a new type of dog food called meal in 100 lb bags; this was the beginning of "Gaines Dog Meal." The food differed from previous food in that a number of dried, ground ingredients were mixed together to form the food.[2] The advantage of this to pet owners was they could buy the food in fairly large quantities, and very little food preparation was necessary before feeding.[2]

In the 1930s the introduction of many new brands including Cadet and Snappy helped to make canned pet foods more popular than dry foods.[1] This continued until World War II, as pet foods were classified as "non essential," the tin used to produce the cans was diverted to the war effort. By 1946, dry foods were about 85% of the total pet food market in the United States.[1]

Marketing of Pet Foods

In the early years for commercial pet foods, primary marketing was through feed stores. The National Biscuit Company (Nabisco) purchased Milk Bones in 1931, and began the first attempt to market its product in grocery stores.[2] At this time, selling pet foods in human markets met with much resistance. Because most pet foods were made from byproducts of human foods, customers and store owners considered it unsanitary to sell such products next to foods that were meant for human consumption.[2] The convenience and economy of buying pet foods at the grocery store rapidly overcame consumer concerns.[2] Improved distribution and availability resulted in increased sales and popularity of commercial pet foods.

Production of Pet Foods

The development of the extrusion process of food production was introduced by researchers at the Purina Laboratories in the 1950s. Extrusion involves first mixing all the food ingredients together and then

Nutrition and Disease Management for Veterinary Technicians and Nurses, Second Edition. Ann Wortinger, Kara M. Burns
© 2015 John Wiley & Sons, Inc. Published 2015 by John Wiley & Sons, Inc.
Companion Website: www.wiley.com/go/wortinger/nutrition

rapidly cooking the mixture and forcing it through an extruder. The extruder is a specialized pressure cooker that allows the food to be rapidly cooked, and then shaped into bite sized pieces. This process also increased the digestibility and palatability of the food produced.[2] After extrusion and drying, a coating of fat or some other palatability enhancer was usually sprayed onto the outside of the food pieces.[2] In 1957, Purina Dog Chow was first introduced to the commercial market. Within a year, it became the best-selling dog food in the United States, and continues to maintain a number 2 position in total dog food sales today.[1,2]

During this same time, General Foods created Gaines Burger, a new food that combined the convenience of dry food with the palatability of canned food. This was the first semi-moist dog food product. Ralston-Purina followed this in the 1970s with the introduction of Tender Vittles, the first semi-moist cat food.[1]

Science Diet produced by Hill's Pet Nutrition was originally produced as a consistent high-quality food for research kennels. In 1968 this became the first specialty product line designed for different life stages.[1] Hill's Pet Nutrition had been producing pet foods in cooperation with Dr Mark Morris Sr. since 1948: this was the Prescription Diet foods that we are all familiar with. The first food produced was Hill's Science Diet K/D diet canned. Originally produced in Dr Morris's office for dogs with kidney disease in his practice, this was the first food designed to aid in the dietary management of disease.[1]

During this time, little was known about the nutrient requirements for dogs and cats. This lack of nutrition knowledge lead many manufacturers to produce the same product for both species, with only the labeling being different.[2] As more knowledge was acquired about different nutrient needs for dogs and cats, separate foods were formulated for each.[2] As knowledge continues to grow, more companies are developing diets that are specifically designed for specific life stages, physiologic states (low activity, moderate activity and performance diets), breed differences (small breed, large breed, long-haired) and health problems.[2]

Regulatory Agencies

A number of agencies and organizations regulate the production, marketing and sales of commercial pet foods in the United States.[2] The American Association of Feed Control Officials (AAFCO) was formed in 1909, and is composed of feed control officials from states and territories within the United States and Canada.[3] AAFCO provides a forum for local, state and federal regulatory officials to discuss and develop uniform and equitable laws, regulations and policies regarding pet foods. AAFCO formed a permanent Pet Food Committee to address the need for information about pet nutrition and pet food regulations.[3] The AAFCO remains the recognized information source for pet food labeling, ingredient definition, official terms and standardized feed testing methodology.[3] Because the AAFCO is an association and not an official regulatory body, its policies must be voluntarily accepted by state feed control officials for actual implementation.[2] Pet food regulations can vary from state to state, and using the AAFCO's policy statements and regulations promote uniformity in feed regulations throughout the United States.[2] Today AAFCO ensures that nationally marketed pet foods are uniformly labeled and nutritionally adequate.[2]

During the 1990s, AAFCO developed the practical Nutrient Profiles to be used as standards for the formulation of dog and cat foods. The profiles are based on ingredients commonly include in commercial foods, and nutrient levels are expressed for processed foods at the time of feeding.[2] Prior to this, nutrient minimums were based on the recommendations of the National Research Council (NRC).[3] The NRC recommendations are based on data obtained from using purified foods, with the assumption of 100% nutrient availability for only one life stage, and only gave minimum levels without any safety margins.[3] The AAFCO's Nutrient Profiles provide suggested levels of nutrients to be included in pet foods rather than minimum levels as do the NRC recommendation, as well as maximum levels of selected nutrients.[2] AAFCO also publishes minimum feeding protocols for dog and cat foods. These minimum feeding protocols are used by pet food manufacturers for substantiating the nutritional adequacy of pet foods using feeding trials and determining the metabolizable energy found in dog and cat food.[3] The NRC provides separate requirements for growth and reproduction in dogs and cats.[4]

The Food and Drug Administration (FDA) requires that all pet food manufacturers provide proper identification of pet foods, a net quantity statement on the label, proper listing of ingredients and the manufacturer's name and address and use acceptable manufacturing procedures.[2,3] Feed control officials within each state inspect facilities and enforce these regulations, although the FDA is authorized to take direct action if necessary to address any violations.[2,3]

The Center for Veterinary Medicine (CVM), a department of the FDA, regulates the use of any health claims on pet food labels. One type of health claim, a drug claim, is defined as the assertion or implication that the consumption of a food may help in the treatment, prevention or reduction of a particular disease or diseases.[2] If a health claim is considered a drug claim, the CVM will not allow its use on the label.[2] An example of a health claim would be "Feeding this food will prevent the development of hypertension in adult dogs" as opposed to a nonhealth claim of "this food may be beneficial in the prevention of blood pressure related issues in adult dogs."

The United States Department of Agriculture (USDA) is responsible for ensuring that pet foods are clearly labeled to prevent human consumers from mistaking these products for human foods and eating them.[2,3] The USDA inspects animal ingredients used in pet foods to ensure proper handling and to guarantee that such ingredients are not used in human foods.[2,3] The USDA is also responsible for inspection and regulation of animal research facilities. All kennels and catteries that are operated by pet food companies, private groups, or universities must fulfill USDA requirements for physical structure, record-keeping, housing and care of animals and sanitation.[2,3] Once these facilities have passed their initial certification, they are subject to unannounced inspections by the USDA at least once yearly.[2,3]

Some pet food manufacturers maintain their own kennels, while other contract their feeding trials out to private research kennels or universities. Long-term feeding trials make up a large portion of the testing conducted on quality commercial pet foods. The USDA ensures that these facilities maintain proper care of their animals and conform to recommended sanitation practices.[2]

The National Research Council (NRC) is a private, nonprofit organization that evaluates and compiles research conducted by others. The NRC functions as the working portion of the National Academy of Sciences, the National Academy of Engineers and The Institute of Medicine.[3] The NRC was created in 1916 in response to the increased need for scientific and technical services

during World War I.[3] The NRC is not part of the United States government, is not an enforcement agency and is not a basic research organization with laboratories of its own.[3] The NRC does not regulate the pet food industry and has requested that its recommendations not be used to substantiate nutritional adequacy of pet foods.[3] The *Nutrient Requirements of Dogs and Cats* was published by the National Academies. The most recent publication was released in 2006, and has not been incorporated into the AAFCO profiles compiled as of 2011.[4]

In 1958 the Pet Food Institute (PFI) was organized to represent manufacturers of commercially prepared dog and cat food in the United States.[2,3] The PFI works closely with the Pet Food Committee of the AAFCO to evaluate current regulations and make recommendations to changes.[2,3] The PFI also works closely with veterinarians, humane groups and local animal control officers to sponsor public and owner education programs that encourage responsible dog and cat ownership.[3] They do not have any direct regulatory powers over production of pet foods, pet food testing or statements included on labels, though they do represent the pet food industry before legislative and regulatory bodies at the federal and state levels.[3]

Individual states are responsible for adopting and enforcing pet food regulations. Many, but not all have adopted regulations that follow those established by AAFCO. Pet food regulation and enforcement in most states is administered by the State Department of Agriculture, Regulatory and Protection Division or State Chemist.[3]

Most of the control over the nutrient content of pet foods, ingredient nomenclature, and label claims is regulated by AAFCO. The Model Feed Bill that the AAFCO developed and implemented is a template for state legislation.[2] Each year the AAFCO publishes an official document that includes a section containing the current regulations for pet foods. These regulations govern the definition and terms, label format, brand and product names, nutrient guarantee claims, types of ingredients, drug and food additives, statements of caloric content and descriptive terms that are to be used with or included in commercial pet foods.[2] The AAFCO sanctioned feeding protocols for proving nutritional adequacy and metabolizable energy is also included in this document.[3]

Regulations

The definition and terms section of the AAFCO's pet food regulations identify the Principal Display Panel (PDP) as part of the container's label and is intended to be displayed to the consumer for retail sales.[2] Statements that are allowed on labels are described and strictly regulated; these are called "statements of nutritional adequacy" or "purpose of the product." If a product states that it is "complete and balanced nutrition for all stages of life" the claim must be substantiated through one of two ways.[2] The first way involves the use of a series of feeding trials to demonstrate that the food satisfactorily supports their health in a group of dogs or cats throughout all life stages of gestation, lactation and growth.[2] The second way requires that the manufacturer formulate the food to contain ingredients in quantities that are sufficient to provide the estimated nutrient requirements for all life stages in the dog or cat.[2] This can be shown through simple calculation of ingredients using standard ingredient tables or through laboratory analysis of nutrients.[2] The AAFCO Nutrient Profiles for dog and cat foods are used as the standard against which nutrient content is measured.[2] The AAFCO also requires that all products labeled "complete and balanced" include specific feeding directions on the product label.[2] The pet food company does not need to include how these numbers were reached. The amount to be fed usually does not specify any information other than animal size, information such as age, activity level or sexual status but does have bearing on the amount to be fed. This is typically measured in standard household measurements such as "cup."

Brand name refers to the name by which a pet food manufacturer's products are identified and distinguished from other pet foods.[2] The AAFCO regulates both brand and product names.[2] Any product claims of "new and improved" are only allowed to be stated on the PDP and can be used for a maximum of 6 months.[2]

The AAFCO identifies acceptable terms for designating the guaranteed analysis for specific nutrients. Comparisons that are made between nutrient levels in the pet food and the AAFCO Nutrient Profiles must be listed in the same units as those used in the published profile.[2] AAFCO also requires that no pet food, with

the exception of those labeled as sauces, gravies, juices or milk replacers, contain a moisture level greater than 78%.[2]

Artificial food colors can only be added to pet foods if they have been shown to be harmless to pets, or "generally recognized as safe" or GRAS.[2] Such additives are approved and listed by the FDA.[2]

In 1994, AAFCO accepted the inclusion of an optional caloric content statement on pet food labels.[2] This statement must be presented separately from the guaranteed analysis table, and the energy must be expressed in ME as units of kcals/kg. The caloric content may also be expressed as kcal/lb, cup or other commonly used household measuring unit.[2] This claim must be substantiated either by calculation using modified Atwater factors or through feeding trials following AAFCO protocols.[2] The method used must be stated on the label.[2]

In 1998 the newest addition to the AAFCO regulations specifies the acceptable use of the terms "light/lite," "less or reduced calories," "lean," "low fat" and "less or reduced fat."[2] Specific maximum energy contents are designated for all pet foods marketed using the term "light/lite." A food designated as "less or reduced calories" must include the percentage of reduction from the product of comparison and a caloric content statement.[2] The terms "lean" and "less fat" must provide the maximum percentages of fat within different categories of dog and cat food and include the percentage of reduction from the product of comparison.[2]

References

1 Cowell CS, Stout NP,; Brinkerman MF *et al.* (2000) Making commercial pet foods. In MS Hand, CD Thatcher, RL Remillard *et al.* (eds), *Small Animal Clinical Nutrition* (4th edn), p. 129, Marceline, MO: Walsworth Publishing.

2 Case LP, Carey DP, Hirakawa DA, Daristotle L (2000) History and regulation of pet foods. In *Canine and Feline Nutrition* (2nd edn), pp. 143–51, St Louis, MO: Mosby.

3 Roudebush P, Dzanis DA, Debraekeleer J, Brown RG (2000) Pet food labels. In MS Hand, CD Thatcher, RL Remillard *et al.* (eds), *Small Animal Clinical Nutrition* (4th edn), pp. 147–50, Marceline, MO: Walsworth Publishing.

4 Delaney SJ, Fascetti AJ (2012) Basic nutrition overview. In AJ Fascetti, SJ Delaney (eds), *Applied Veterinary Clinical Nutrition*, pp. 20–1, Ames, IA: Wiley-Blackwell.

12 Pet Food Labels

Introduction

Pet food labels are legal documents regulated primarily at the state level with state feed control officials making sure that the labels found on pet foods are in compliance with guidelines published in the most current *Official Publication* of the Association of American Feed Control Officials (AAFCO).[1,2] State feed control officials operate under the jurisdiction of the Food and Drug Administration (FDA) in the United States. Regulations that apply to pet food labeling and testing of foods for nutritional adequacy are published in the AAFCO manual.[1] This manual is updated yearly and also provides definitions for the various terms used in pet food labeling.[1]

Definition of Terms

Complete

a nutritionally adequate feed for animals other than man; by specific formula it is compounded to be fed as a sole ration and is capable of maintaining life and/or promoting production without any additional substance being consumed except water.[1]

Balanced

a term that may be applied to a diet, ration, or feed having all the required nutrients in proper amount and proportion based upon recommendations of recognized authorities in the field of animal nutrition, such as the NRC, for a given set of physiological requirements. The species for which it is intended and the functions such as maintenance or maintenance plus reproduction shall be specified (Table 12.1).[1]

Regulations

Current regulations require that all labels for all pet foods manufactured and sold in the United States

contain the following items: product name; net weight; name and address of the manufacturer; guaranteed analysis for crude protein, crude fat, crude fiber and moisture; list of ingredients in descending order of predominance by weight; the terms "dog food" or "cat food"; and a statement of nutritional adequacy or purpose of the product.[1,3] A statement must also be included that indicates the method used to substantiate the nutritional adequacy claim. This can either be through the AAFCO feeding trials or by formulating the feed to meet AAFCO *Nutrient Profiles*. An expiration date indicating the time span from the date of production to the date of expiration of the product is optional, as is a "best if used by" date.[1,3]

Principal Display Panel

The required information can be found on either the principal display panel (PDP) or on the information panel. The PDP is defined by the FDA as "the part of the label that is most likely to be displayed, presented, shown or examined under customary conditions of display for retain sale."[4] This is the primary means of attracting the consumer's attention to a product and should immediately communicate the product identity. AAFCO requires that the PDP contain only three things: the product name, the intended species to be fed to, and the net quantity of the product contained within the package.[2] The information panel is defined as "that part of the label immediately contiguous and to the right of the PDP" and usually contains information about the product.[4] Any information contained on the label must be both truthful and substantiated or proven (Figure 12.1 and Table 12.2).[2]

The product identity is the primary means of identification of pet foods by consumers.[4] In the United States, the product identity must legally include a product name, but may also include a manufacturer's name, a

Nutrition and Disease Management for Veterinary Technicians and Nurses, Second Edition. Ann Wortinger, Kara M. Burns
© 2015 John Wiley & Sons, Inc. Published 2015 by John Wiley & Sons, Inc.
Companion Website: www.wiley.com/go/wortinger/nutrition

Table 12.1 Percentage of content in a food (using chicken as an example)[4]

Chicken	Chicken must be at least 70% of the total product
Chicken dinner, chicken platter, chicken entree	Chicken must be at least 10% of the total product
With chicken	Chicken must be at least 3% of the total product
Chicken flavor	Chicken must be recognizable by the pet, usually less than 3% of the total product
Canned foods	Moisture not greater than 78%
Gravy, stew, broth, sauce, juice or milk replacer	Moisture can be greater than 78%

Sample Label

**Dr K's
Natural Food**

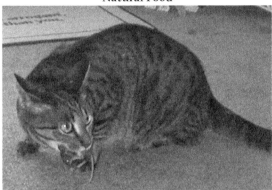

Field Mouse
For Cats

Complete and Balance as
Nature Designed for adult
maintenance

INGREDIENTS: Water sufficient for processing, Michigan grown whole ground wild field mouse.

GUARANTEED ANALYSIS: Crude protein min. 20%, crude fat min. 10%, crude fiber max. 1%, moisture max. 65%, ash max. 4%

AAFCO feeding studies substantiate complete and balanced for adult maintenance

Manufactured by MVS, Southfield MI USA (248) 354–6660

Feeding Recommendations:

Size	1–5#	6–10#	11–15#	16–20#
Amt fed	.5–.6 can	.6–1 can	1–1.5 can	1.5–2 can

Figure 12.1 Sample label.

brand name or both.[4] The brand name is the name by which the pet food products of a given company are identified.[4] The product name provides information about the individual identity of a particular product within that brand.[4]

The PDP must identify the species for which the food is intended, such as "dog food" or "cat food." This statement is intended to help guide consumer purchases.[1] This does not mean that the food can not be fed to an alternate species, but that it has only been tested and formulated for the indicated species. This is called the "designator" or "statement of intent."[4]

The net weight indicates the amount of food in the specific container, often given in pounds or grams or

both.[1] This is found on the PDP and must be placed within the bottom 30% of panel.[4]

A product vignette refers to any vignette, graphic or pictorial representation of a product on a pet food label.[4] The product vignette should not misrepresent the contents of the package by looking better than the actual product or ingredients.[4]

Nutrition statements on the PDP include the terms "complete and nutritious," "100% nutritious," "100% complete nutrition" or similar designations. Nutritional adequacy statements indicate which species the food is formulated for and also what life stage of that species the food is appropriate to feed.[2] The terms "all life stages" indicates that it can be fed to gestating or lactating females, growing animals and adults. These claims must be substantiated by a nutritional adequacy statement on the information panel.[4]

Nutritional adequacy can be established using one of three methods; the first is to conduct a feeding trial or protocol using the food fed to the designated species in a controlled setting using a defined protocol.[2] Alternately, adequacy can be established using a computer formulation to a specific nutritional profile established by AAFCO. Finally, adequacy can be established following the "family product rule," which allows foods which are similar in ingredients and that have been tested to match or exceed key nutrient levels of another food that has passed a feeding trial or protocol to claim that the unfed "family member" food has passed a feeding trial or protocol for the same life stage.[2] There is no way to tell from the label if the "family product rule" has been used.

Bursts and flags are areas of the PDP that are designated to highlight information or provide specific information with visual impact.[4] New products, formula or ingredient changes and improvements in taste are most often highlighted.[4] "New" or "new and improved" can only appear on the label for six months, while comparisons such as "preferred 5 to 1 over the leading national brand" can appear on the label for 1 year, unless it is resubstantiated.[4]

Information Panel

The information panel is usually the second place that consumers look for information about a food they are buying.[3] The list of ingredients must be arranged in decreasing order by predominance by weight. The terms used to describe the products must be those assigned for that product by the AAFCO, or names that are commonly accepted as a standard in the feed industry.[3] No single ingredient can be given undue emphasis nor can designators of quality be included.[3]

Most grocery store and generic brands are formulated as "variable formula diets."[3] This means that the ingredients used in the food will vary from batch to batch, depending on market availability and pricing. In contrast, most premium foods sold in feed stores, pet stores and through veterinarians (i.e. therapeutic diets) are produced using fixed formulas.[3] Although the cost for a fixed formula food may be more than a variable formula diet, the consistency between batches of food is a distinct advantage to the dog or cat consuming the food.[3] This will help to eliminate the GI distress that can often accompany a diet change, even if the brand of food itself has not changed.

The ingredient list must be listed on the packaging and is listed in decreasing order of inclusion based on weight before cooking; drying or other processing has taken place.[2] It also gives no indicator of the quality of the ingredients used in the food. These ingredients can vary

Table 12.2 Important elements found on pet food labels in the US and Canada[4]

Principal display panel	Information panel
Product identity (required)	Ingredient statement (required)
Manufacturer's name	
Brand name	
Product name	
Designator or statement of intent (required)	Guaranteed analysis (required)
Net weight (required)	Nutritional adequacy statement (required)
Product vignette or picture (optional)	Feeding guidelines (required)
Nutritional claim (optional)	Manufacturer or distributor (required)
Bursts or flags (optional)	Universal product code (optional)
	Batch information (optional)
	Freshness date (optional)
	Caloric content (optional)

in digestibility, amino acid content and bioavailability, mineral availability and the amount of indigestible materials they contain.[3] Unfortunately, there is no way to determine quality of the ingredients from the ingredient list. In fact, some premium foods with very high-quality ingredients may have an ingredient list that is almost identical to a generic food that contains poor-quality ingredients with low digestibility and poor nutrient availability.[3] This can be seen in products that claim to be "the same as" another higher priced product. As with most anything else, you get what you pay for. Ingredients must be listed using their AAFCO or FDA defined names using generic name only. Brand or trade names cannot be used.

References to the "quality, nature, form, or other attributes of an ingredient shall be allowed when the designation is not false or misleading; [and] the ingredient imparts a distinctive characteristic to the pet food because it possesses that attribute; [and]the reference to quality or grade of the ingredients does not appear in the ingredients statement." We are commonly seeing references on the ingredient panel stating that chicken is a natural source of glucosamine. We will not see references stating that the ingredient is "USDA choice beef."[2]

Another misleading practice is the splitting of ingredients to place them lower on the ingredient list. This occurs when several different forms of the same product are listed separately (e.g. wheat germ meal, wheat middlings, wheat bran, wheat flour). Because the requirement is to list by weight, by splitting the ingredients, they each weight less and can be placed further down the ingredient list when in fact they compromise a major portion of the product. Dry ingredients also appear lower on the list than those that are naturally higher in moisture. This allows most "meat" products to appear higher on the ingredient list than the dry grains and starches which may actually be found in a higher percentage in the diet.[4] By their very nature, meats, which contain a higher portion of water than other ingredients, will appear higher on the ingredient label. Consumers are continually told that meat-based products are more desirable ingredients than plant-based products, so there is a lot of incentive for manufacturer to manipulate the label to appeal to consumers.

Pet food additives such as vitamins, minerals, antioxidant preservatives, antimicrobial preservatives, humectants, coloring agents, flavors, palatability enhancers and

emulsifying agents that are listed by the manufacturer must also be included on the ingredient list (Table 12.3).[4]

In the United States, pet food manufacturers are required to include minimum percentages for crude protein and crude fat, and maximum percentages for crude fiber and moisture.[4] These percentages generally indicate the "worst case" levels for these nutrients in the food and may not accurately reflect the exact or typical amounts included.[4] Also notice that these indicate only minimums or maximums found in the foods. Actual values may differ dramatically.

Crude protein is the estimate of the total protein in a food that is obtained by multiplying analyzed levels of nitrogen by a constant numerical value.[3,4] Crude protein is an index of protein quantity, but does not give an indication of amino acid content, protein quality or digestibility.[3,4]

Crude fat is an estimate of the lipid content of a food that is obtained through extraction of the food with ether.[3,4] This procedure also isolates certain organic acids, oils, pigments, alcohols, and fat-soluble vitamins. But it may not be able to isolate some complex lipids such as the phospholipids.[3,4]

Crude fiber represents the organic residue that remains after the plant material has been treated with dilute acid and alkali solvents and after mineral components have been extracted.[3,4] Although crude fiber is used to report the fiber content of commercial foods, it usually underestimates the true level of fiber found in the food.[4] The values also do not indicate the solubility or fermentabilty of that fiber by the intestinal bacteria, which release additional energy from the food.

The amount of water found in an individual product can significantly affect the values of the other nutrients listed on the guaranteed analysis because most pet foods display nutrients on as "as-fed" basis, rather than on a "dry-matter" basis.[3,4] "As-fed" means that the percentages of nutrients were calculated directly, without accounting for the proportion of water in a product.[3,4] It is important to convert these guarantees to dry-matter basis when comparing foods of differing moisture contents, such as canned versus dry foods to get an accurate representation of the actual nutrients.[3,4] Most dry foods contain 6–10% water, while canned foods can contain up to 78% water.[3,4] It is also possible to use metabolizable energy when comparing different foods; this will give you the percentage of each nutrient in the food on an as fed basis, taking into account the

Table 12.3 Common pet food ingredients[5]

Description	Example	Contribution to diet
Meat (muscle)	Skeletal muscle, tongue, diaphragm, heart	Animal fat, protein, energy
Meat by-products	Lung, spleen, kidney, brain, blood, bone, intestine	Animal fat, protein, energy
Meat meal, meat and bone meal, fish meal, blood meal	Dry rendered product from animal tissue	Animal fat, protein, energy
Cereals	Corn, wheat, oats, barley, corn gluten meal	Carbohydrate, protein, fiber, energy
Soy flour, soy meal	Vegetable protein source including Textured Vegetable Protein (TVP)	Protein, texture/chunks (usually the meaty chunks in foods)
Animal fat, vegetable oil	Tallow, chicken fat, corn oil, soy oil	Fats, fatty acids, essential fatty acids, energy
Egg	Egg powder	Protein of high biologic value
Milk	Skim milk powder, whey	Milk protein
Grain hulls, root crops	Bran, beet pulp, chicory root	Dietary fiber
Humectants	Sugars, salt, glycerol	Reduction in water availability, energy
Digest	Hydrolyzed liver or intestine	Flavor and palatability enhancer, some protein and fat
Preservatives	Sodium benzoate, sodium and potassium sorbate	Retard spoilage from molds and bacteria
Flavors	Natural and artificial and "nature identical" flavors, process reacted flavors, key character compounds	Improvement in taste, smell and mouth feel
Coloring agents	Natural and artificial colorings	Improvement in owner appeal
Aromas	Natural and artificial aromas and tones	Improvement in owner and animal appeal
Vitamins, minerals	Vitamin and mineral premixes	Nutrients and dietary balance
Antioxidants	BHT, BHA, ascorbic acid, mixed tocopherols (vitamin E)	Prevents fat rancidity

different caloric amounts of each nutrient in the food. Metabolizable energy proves the percent of protein, fat and carbohydrates found in the food, as these are the only energy containing nutrients.

Maximum ash guarantees are not required in the United States, but are often included on pet food labels.[4] Ash consists of the noncombustible materials in food, usually composed of salt and other minerals. This is determined by burning the food in a bomb calorimeter, incinerating all nonmineral based components. High ash content in dry and semi-moist foods generally indicates high mineral content, specifically magnesium.[4] The ash content of canned cat foods usually correlates poorly with the magnesium content of that food.[4]

With the exception of treats or snacks, all pet foods that are in interstate commerce must contain a statement and validation of nutritional adequacy.[3,4] Current AAFCO regulations allow four primary types of nutritional adequacy statements:

Complete and balanced for all life stages
the food has been formulated to provide complete and balanced nutrition for gestation, lactation, growth and maintenance.

Limited claim
the food provides complete and balanced nutrition for a particular life stage such as adult maintenance or growth.

Intermittent or supplemental
the food has been formulated for only intermittent or supplemental use and is not intended for full time feeding.

Therapeutic
the food is intended for therapeutic use under the supervision of a veterinarian.[3,4]

The foods must also indicate what method was used to establish the nutritional adequacy claims. The use of feeding trials is the most thorough and reliable method of evaluation. The terms "feeding tests," "AAFCO feeding test protocols" or "AAFCO feeding studies" all validate that the product has undergone feeding tests with dogs or cats. If the substantiation claim states only that the food has met the AAFCO's *Nutrient Profiles*, this indicates that feeding trials were not done on the food.[3,4] The nutrient levels can be calculated in a laboratory after production or the diet can merely be formulated using a standard table of ingredients.[3] Neither of these methods takes into account digestibility or availability of individual nutrients or loss of nutrients through processing or excesses found in the ingredients.

Feeding guidelines are required on all foods labeled as completed and balanced for any life stage.[4] These directions must be given in common terms and must appear prominently on the label. At a minimum, these should state "feed (weight/unit of product) per (weight unit) of dog or cat" with a stated frequency. The guidelines are general at best and do not take into account the individual pet's sexual status, activity level or environmental factors like exposure to heat and cold. Because of individual variations, specific animals may require more or less food than recommended on the label to maintain optimal body condition and health.[4] An exception to this rule is therapeutic diets, which can state "use only as directed by your veterinarian."[2]

A statement of caloric content may be included in the information panel, but is not required. It must be separate from the guaranteed analysis, and appear under the heading of "caloric content." The statement is usually based on kilocalories of metabolizable energy (ME) on an as fed basis and must be expressed as kilocalories per kilograms of product. It may also be given as kilocalories per familiar household measure such as kcal/cup or kcal/can.[4]

In the United States, the name and address of the manufacturer, distributor or dealer of the pet food must be found on the label, usually on the information panel.[4] This information is not required to be complete, and may only include the distributor and city of origin. Most premium foods include their name, mailing address, phone number with hours of operations and possibly a website address. This makes it much easier on the consumer to contact the manufacturer with any problems or questions regarding the product.

Although not a legal requirement, most manufacturers include the Universal Product Code (UPC) or bar code on the label. Other information, such as batch numbers and date of manufacture can also frequently be found on the labels. There may also be a freshness date included on the label.[4]

References

1 Buffington CA, Holloway C, Abood SK (2004) Diet and feeding factors. In *The Manual of Veterinary Dietetics*, pp. 43–8, St Louis, MO: Elsevier.

2 Delaney S, Fascetti A (2012) Using pet food labels and product guides. In S Delaney, A Fascetti (eds), *Applied Veterinary Clinical Nutrition*, pp. 69–74, Ames, IA: Wiley-Blackwell.

3 Case LP, Carey DP, Hirakawa DA, Daristotle L (2000) Pet food labels. In *Canine and Feline Nutrition* (2nd edn), pp. 153–63, St Louis, MO: Mosby.

4 Roudebush P, Dzanis DA, Debraekeleer J, Brown RG (2000) Pet food labels. In MS Hand, CD Thatcher, RL Remillard *et al.* (eds), *Small Animal Clinical Nutrition* (4th edn), pp. 151–7, Marceline, MO: Walsworth Publishing.

5 Kelly NC (1996). Food types and evaluation. In N Kelly, J Wills (eds), *Manual of Companion Animal Nutrition and Feeding*, p. 34, Ames, IA: Iowa State University Press.

13 Nutrient Content of Pet Foods

Introduction

Nutrient content refers not only to the exact levels of the various nutrients in the food but also to the digestibility and availability of all of the essential nutrients.[1] Since we are feeding a specific food to provide nutrients, knowledge of the levels of these nutrients is important to know. There are four different ways that the nutrient content of a product can be determined.[2]

1 Laboratory analysis of the final product can be done.
2 The target values can be obtained from the manufacturer.
3 Nutrient content can be calculated based on published values for the ingredients.
4 The information found on the label guaranteed analysis and typical analysis can be used.[2]

Laboratory Analysis

Laboratory analysis or proximate analysis is used to provide information on a specific group of nutrient and will not usually contain all the nutrients found in a food. The nutrients typically looked at are expressed as percentages: Moisture, crude protein, crude fat ash (minerals) and fiber.[3] The guaranteed analysis found on the product label is generated from the proximate analysis. If a company wants to provide additional material to the consumer or veterinary professional above what is allowed on the label, product information can be found online, through product brochures and in product reference guides.[3]

If contact information is provided for the product, contacting the manufacturer can also be a source of additional information. Of course this is dependent on the level of customer support provided by the manufacturer. Using the label guaranteed analysis to determine actual nutrient levels in the food is the least accurate method due to the way these values are given. Moisture, fiber and ash as reported as maximum levels, which may or may not be close to what is actually found in the product, and protein and fat are reported as minimum levels.

If a food is formulated to meet the nutrient profile of a specific life stage, nutrient levels should be equal or greater than the nutrient profiles minimums and equal or less than the nutrient profile's maximums.[4] This method of evaluating nutrient content is not recommended due to severe limitations and discrepancies in the calculated values.[2]

Calculation

Calculating nutrient content based on published values of ingredients also has limitations; there is a lack of complete and accurate data for the nutrient content of many ingredients used in commercial pet foods. Because of this, manufacturers rely on lists that contain approximations of the types of ingredients that are used.[1] These lists may also contain information that is outdated or misleading resulting in inaccurate values being used.[1] The National Research Councils (NRCs) published values are often used to evaluate the level of nutrients in pet foods.[3]

The quality of the ingredients is not taken into account when using the calculation method; this can affect the level and availability of nutrients in the finished product.[1] The standardized tables represent average nutrient content for individual ingredients, and therefore may not represent ingredient quality among various raw ingredients.[3] Processing methods can further affect ingredient quality with nutrient losses occurring during both processing and storage.[1] Studies have shown that digestibility and nutrient availability of animal-based and plant-based ingredients are

Nutrition and Disease Management for Veterinary Technicians and Nurses, Second Edition. Ann Wortinger, Kara M. Burns
© 2015 John Wiley & Sons, Inc. Published 2015 by John Wiley & Sons, Inc.
Companion Website: www.wiley.com/go/wortinger/nutrition

significantly affected by processing methods.[1] This method would likely be used for determining the nutrient content of homemade diets, though adequate time and knowledge to perform the calculations would be a major limitation.[2]

Most pet food manufacturers will supply target values for the nutrient content of their foods upon request.[2] Though these values often reflect actual average nutrient levels, occasionally they will vary significantly from the actual values found in the food.[2] Since there are no laws governing the accuracy of target nutrient levels, the manufacturer does not have to have the food within these levels.[2] Remember, the manufacturer only has to ensure the food is within the stated maximum and minimum levels. Overall, these values should be a reasonable approximation of nutrient levels, and will be adequate for most instances.

Final Product Analysis

Of the methods listed above, the most accurate way to determine nutrient content of a food is through laboratory analysis of the final product; this provides the proximate analysis.[1] A proximate analysis tests for a limited number of parameters, including moisture content, crude protein, crude fat, ash (minerals) and fiber contents.[1] Nitrogen-free extract (NFE) represents a rough estimation of the soluble carbohydrate content of the food and can be calculated by simple subtraction. Starting at 100%, subtract the percentages given for moisture, protein, fat, ash and fiber. What is left is the NFE.[2] The guaranteed analysis panel is generated from the proximate analysis results, and reports only the maximum or minimum levels.[1]

Digestibility

Digestibility provides a measure of the final diet's quality because it directly determines the proportion of nutrients in the food that are available for absorption into the body.[1] Currently, AAFCO regulations do not require companies to determine or provide digestibility levels for their foods.[3]

Digestibility should always be considered when evaluating various pet foods. Digestibility is a measure of the actual level of nutrients that are available for the body

for use.[3] Feeding trials are the most accurate method used to determine digestibility of nutrients and measures the disappearance of nutrients as they pass through the animal's digestive system and are absorbed by the body for use.[3] Information about the nutrient content of a diet has little meaning if the digestibility is unknown.[1]

For example, you have two diets that each contains 28% protein, if the digestibility of one diet is 70%, and the digestibility of the second diet is 85% the actual protein available to the animal is less than 20% in the first diet, and over 24% in the second diet.[1] While this difference may not seem significant, the amount of protein provided to the animal can become significant over time. Even though laboratory analysis would show that they have similar protein contents, digestibility shows that the second diet provides significantly more digestible protein than would the first diet.[1]

Digestibility also affects fecal volume, form and frequency. As a diets digestibility increases, fecal volume decreases significantly, additionally a highly digestible diet produces firm and well-formed feces.[1]

Manufacturers are not required to conduct feeding trials to determine digestibility of their foods. Reputable companies that produce quality products always conduct these trials to ensure that their foods contain levels of nutrients that will meet an animal's daily requirements for absorption into the body.[1] It is possible for a food to pass a feeding trial without meeting a nutrient profile's values. Because of this, you should not make assumptions on nutrient levels of food based solely on the absence or presence of feeding trials. Examples of this can be seen in many therapeutic diets that do not meet AAFCO nutrient profiles, but have undergone feeding trials. This also explains why these foods are prescription diets, which should only be fed when the animal in under the supervision of a veterinarian who would be monitoring for any nutrient deficiency caused by restricted diets.[4] This is also why OTC foods for specific disease management do not exist, as the animals would not be monitored to determine if nutrient deficiency or excesses exist.

Feeding Trials

In the United States, the AAFCO testing procedure for adult maintenance diets are done over a period of six months, require only eight animals per group and monitor only a limited number of parameters.[2] The food being evaluated is fed to a group of animals, and feces and urine are collected throughout the testing period. The energy found in the feces and urine is subtracted from the total energy found in the food before feeding to evaluate actual digestibility.[5] This data provides digestibility energy (DE) or metabolizable energy (ME) of that specific food. Passing such tests does not ensure that long-term nutrition or health related problems will not occur, or that problems with an occurrence rate less than 15% won't be seen.[2] The protocols are also not designed to ensure optimal growth or maximize physical activity.[2]

Digestible energy (DE) measures the amount of energy found in a food that is absorbed across the intestinal wall. Metabolizable energy (ME) accounts for any energy lost in the urine and feces, as well as what is absorbed across the intestinal wall.[3] Metabolizable energy provides a more accurate assessment of the energy that is actually available to the animal for use, rather than measuring the total amount of energy found in the food (gross energy). Digestion is not 100% efficient, and ME reflects the degree of inefficiency seen in a specific species. Remember that each individual animal may be more or less efficient at digestion than their species average, especially when we factor in disease processes.

If these factors are of concern due to disease, additional long-term feeding trials need to be evaluated. Numerous premium pet food manufactures conduct long-term studies looking at optimizing the response to various nutrients as well as therapeutic treatment protocols.

Food Comparisons

When trying to compare various foods or different types, what method is best to use? If foods are compared on a dry-matter basis (DMB), differences seen with different food types can be eliminated, but differences in energy content are not addressed. The energy content for protein and carbohydrates is calculated at ~3.5 kcal/g while fat is calculated ~8.5 kcal/g. To accurately evaluate different diets the nutrient density should be evaluated as a proportion of metabolizable energy (ME).[1] Nutrient density accounts for differences in both water content and energy content, and expresses nutrient levels in pet foods based on the energy available for the animal to use as metabolizable energy.[1]

Nutrient density is expressed as grams/100 kcal of ME for each nutrient.[1] Since all animals are fed to meet their energy requirements, the amount of food consumed and the amount of nutrients received depends on the energy density of the food.[1] When an animal is fed a calorically dense food, the percentage of nutrients by weight in these foods must be higher to meet the needs for all of the essential nutrients since less food will be consumed by the animal.[1] The inverse is also true, when feeding a food that is calorically dilute, the amount of nutrients provided in that food must be available in a level that the animal can meet when consuming the volume of food that meets their energy requirements.

Metabolizable Energy

The easiest way to express nutrients is as a percentage of ME or as units per 1000 kcal of ME, instead of a percentage of weight. Nutrient densities of foods with different moisture contents can be compared because water does not contribute any calories to the distribution.[1] Unfortunately, this method does not take into account the calories in the foods or the amount that must be consumed by the animal to meet energy requirements.[1]

Caloric distribution is helpful when trying to find a diet that is higher or lower than another diet in certain nutrients. The three primary nutrients that are evaluated are protein, fat and carbohydrates. These are usually expressed as a percentage, and given as pie charts or line charts in the product reference guides available from the manufacturers (Table 13.1).

Table 13.1 Examples of nutrient density and caloric distribution (Iams Veterinary Formula)

Diets Product Reference Guide[3]

Diet A – dry food (renal diet)

Nutrient density (gm/1000 kcal ME)

Crude protein	54.79
Crude fat	34.40
Crude fiber	5.53
Carbohydrate	149.80

Guaranteed analysis

Crude protein	18% DM
Crude fat	12%

(continued)

Table 13.1 (*Continued*)

Crude fiber	4%
Moisture	10%
% Metabolizable calories	
Protein	18%
Fat	31%
Carbohydrate	51%

Caloric distribution

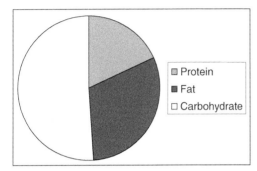

Diet B – canned food (recovery diet)

Nutrient density (gm/1000 kcal ME)

Crude protein	71.80
Crude fat	63.84
Crude fiber	4.56
Carbohydrate	21.49

Guaranteed analysis

Crude protein	14%
Crude fat	12%
Crude fiber	1%
Ash	3%

Metabolizable calories

Protein	29%
Fat	68%
Carbohydrate	3%

Caloric distribution

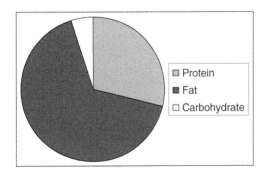

Diet C – dry food (intestinal diet)

Nutrient density (gm/1000 kcal ME)

Crude protein	66.10
Crude fat	28.70

Table 13.1 (*Continued*)

Crude fiber	6.34
Carbohydrate	150.00
Guaranteed analysis	
Crude protein	22%
Crude fat	9%
Crude fiber	4%
Moisture	10%
Metabolizable calories	
Protein	23%
Fat	24%
Carbohydrate	53%

Caloric distribution

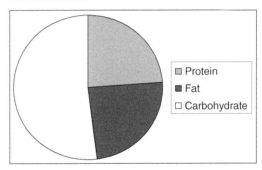

Diet D – canned food (intestinal diet)

Nutrient density (gm/1000 kcal ME)

Crude protein	80.50
Crude fat	45.20
Crude fiber	2.30
Carbohydrate	95.40

Guaranteed analysis

Crude protein	7%
Crude fat	2.8%
Crude fiber	1%
Moisture	78%

Metabolizable calories

Protein	28%
Fat	38%
Carbohydrate	34%

Caloric distribution

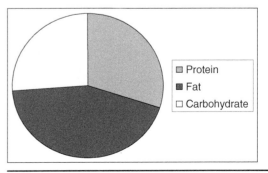

Table 13.2 Nutrients as a percentage of metabolizable energy[1]

Total calories in 100 grams of food

Protein = 3.5 kcal/gram × grams in food

Fat = 8.5 kcal/gram × grams in food

Carbohydrate = 3.5 kcal/gram × grams in food

Total calories/100 gram = protein calorie + fat calorie + carbohydrate calorie

Percentage of ME contributed by each nutrient (caloric distribution)

Protein = (protein calories/100 gram divided by total calories/100 gram) × 100 = % ME

Fat = (fat calories/100 gram divided by total calories/100 gram) × 100 = % ME

Carbohydrate = (carbohydrate calories/100 gram divided by total calories) × 100 = % ME

Table 13.3 Finding energy density from guaranteed analysis [2, 3]

Energy density from guaranteed analysis

% in diet of nutrient × mod. Atwater factor = kcal/100 gm of food

Divided % nutrient by total calories to get nutrient distribution

Work sheet examples

No name dog food guarantee analysis

Protein	21%
Fat	5%
Moisture	12%
Insoluble fiber	12%
Ash	3%
Protein	21% × 3.5 = calories from protein
per 100 g of food	
	73.5 protein calories

Fat 5% × 8.5 = calories from fat
per 100 g of food

42.5 fat calories

Carbohydrate need to be calculated from
given values, usually not provided
(100 − (protein + fat + insoluble fiber
+ moisture + ash)
Carbohydrate = (100 − (21 + 5 + 12 + 12 + 3)
= 47% × 3.5 = calories from carbohydrate
per 100 g of food

164.5 carbo calories

Total calories = 73.5 + 42.5 + 164.5
= 280.5 kcal/100 g

Metabolizable calories equals

Protein	73.5/280.5 × 100 = 26.2%
Fat	42.5/280.5 × 100 = 15%
Carbohydrate	164.5/280.5 × 100 = 58.6% (2, 3)

These two last diets are the same brand; notice the different caloric distribution between the canned and dry foods (Table 13.2).

If the grams of nutrient/100 gram of food is not given, then using the guaranteed analysis and kilocalories/100 grams the following formula can be used. Because you are not accounting for metabolic or fecal/urine losses, these values are not as accurate as the metabolizable energy values (Table 13.3).

By converting the nutrients into percentage of metabolizable energy, we can compare dry foods to canned foods by any manufacturer. This is the most accurate way to compare foods. It will also allow us the best way to find a food that meets a specific nutrient profile (i.e. low fat or high protein).

References

1 Case LP, Carey DP, Hirakawa DA, Daristotle L (2000) Nutrient content of pet foods. In *Canine and Feline Nutrition* (2nd edn), pp. 165–86, St Louis, MO: Mosby.

2 Hand MS, Thatcher CD, Remillard RL, Roudebush P (2000) Small animal clinical nutrition: An iterative process. In MS Hand, CD Thatcher, RL Remillard *et al.* (eds), *Small Animal Clinical Nutrition* (4th edn), pp. 7–11, Marceline, MO: Walsworth Publishing.

3 Iams Veterinary Formula Diets (2011) *Product Reference Guide*, pp. 10, 32, 37.

4 Case LP, Daristotle L, Hayek MG, Raasch MF (2011) Nutrient content in pet foods. In *Canine and Feline Nutrition* (3rd edn), pp. 141–60, St Louis, MO: Mosby.

5 Delaney S, Fascetti A (2012) Using pet food labels and product guides. In Delaney S, Fascetti A (eds), *Applied Veterinary Clinical Nutrition*, pp. 69–74, Ames, IA: Wiley-Blackwell.

14   Types of Pet Foods

Introduction

Until the early 1900s, there were few options on what to feed our companion animals: They ate what we ate. After the start of commercial pet food production, the options available have continued to expand at an alarming rate to encompass the amazing variety of foods and flavors that we see today.

While clients typically make the decision on what food to feed their pet themselves, many clients wish that their veterinary team would recommend a specific diet.[1] American Animal Health Association (AAHA) and the World Small Animal Veterinary Association (WSAVA) have made the recommendations and developed guidelines to make nutritional assessments and recommendations the 5th vital assessment, along with temperature, pulse, respiration and pain on our routine physical exams.[2,3] While every veterinary professional cannot hope to know about the estimated 175 pet food manufacturers in the United States, developing a working knowledge of the most popular or your favorite foods is essential.[1]

Pet Food Library

Making a "pet food library" of the foods that are commonly available in your area, and those on which your clients routinely feed can be very helpful. Depending on where you live, you could easily fill a 4 inch, 3 ring binder with product reference guides, ingredient lists and nutritional information on these foods. You can set this binder up according to manufacturer, alphabetically or by category, whatever system works best for you. Maintaining product reference guides for those manufacturers who's products you use most commonly is especially helpful. It is also important to maintain a list of those manufacturers about whom you can't find information, who won't provide you complete product information or those that you can't reach through the available means. This can be your "thou shalt not" list. Having this information can be very helpful when discussing diet changes or diet related problems with clients; it will provide you with concrete information to back up your views and recommendations.

Commercial Diets

It has been reported that over 90% of dogs and cats in the US consume more than half of their daily calories in the form of commercial pet foods.[1] These commercial diets are available in several forms that vary according to their processing methods, the ingredients used and the method of preservation.[4] The foods can be further classified based on their nutrient content, purpose of use, the quality of the ingredients and the water content of the diet.[4,5]

Commercial pet foods are available in four basic forms: these would be dry, canned, semi-moist and raw diets.[1,4] Knowing what the potential advantages and disadvantages each of these types of diets have to offer is helpful for client communication and when making diet recommendations.[1]

Dry Pet Foods

Dry or kibble foods are the most common type of pet food fed to dogs.[1] Dry pet foods contain between 3% and 11% moisture, and 90% or more dry matter (DM).[1,4] They are generally sold in the form of kibbles, biscuits, meals and expanded, extruded pellets.[4−6] These may be "complete and balanced" for all life stages or designed for a specific life stage. They may also be formulated to only be a treat or snack.[4−6] This is the food of choice, when the owners choose to feed free choice.[1] This type of food also tends to be the most economical to feed.[1]

Nutrition and Disease Management for Veterinary Technicians and Nurses, Second Edition. Ann Wortinger, Kara M. Burns
© 2015 John Wiley & Sons, Inc. Published 2015 by John Wiley & Sons, Inc.
Companion Website: www.wiley.com/go/wortinger/nutrition

A certain level of starch content must be included in expanded products to allow for proper processing of the product. This generally is met through the inclusion of cereals, cereal by-products and soy meals.[4] The loss of nutrients, particularly vitamins, through processing is limited because the baking or extrusion processes do not require excessive temperatures or time, and sufficient supplements are added to counterbalance processing and storage losses.[5]. Because of the low moisture content of the food, they usually do not contain enough water for bacterial or fungal growth, and have a long shelf-life if kept in cool, dry storage conditions.[5]

Kibbles and biscuits are prepared in much the same way, though the final shapes are different.[4] In both cases, the ingredients are mixed together to form a dough similar to cookie dough, which is then baked. When biscuits are made, the dough is formed or cut into desired shapes and the individual biscuits are baked like cookies.[4] With kibbled foods, the dough is spread onto large sheets and baked. After cooling, the large sheets are broken into bite-sized pieces and packaged.[4] Most dog and cat treats are baked biscuits, though a few companies still produce complete and balanced kibble.[4] Dry meal foods are prepared by mixing together a number of dried, flaked and granular ingredients to form a dog and cat version of "trail mix."[4,6]

The development of the extrusion process by Purina in the 1950s resulted in the almost complete replacement of meals and kibbles with extrusion in commercial foods.[4] The extrusion process produces expanded pet foods and involves the mixing of all the ingredients together to form dough. This dough is then cooked under conditions of high pressure and temperature in an extruder. When the cooked dough reaches the end of the extruder (within 20–60 seconds), it exits through a small die. This die forces the soft product into the desired shape(s) and a rotating knife cuts the pieces into the desired kibble size.[4] The extrusion process causes rapid cooking of the starches within the product, resulting in increased digestibility and palatability. After cooling, a coating of fat or digest (a type of flavor enhancer produced by chemical or enzymatic breakdown of proteins) is usually applied to the outside of the food in a process called enrobing. The enrobing further enhances the palatability of the food. Hot air drying reduces the total moisture content to 10% or less.[4]

Dry foods contain a greater concentration of nutrients and energy per unit weight than do foods of higher moisture content. Because of this, relatively small amounts are needed to provide a particular quantity of nutrients.[5,6] Unless they contain a large amount of nondigestible fiber such as cellulose or hemicellulose, the overall digestibility of dry foods is good, but often lower than that of meats or canned foods.[5] Dry foods are considered to be better digested by dogs than by cats due to the higher carbohydrate content found in the diets.[5] Since most cat foods have higher protein and lower carbohydrate levels than do dog foods, this difference is negligible.

Dry foods also tend to be less expensive than canned or semi-moist diets, but this can vary based on the ingredients used, and the quality of those ingredients.[6] The primary disadvantage of dry diets is that they are less palatable than meats or canned diets, but the process of enrobing the finished kibble can affect this by increasing palatability.[1,5] Decreased palatability can be an advantage in animals that are overweight or obese, but can be problematic in finicky or underweight animals.[1] The major advantage to dry foods would be cost and convenience.

Most popular or premium brands of dry foods may be lower in nondigestible fiber than less expensive brands and are comparable to quality canned foods in digestibility of nutrients.[6] The stools produced will help to indicate the quality of the food, with a high quality food producing well formed, firm stools 1–2 times/day, while a poor quality food may result in bulky, less formed stools produced more often.[6]

The availability of essential fatty acids (EFAs), especially linoleic acid for the dog and arachidonic acid for the cat can be affected by prolonged storage, in less than optimal conditions for some complete dry foods. This would include those foods stored in warm, damp environments (kitchens) or exposed to sunlight. This is a particular problem if beef tallow (fat) is used as the fat source.[4,6] This can also be seen in those situations where food is bought in bulk, especially with a small dog or cat and stored in an open container in the kitchen for prolonged periods of time (6 months or more).[4,6]

Moist Pet Foods

Moist diets are not longer just found in "cans," but also in plastic trays, foil containers, plastic cans and pouches. All of these products have a moisture range of 60–87% on an "as fed" basis.[1,6] Moist diets can either be "complete and balanced" or designed to be used for supplemental feeding, as with a treat.[4] Cats, unlike dogs, are more likely to receive the majority of their calories from moist diets.[1]

Moist diets are prepared by first blending the meat and fat ingredients with measured amounts of water. Measured amounts of dry ingredients are then added and the entire mixture is heated.[4] Canning occurs on a conveyer line. After filling, the cans are sealed, washed and labeled. Pressure sterilization of canned products is called retorting.[4] Temperatures and times can vary with the product and can size, but typically is done at 250°Celsius for 60 minutes.[4] After exiting the retort, the cans are cooled under controlled conditions to ensure sterility of the food and the integrity of the sealed product. After cooling, paper labels are then applied.[4]

For processing methods, there are three main types of moist foods: loaf, chunks or chunks in gravy, and a chunk-in-loaf combination (Table 14.1).[4]

Depending on the ingredients used, these products can vary greatly in nutrient content, digestibility, and nutrient availability.[4] These diets are often higher in fat, sodium and phosphorus when compared to dry foods.[1] Many owners assume that the "meaty chunks" found in the food are indeed meat, but more commonly these chunks are textured soy product (TSP) similar to tofu. These chunks provide the owners with the visual appeal that they are looking for while keeping the cost down for the manufacture.[4]

Moist diets tend to be more palatable and digestible than many dry foods, but a poor quality moist diet would not be more digestible than a good quality dry food.[4] The high heat and pressure used in processing moist diet kills harmful bacteria and causes some nutrient losses.[4]

Manufacturers that conduct feeding trials adjust their formulas to compensate for these losses. Companies that use the calculation method to substantiate their label claims are not required to compensate for losses because the calculation method is used before processing of the ingredients.[4]

The high moisture content of these foods affects the nutrient density, meaning that these foods have less nutrients per 100 grams of food that do other food types so that more food must be eaten to satisfy energy and nutrient needs.[6] The higher moisture content and lower energy density can be helpful in providing satiety and reducing calorie intake. The higher moisture content can also be helpful when dealing with a patient where increased water intake is desirable, such as urinary tract health concerns, and chronic renal failure.[1]

The most palatable diets are those that contain little or no cereal products and are presented as meaty or fishy chunks in gravy or jelly.[5] Protein content can range from 7–9% in dog foods and 8–11% in cat foods on an "as fed" basis.[5] Digestibility of moist foods for both dogs and cats is high, being 80–85% for most nutrients in quality products.[5] Energy density is highest in moist diets on a dry matter basis of all commercially available diets. Palatability is directly related to the meat and fat content, with the foods higher in cereal being less palatable.[5]

Moist foods offer extremely long shelf life with high acceptability by the pet. Because of their nutrient content and texture, canned foods tend to be highly palatable. If moist diets are fed free choice to an animal with low energy requirements they can override their tendency to eat to meet energy requirements, resulting in overeating and obesity.[4]

Because the diets are sterilized using steam and heat, no other preservative are needed. This makes them ideal for a client concerned about the use of preservatives in

Table 14.1 Three main types of moist foods[5]

Loaf	Ground cereal and chopped meat, fish, poultry. Has a solid meatloaf-like appearance
Chunks, chunks in gravy	Ground cereal and chopped or pre-formed meat. May be meat-based, fish-based or meat & cereal based. May appear as balls, shapes or chunks together with gelling agents and mineral/vitamin supplements in gravy or jelly.
Chunk-in-loaf	A combination of the chopped loaf appearance and the chunks in gravy foods.

their pets' food.[1] Though many owners do not like the smell or mess associated with moist diets or the fact that unsed portions need to be stored in the refrigerator.[1]

Not all moist foods are complete and balanced; many are designed to be used for supplemental feeding only. Many clients use these foods to "top dress" their pets' dry foods to improve palatability. This is what they are supposed to be used for, but many animals, especially cats can easily develop "fixed food preferences" and will only eat this one food item and refuse all others irregardless of nutrient balance (cats aren't very good at math).[4]

Semi-moist Foods

A third class of food product is the semi-moist or soft-moist foods. These foods generally contain between 15% and 30% water and can include fresh or frozen animal tissues, cereal grains, fats and simple sugars as their main ingredients.[4] Semi-moist foods more closely resemble dry foods in nutrient content; they do tend to have higher proportions of animal protein and a higher energy density on a dry matter basis.[5] The carbohydrate portion of the diet is mainly disaccharides (sucrose).[5] Digestibly can be as high as 80–85%.

Preservation is achieved through the use of humectants and certain preservatives.[4,5] Humectants such as sugars, salts and glycerol are included in the foods to decrease the availability of water for use by invading microorganisms.[4,5] This helps to retard microbial spoilage. The addition of potassium sorbate is used to inhibit the growth of yeast and molds, and small amounts of organic acids can be included to decrease the pH and further help in inhibiting bacterial growth.[4,5]

The high sugar content of many semi-moist products contributes to the palatability and digestibility of these products, especially for dogs. Cats are less likely to select a sweet food than are dogs.[4] Semi-moist diets that contain high levels of simple carbohydrates have digestibility similar to those of moist products, though because of their lower fat content the energy density tends to be lower.[4] The carbohydrate content of semi-moist diets is similar to that found in dry food diet, but the carbohydrate type found is largely in the form of simple carbohydrates, with relatively small proportions of starch or complex carbohydrates.[4] Because of the use of simple carbohydrates for preservation, these diets would not be recommended for use by diabetic animals, and the use

of semi-moist treats should be limits to less than 10% of the overall diet.

Semi-moist foods do not require refrigeration prior to use and have a relatively long shelf-life. The overall cost of the foods tends to be in between dry foods and moist foods.[4] Because they are usually sold in single-serving packets though, the price is usually closer to that of moist diets.[4] Some owners prefer the semi-moist diets due to the relative lack of odor and mess associated with moist foods and because they come in shapes similar to foods that they eat (e.g., burgers, vegetables, etc.). These diets can become hard and dry out if left exposed to room air for extended periods of time.[1]

On an "as fed" basis, semi-moist diets have the highest caloric density when compared to dry or moist diets. They have lower moisture content than do canned foods and fewer air pockets than do extruded products.[4]

Raw

Raw food diets can either be commercially prepared, or homemade by the owner.[7] These may be referred to as "BARF" diets, which stands for either "bones and raw foods" or "biologically appropriate raw food" diets.[1] Some advocates for this tye of diet present the theory that dogs should be fed raw meat because their wild ancestors survived and present-day relatives continue to survive on uncooked food.[7] There is no compelling scientific evidence to support statements that dogs should eat uncooked food as did their wild ancestors.[7] There are numerous studies that present evidence that raw diet tend to be unbalanced and can present significant parasite and microorganism risk to pets consuming them as well as their families.[7]

The two most common forms of raw food diets fed include commercially complete foods that are intended as sole source nutrition and combination diets here the owner purchases a supplement mix that is then combined with the raw meat they provide.[1] For the complete diets, they are available as fresh raw food, frozen raw food and freeze-dried raw diets that the owner can rehydrate before feeding.[1] With the combination diets, the owner has more flexibility in what source of meat is being fed as they purchase that to mix with the supplement.[1]

Proponents of this type of diet claim many health benefits associated with feeding raw foods. Some of these include improved coat health and dental benefits (less gingivitis and tarter). The high fat content (>50%) of these diets can account for the improved coat health. Increased incidence of periodontitis and tooth fractures have been associated with feeding of raw meats, and bones. In a study conducted by Drs Freeman and Michel, none of the homemade and commercially available raw food diets analyzed was appropriate for long-term feedings, each diet having deficiencies or excesses in nutrient levels, some of these significant.[7]

Significant health problems have been associated with feeding pets raw food diets; these include: risk of nutritional imbalances, cracked or fractured teeth, gastrointestinal obstruction and perforations, bacterial contamination of not only the pet's GI tract but also of the environment the food is prepared and fed in, and the potential for parasitic infections from contaminated meat.[1]

The overwhelming majority of raw food diets have not undergone feeding trials to detect any nutritional imbalances in their formulations. They count on the owners, ability to detect any imbalance and institute a corrective program, or to maintain a varied enough diet to prevent imbalances over a period of time rather than over each meal.

Snacks and Treats

Snacks and treats have become increasingly popular with pet owners in recent years. Snacks and treats are usually not purchased for their nutritional value, but as a way of showing love and affection for the dog or cat. Many pet owners also use snacks and treats as training aids to reinforce positive behaviors, and as an aid to proper dental health,[4] though most pet owners buy treats for emotional reasons.

Because of this emotional connection, palatability is of chief importance.[4] In the early years, all dog treats were in the form of baked biscuits. Since the buying of treats is usually an impulse buy on the owner's part and intended as a means of showing affection or as a training aid, the design is geared primarily to the owner. Today treats can be categorized into four basic types: semi-moist, biscuits, and jerky and rawhide products. Cat treats are usually in the form of either semi-moist or biscuit products, with dogs preferring rawhide and jerky treats.[4]

Although treats and snacks do not have to be nutritionally complete, a significant proportion of the products are formulated to be complete and balanced, and some may carry the same nutritional claim as dogs and cat foods.[4] In general, treats and snacks are highly palatable and cost significantly more than other types of pet foods when compared on a weight basis.[4] A large portion of this cost is due to the larger amounts of money directed towards marketing.[4] Clients should be advised that treats do contribute significant calories to the pet, and should not be more than 10% of the total caloric intake per day.

References

1 Delaney S, Fascetti A (2012) Commercial and home-prepared diets. In Delaney S, Fascetti A (eds), *Applied Veterinary Clinical Nutrition*, pp. 95–105, Ames, IA: Wiley-Blackwell.

2 http://www.petnutritionalliance.org/PDFS/PNA-Nutritional Assessment.pdf (accessed 3/9/13).

3 https://www.aahanet.org/Library/NutritionalAsmt.aspx (accessed 3/9/13).

4 Case LP, Carey DP, Hirakawa DA, Daristotle L (2000) Types of pet foods. In *Canine and Feline Nutrition* (2nd edn), pp. 187–97, St Louis, MO: Mosby.

5 Burger I (1995) Balanced diets for dogs and cats. In JM Wills. KW Simpson (eds), *The Waltham Book of Companion Animal Nutrition*, pp. 52–5, Tarrytown, NJ: Elsevier.

6 Kelly NC (1996) Food types and evaluation. In N Kelly, J Wills (eds), *Manual of Companion Animal Nutrition and Feeding*, pp. 22–42, Ames, IA: Iowa State Press.

7 Miller EP, Ahle NW, DeBey MC (2010) Food safety. In MS Hand, CD Thatcher, RL Remillard, *et al.* (eds). *Small Animal Clinical Nutrition* (5th edn), pp. 227–9, Marceline, MO: Walsworth Publishing.

15 Raw Food Diets: Fact versus Fiction

Introduction

It is generally accepted that dogs were domesticated from wolves; the period of this evolution ranges from 10,000 to 135,000 years ago. Accordingly, some recent DNA research shows that this occurred in stages in different areas, not all dogs breeds came from the same wolf or from the same geographic area.[1] Ben Sacks from the University of California Davis, School of Veterinary Medicine has found genetic evidence that 6000–9000 years ago, ancient farmers brought wolf-dogs from Europe and the Middle East to an area of present-day China south of the Yangtze River. It is in this area that dogs evolved separately from wolves.[2]

Early dogs in Europe and the Middle East continued to interbreed with wolves, while the dogs that had moved to China "apparently underwent a significant evolutionary transformation in southern China that enabled them to demographically dominate and largely replace earlier western forms." Dr Sacks and his team also suggest that the ability of dogs to digest starch occurred during the domestication in China associated with the development of agriculture, specifically rice farming that had become a major source of food for humans.[2]

The primary ancestor of the domestic cat is believed to have been the African wild cat, *Felis libyca*. Domestication started for cats much later then it did for dogs, ~8000 years ago with full domestication taking place only 4000 years ago.[3] The time difference between these two species is reflective in what these animals were domesticated for: dogs were hunters and protectors, while cats were vermin killers on the farms. As we evolved from a hunting society to a farming society, our needs changed.

With this history in mind, we need to look at what food these animals have consumed since they joined us in our farms and homes. Dogs did not continue to hunt and eat raw foods once domesticated; they primarily ate our leftovers and scraps. Since we have not consumed a raw food diet since fire was discovered, our dogs did not eat raw food either. Since cats were domesticated for their ability to control small vermin, they have continued to eat a raw food diet for a much longer period of time.

Myth: Raw Food Diets Are Nutritionally Superior to Processed Diets, and Are "What Nature Intended Dogs and Cats to Eat"

There is no scientific evidence showing that raw food diets are nutritionally superior to processed foods. All processed foods are required to conform to American Association of Feed Control Officials (AAFCO) standards for sale in the United States. These standards can be met in one of two ways. The food can be "formulated" to meet AAFCO standards, or feeding trials can be done. Feeding trials are the preferred method of substantiating AAFCO certification.[4] This takes into account not only nutrient content, but nutrient loss due to processing and digestibility.

Raw food diets overall are not marketed as "complete and balanced" and therefore do not need to meet AAFCO standards. Some of the frozen diets, however, are marketed as "complete and balanced" and have AAFCO statements on the labels, but the majorities have not undergone feeding trials. The claim is that

Nutrition and Disease Management for Veterinary Technicians and Nurses, Second Edition. Ann Wortinger, Kara M. Burns
© 2015 John Wiley & Sons, Inc. Published 2015 by John Wiley & Sons, Inc.
Companion Website: www.wiley.com/go/wortinger/nutrition

these diets are "complete and balanced" over a period of time, but not for each meal.

There are three main types of raw food diets.

- Commercially available complete raw food diets.
  - These diets are intended to be complete and balanced without the need for additional supplements. They are typically sold in frozen form.
- Homemade complete raw food diets (many recipes for homemade raw food diets are available in books, articles and on the Internet).
  - These diets expect the owner to balance the diets out in the long term as each meal is not in itself balanced.
- Combination diets.
  - These consist of commercially available mixes of grains and supplements. This mix is in turn combined with raw meat.[5]

Granted, raw food diets may be nutritionally superior to some commercially processed foods. Those would be the poor quality foods that have not gone through feeding trials, use lower grade ingredients, and have high cereal contents. Feeding any premium quality food would show an improvement in the animal's hair coat, activity and overall health, just due to the increased quality of the ingredients used.

Since the majority of raw food diets have not gone through feeding trials, it is difficult to know if they are nutritionally balanced or not. One study done by Drs Freeman and Michel looked at the nutrient content of a variety of raw food diets, both home-prepared and commercially available. None of the diets studied was balanced, and all had nutrient deficiencies or excesses. The authors note that these deficiencies and excesses may have been balanced out in the long term, but this is not guaranteed.[5]

Pet food manufacturers know what changes occur with their foods with the various processing methods, and supplement them as needed to maintain optimum nutrient levels. As with any science, we continue to discover every day new ways to use diets to modulate various diseases or conditions-and the pet food manufacturers continue to change and improve their foods.

Myth: Domesticated Species Tolerate Bacterial Contamination in Food without Problems, Even If They Are Pediatric, Geriatric, or Critically Ill Animals

There is no scientific evidence to support this claim, and in fact numerous studies have found either bacterial contamination in the food or dishes, or death related to pathogenic bacteria directly linked to the diet being fed.[5-8]

The study done by Drs Freeman and Michel that looked at nutrient content of the raw food diets also looked at microbial analyses. One of the diets yielded growth of *E. coli 0157:H7*.[5,8] This strain of *E. coli* has been connected to *E. coli* infections in people, and is one of the more pathogenic strains.

Another study presented in JAAHA reported two cats presenting for necropsy that died from septic *Salmonellosis*. In one of the cases it was directly traced back to the raw food diet fed. The two cases were 9 months apart in presentation, but from the same household. Healthy adult cats appear to have high immunological resistance to the development of clinical *Salmonellosis*. Cats that are immune compromised or otherwise ill would be at increased risk of infection due to contaminated food stuffs.[6]

Animals that are not sick themselves can also pose a public health concern due to shedding of bacteria into the environment. There are a number of bacteria that can be found on raw meat and transmitted to animals and subsequently to their owners or others in contact with the animal or their stool.[8]

20–25% of poultry carcasses intended for human consumption test positive for *Salmonella* organisms, the raw meat used for feeding dogs is even more frequently contaminated. Most raw poultry is also contaminated with *Campylobacter* species, primarily *Campylobacter jejuni*, food borne infection is highly probable for dogs fed raw chicken.[7]

Shiga toxic *Escherichia coli* strains are routinely isolated from fresh ground hamburger. *Escherichia coli* 0157:H7 has been identified in dog feces and would pose a hazard for environmental contanimation.[7]

Yersinia enterocolitica can frequently be isolated from raw meat, especially pork. As much as 89% of the commercially available raw pork may be contaminated with this organism.[7]

Numerous food-borne parasitic infections can also affect dogs and cats. Feeding raw fish can result in infection with a variety of organisms including *Diphyllobothrium latum,* the fish tapeworm; *Opisthorchis tenuicollis,* a trematode that infects the bile duct, pancreatic ducts and small intestines; *Dioclophyme renale,* the giant kidney worm; and *Nanophyetus salmincola,* the vector for *Neorickettsia helminthoeca,* the agent responsible for salmon poisoning in dogs.[7]

Dogs routinely fed raw meat are commonly infected with the protozoan *Sarcocystis* spp., and infected dogs may excrete sporocysts in their feces and contaminate the environment. Dogs can become infected with *Toxocara canis* and with the raccoon ascarid, *Baylisascaris proconis* as a result of eating raw meat. Infected dogs can develop enteritis and shed infective eggs into the environment. In humans these two parasites cause visceral larval migrans. Dogs are also susceptible to infection with *Trichenella spiralis* whose larvae is found encysted in meat. Undercooked or raw pork is occasionally contaminated with this parasite.[7]

Raw Food Diets Improve the Health of the Pets

The primary claim from raw food proponents is that this diet improves the health of their pets. While this is fairly nebulous and hard to prove, very few medical conditions can be directly traced back to nutrition other than specific nutrient excesses or deficiencies.

On average a wolf in the wild only survives to 8 years old, wolves in captivity can survive up to 16 years. Most deaths in the wild are attributed to predation, disease and starvation. As Darwin showed us, life in the wild is survival of the fittest. An animal with many of the diseases we treat for commonly in small animal medicine would not survive in the wild. That, to our pets would be the benefit of domestication. Until fairly recently, we did not have the medical knowledge to treat these conditions either, but as human medicine progresses, so does veterinary medicine.

It would be presumptuous to think that the conditions that we see and treat our cats and dogs for do not exist in the wild, and that this is solely due to the diet they consume. Furthermore, what would be the hunting ability of many of our current breeds? Could a Persian administer a cervical bite to a mouse, or is their breeding induced malocclusion too severe to do this? What are the chances that a Yorkie would be able to catch and kill anything to eat, and considering the variety of foreign objects that a Labrador eats, would it be able to find the right food to kill and eat without developing a GI foreign body that results in its death?

Myth: Raw Food Diets Improve Dental Health

There is significant concern among veterinarians that consumption of raw bones can lead to oral and dental trauma, as well as esophageal and GI obstructive foreign bodies.[8] When compared to cooked bones, raw bones have a lesser potential of splintering and causing tooth fractures, but there is still the strong possibility of sharp bone fragments being produced that can cause injury at any point along the GI tract from the mouth to the colon.[8] Grinding of bones included in the raw diets has been suggested as a way to decreased the incidence of GI trauma, but the bioavailability of the calcium from these sources is still unknown.[8] Bones can also pose a significant risk of bacterial contamination, especially is they are allowed to remain at room temperature for extended periods of time.

Myth: Uncooked Food Is More Easily Digested Because It Contains Enzymes that Cooking Destroys

Some nutrients are destroyed by heat, but not all heat-sensitive nutrients are eliminated during cooking. This is dependent on what the nutrient content of the food was initially and how the food is processed, stored and cooked.[2]

Heat can also affect proteins. Proteins can be "denatured." Their physical and chemical properties can be changed or altered. This happens with egg whites when they are cooked: the albumin becomes denatured and easier for the body to digest. Some proteins in meat also exist as enzymes; proponents of raw food diets contend that these enzymes become inactive when the meat is cooked. These proteins would also become inactive in the stomach when they meet up with the digestive enzymes. There are also other enzymes that are resistant to digestion (digestive enzymes) and may or may not be affected by stomach acid or heat from cooking. For the enzymes that are affected by heat, there is little evidence to suggest that they are more beneficial to animals that eat them raw.[2]

Due to the cellulose layer found in all plant-based compounds, digestion of these nutrients is reduced until the cellulose layer is broken down allowing the digestive enzymes assess to the cell contents. This can be accomplished either through chewing, grinding of the food or cooking. As anyone who has watched a dog or cat eat or cleaned up vomited food, there is little grinding of their food stuffs before it enters the stomach for continued digestion.

Plant-based materials are the primary source of carbohydrates for the body; these carbohydrates in turn are used for glucose production. If insufficient carbohydrates are available for energy, the body can also use glucogenic amino acids or glycerol from fats. If adequate dietary carbohydrates are not available, amino acids will be directed away from muscle growth, fetal growth and milk production to be used for glucose production.[4]

As carbohydrates are heated or cooked with water the starch contained within the cells undergoes a process called gelatinization. The greater the degree of gelatinization that occurs in the starch with cooking, the greater the digestibility for the food. The central nervous system and the red blood cells require glucose for their energy needs, and they will not use alternate fuel sources such as ketones unless absolutely necessary. Glucose consumed in excess of energy needs can be stored as glycogen. After glycogen stores are filled, any extra carbohydrates are converted into long-chain fatty acids and stored as fat.[4]

Since feeding trials have not been done on the majority of raw food diets, their nutrient content, digestibility and supplementation levels are for the most part unknown. By using raw meats, clients are leaving their pets and themselves open to bacterial and parasitic infection from possibly contaminated meats. And there is also no guarantee of improved health.

What other options are available to client in feeding their pets if they do not want to feed foods with preservatives, fillers, gluten or processing? There are numerous commercial diets available that provide similar nutrient profiles to that seen with raw food diets or that do not contain grain, preservatives or offer natural ingredients.[8] If the owner is determined to feed a homemade diet, a cooked formula designed by a trained veterinary nutritionist would provide an excellent option, and ensure that adequate nutritional needs are being met.[8]

First and foremost, do not ostracize these clients; most people opting to feed a raw food diet are conscientious owners looking to do the best thing for their pets. They unfortunately do not have a veterinary nutritionist in their kitchens. Most importantly, try to get them to cook the food being fed to their pet. This will at least address the bacterial and parasitic problems.

Find out what they don't like about commercially available diets. If they are misinformed on any issues gently guide them in the right direction. If clients insist on continuing to feed raw food diets, or homemade cooked diets, recommend 2–4 yearly visits for complete physical exams and blood screens to detect any problems before they become severe. These screenings and exams should include a complete serum biochemistry profile including T4 levels CBC with differential and complete urinalysis.

References

1 Derr M (2004) *DNA identifies dog breeds with 99% accuracy. New York Times News Service*, May 20.
2 Sacks B (2013) Agriculture and parting from wolves shaped dog evolution. VetLearn, 2/22/2013. https://www.vetlearn.com/_preview?_cms.fe.previewId=4c1c53d0-7529-11e2-8da9-005056ad4736 (accessed 3/15/13).
3 Bisno J (1997) Cats in Ancient Egypt. *Natural History Museum of Los Angeles County*, May 10. www.lam.mus.ca.us/cats
4 Roudebush P, Dzanis DA, Debraekeleer J, Brown RG (2000) Pet food labels. In MS Hand, CD Thatcher, RL Remillard *et al.* (eds), *Small Animal Clinical Nutrition* (4th edn), pp. 147–50, Marceline, MO: Walsworth Publishing.
5 Freeman LM, Michel KE (2001) Evaluation of raw food diets for dogs. *JAVMA* **218** (**5**): 705–9.
6 Stiver SL, Frazier KS, Mauel MJ (2003) Septicemic Salmonellosis in two cats fed a raw meat diet. *JAAHA* **39**(**6**): 538–42.
7 LeJeune JT, Hancock DD (2001) Public health concerns associated with feeding raw meat diets to dogs. *JAVMA* **219**(**9**): 1222–4.
8 Delaney S, Fascetti A (2012) Commercial and home-prepared diets. In S Delaney, A Fascetti (eds), *Applied Veterinary Clinical Nutrition*, pp. 104–5, Ames, IA: Wiley-Blackwell.

16 Additives and Pet Food Preservatives

Introduction

Preservatives are added to foods to help prevent microbial growth and oxidative damage to a food or food product. They also function to retard spoilage or help maintain certain desired qualities in foods such as softness or crunchiness.[1-4] Additives on the other hand can be used to make the food more appealing to the consumer by the use of various colors, flavor enhancers either artificial or natural that can make the food more palatable to the animal, texture enhancers and nutrient additives used to fortify or maintain the nutritional quality of foods.[4] In general, additives other than vitamins and minerals are found in the smallest amounts in moist foods, and in the largest quantities in dry foods, semi-moist foods, treats and snacks.[3]

Antimicrobial agents are designed to prevent microbial growth in or on pet foods.[4] Colors are used to increase the eye appeal to the consumer and offer little to the pet as they are not able to differentiate the colors that are used.

Food manufacturers are responsible for ensuring that their foods remain free from bacterial contamination and harmful toxins and are protected from nutrient loss during storage.[1] The FDA is concerned with additives and their safety in foods. A manufacturer must be able to ensure that the additives is effective, is detectable and measurable in the final product, and is safe.[4]

Safety is defined as not causing cancer, birth defects or other injury when consumed in large quantities to animals under controlled conditions. Many substances are exempted from FDA compliance because they are Generally Recognized as Safe (GRAS). This designation is based either on their extensive, long-term use in foods or on current scientific evidence.[4] Several

Table 16.1 Methods of preservation[1]

Dry foods	Low moisture content helps to inhibit growth of most organisms
Moist foods	Heat sterilization and anaerobic environment kill all microbes
Semimoist foods	Low pH and humectants bind water in the food, making it unavailable to bacteria and fungi
Frozen foods	Protected by storage conditions and low temperatures
Irradiated foods	Sterilized by radiation

hundred substances are on the GRAS list, and include such substances as sugar, salt, caffeine and many spices (Table 16.1).[4]

Antioxidants

An antioxidant is any substance that when added to a food significantly delays or prevents oxidation of that food product.[5] Foods that have no added antioxidant preservatives at the time of processing may contain ingredients such as animal fat, fish meal and fat-soluble vitamins that are preserved with antioxidants.[6]

The primary nutrients that require protection during storage are fats in form of vegetable oils or animal fats and the fat-soluble vitamins A, D, E and K.[1] It takes as little as 0.05% of the fat to react with oxygen to produce rancidity.[6] Oxidation of fats results in loss of calorie content and formation of toxic forms of peroxides that can be harmful to health.[1] Antioxidants do not reverse the effect of oxidation once it has started, but they retard the oxidative process and prevent further destruction of fats.

Nutrition and Disease Management for Veterinary Technicians and Nurses, Second Edition. Ann Wortinger, Kara M. Burns
© 2015 John Wiley & Sons, Inc. Published 2015 by John Wiley & Sons, Inc.
Companion Website: www.wiley.com/go/wortinger/nutrition

Therefore, to be fully effective, they must be included in the diet when it is initially mixed and processed.[6] Ingestion of inadequately preserved rancid fats may be more harmful to the health of the pet than any adverse effects of the preservatives.[6]

Naturally Derived Antioxidants

Naturally derived antioxidants are commonly found in certain grains, vegetable oils and some herbs and spices.[1] These antioxidants have been processed to make them more available for use.[1] There are no naturally derived antioxidants that do not undergo extensive processing to make them usable.

Mixed tocopherols, incorrectly called vitamin E, are obtained primarily from distilling soybean oil residue. Further processing separates out α (alpha), λ (delta), and δ (gamma) fractions. Alpha-tocopherol, accurately called vitamin E, is the most biologically active form but provides little protection against oxidation in foods. Delta and gamma tocopherols have lower biologic activity than alpha-tocopherol but are more effective as antioxidants.[1] Mixed tocopherols using both alpha and delta-tocopherols are the most effective naturally derived antioxidants and show the greatest efficacy in protecting fats in pet foods.[1] Because tocopherols rapidly decompose as they protect fats from oxidation, the shelf-life of foods preserved with tocopherols alone is shorter than that of foods stabilized with a mix of several different antioxidants.[1]

Ascorbic acid, more commonly called vitamin C, functions as an antioxidant by scavenging oxygen; however, it is water soluble and not easily mixed with the fat found in foods. It does work synergistically with other antioxidants such as the mixed tocopherols, buylated hydroxytoluene (BHT) and is included in foods for this reason.[1]

Ascorbyl palmitate is similar in structure to ascorbic acid but is not normally found in nature. It undergoes hydrolysis to form ascorbic acid and the fatty acid palmitic acid, both of which are found in nature. Citric acid is often used in combination with other naturally derived antioxidants.[1]

Dried leaves from the shrub *Rosemarius officinalis* (common rosemary) are used to make a refined extract (rosemaric acid/rosemarequinone). The extract is used to avoid the influence of the herb on the taste and odor of the food.[1,2] This extract is effective in high-fat diets and has been shown to enhance the antioxidant efficiency when included in combination with mixed-tocopherols, ascorbic acid and citric acid.[1]

Effective antioxidants must have good carry-through. This is the retention of antioxidant functions after being subjected to the high heat, pressure and moisture of pet food processing.[1] Because most naturally derived antioxidants have poor carry-through, excessive amounts must be included to compensate for the high losses that occur during processing.[1] Since naturally derived preservatives tend to be significantly more expensive than synthetic ones, it is difficult to achieve necessary levels of protection using only naturally derived products without production becoming cost prohibitive.[1]

Lecithin, modified starches, monoglycerides and diglycerides are naturally derived compounds that act as emulsifying agents, preventing separation of fats from other dietary components and allowing greater contact between antioxidants and fats.[1]

Potassium sorbate is used to prevent the formation of yeast and molds in foods. Glycerol and certain other sugars are used as humectants to keep foods soft and moist.[1]

Synthetic Antioxidants

Synthetic antioxidants are made in laboratories and not from naturally derived products. The Food and Drug Administration (FDA) has approved butylated hydroxyanisole (BHA) and butylated hydroxytoluene (BHT) for use in both human and animal foods. They have a synergistic antioxidant effect when used together and exhibit good carry-through and increased efficiency compared with naturally derived antioxidants in protecting animal fats, but have slightly lower efficacy in protecting vegetable oils.[1]

Tertiary butylhydroquinine (TBHQ) is an effective antioxidant for most fats and is approved for human and animal use in the United States. However, TBHQ has not been approved for use in Canada, Japan or the European Union, so it is not used in foods for the international market.[1]

Ethoxyquin is approved for use in human and animal foods and has been in use for over 30 years.[1,7] Its mechanism of action is similar to those of BHA and BHT in that it reduces oxidative damage of polyunsaturated fatty acids, vitamins A and E, and other fat-soluble substances by stopping free radical formation.[7] Ethoxyquin is more efficient that either BHA or BHT in protecting oils with high levels of polyunsaturated fatty acids such as linoleic, alpha-linolenic and arachidonic acids. This allows for lower levels of antioxidants to be added to the final product.[1]

Ethoxyquin has a toxicity rating of 3 and is considered to be moderately toxic. This rating is slightly higher than that for tetracycline or penicillin and is lower than that for aspirin or caffeine.[6] Ethoxyquin is readily absorbed, metabolized and excreted in the urine and feces. Residual levels are found in the liver, gastrointestinal tract and adipose tissue.[6] Before ethoxyquin gained FDA approval, the manufacturer (Monsanto, St Louis MO) conducted a 1-year chronic toxicity study in dogs in which "no observable effect level" was determined to be 3 mg/kg administered on a 5 day/week schedule.[7] Mild changes were seen histopathologically in the liver and kidneys at much higher doses (10 mg/kg), with more pronounced signs of toxicity observed at 50 and 100 mg/kg.[7] The Center for Veterinary Medicine requested as of July 31, 1997, that manufacturers voluntarily lower the maximum level of ethoxyquin in complete dog food to 75 parts per million (ppm) from the allowed 150 ppm to further increase the margin of safety for lactating females and puppies.[8]

Ethoxyquin and other synthetic preservatives have been blamed for widespread infertility, neonatal illness and death, skin and coat problems, immune disorders, dysfunction of the thyroid, liver and pancreas and behavioral problems.[2,3,7] Reports of adverse reactions have been almost exclusively in dogs, the majority of these being purebred or inbred ones.[3,7] To date, the FDA has found no scientific or medical evidence that ethoxyquin used at approved levels is injurious to human or animal health.[2] After gaining FDA approval for ethoxyquin, Monsanto conducted an additional study of a multigenerational group of dogs over a 5-year period using foods with two times the approved level of ethoxyquin at that time (i.e. 300 ppm).[7] No adverse effects, especially those noted by breeders, were found in these dogs (Table 16.2).

Antimicrobials

Bacteria can affect foods in two ways; one way is relatively harmless – causing the food to lose flavor and

Table 16.2 Characteristics of some antioxidants[1]

Antioxidant	Carry-through	Effectiveness
Naturally derived		
Mixed tocopherols	Poor	Low
Ascorbic acid	Poor	Low
Ascorbyl palmitate	Poor	Low
Synthetic		
Butylated hydroxyanisole	Good	High
Butylated hydrosytoluene	Good	High
Tertiary butylhydroquine	Good	High
Ethoxyquin	Excellent	High

attractiveness. The other way bacteria can affect food is by causing food borne illnesses such as food poisoning.[4]

The most widely used antimicrobials found are ordinary salt and sugar. Salt has been used throughout history to preserve meat and fish, sugar serves the same purpose in semi-moist foods.[4] Both of these products work by capturing water and making it unavailable to the bacteria.

Nitrites are also added to foods to preserve color, to enhance flavor by inhibiting rancidity of fats and to protect against bacterial growth.[4] Because of the concerns over nitrosamine formation when nitrites are heated, minimal amounts are used in food products to achieve the desired results.[4]

Food-borne infections can be caused by microorganisms such as *Escherichia coli* and species of *Salmonella, Neorickettsia, Vibrio, Yersinia* and *Campylobacter*. Illness can also be caused by ingestion of the toxins produced by such microorganisms as *Clostridium botulinum, Bacillus cereus, Staphylococcus aureus* and various mycotoxins.[2] Properly preserved foods kill most microorganisms by cooking/sterilization and prevent the proper conditions for growth in the final product. While cooking and sterilization can effectively kill bacteria contaminating a food, they have no effect on the toxins potentially produced by these bacteria.

Colors

Only a few artificial colors remain on the FDA's approved list of additives for pet foods. Colors derived from natural sources must also meet the same standards of purity and safety as the synthetic colors do.[4] Food color additives are common in pet foods, and are used primarily for the consumers benefit.[9]

Artificial Flavors and Flavor Enhancers

Natural and artificial flavors as well as flavor enhancers are the largest single group of food additives.[4] In people, taste is confined to four basic groups: sweet, salty, bitter and acidic. Dogs and cats can also taste several amino acids that taste only weakly bitter or acidic to people.[5] These amino acids contribute to the meaty and savory aromas in pet foods.

Dogs are able to taste and demonstrate a preference for simple sugars, while cats show little interest in sweet flavors.[5] Foods acidified with phosphoric or citric acid seem to appeal to cats, though this is decreased in moist cat foods. Dogs do not seem to appreciate any significant changes in pH of their foods.[5]

Texture and Mouth Feel

Mouth feel of a particular food has a tremendous effect on food preferences for both dogs and cats.[5] The size and shape of expanded kibbles can be important in food acceptance. Dogs prefer larger kibbles over smaller kibbles of the same formula. Cats prefer one specific shape to others in identical formulas, and may develop strong preferences for mouth feel, and can be found with a pile of sorted out shapes sitting next to their food dishes.[5]

In moist diets, gums can be added to thicken sauces and help form gels that may appeal to certain animals.[4] Neither cats nor dogs like sticky foods.[5]

Smell

We know that dogs and cats have highly developed senses of smell, when compared to people. Despite this fact, foods must also provide taste for animals to maintain a sustained interest in a particular diet.[5] The smell of moist foods can be intensified by heating to slightly below body temperature. This can be used to interest an animal in a particular food, but obviously cannot be relied on to maintain interest (Table 16.3).

Table 16.3 Common food additives[4,5]

Antioxidant – natural derived	Mixed tocopherols (vitamin E)
	Ascorbic acid (vitamin C)
	Ascorbyl palmitate
	Citric acid
	Rosemary extract
Antioxidant – synthetic	BHA
	BHT
	TBHQ
	Ethoxyquin
Antimicrobial	Sugar
	Salt
	Nitrite
	Potassium sorbate
	Glycerol
	Sterilization
Texture enhancer	Guar gum
	Lecithin
Artificial color	GRAS colors
	Sodium nitrite
Flavor enhancer	Phosphoric acid
	Citric acid

Need for Additives

The need for antioxidants in pet foods is obvious. Therefore, questions about the safety of preservatives need to be balanced against the needs of the pets. Canned or frozen foods have the lowest levels of antioxidants because they are preserved by either heat or cold – not antioxidants. Some pet food manufacturers produce dry foods that are preserved with naturally derived antioxidants, although they may contain small amounts of synthetic antioxidants in the vitamin premix. When buying a food preserved with only naturally derived antioxidants, look for a "best if used by" date, and use the food within this time frame. If no date is included on the package label, contact the manufacturer for information on when the product was manufactured and its shelf-life.

The FDA requires that preservatives in quantities high enough to affect the final product must be listed on food labels. If the preservative is present in trivial amounts or no longer serves a technical or functional effect, it may be exempt from inclusion on the label.[10] This applies to premixes or vitamin additives in foods. Ethoxyquin is an exception to this regulation; the FDA Center for

Veterinary Medicine has stated that ethoxyquin should be declared on labeling regardless of the source or final level in the food.[10]

Manufacturers of premium pet foods conduct feeding trials on their products to detect deficiencies or other problems before foods are released for sale. Check the labels on the foods to see whether feeding trials have been done. Manufacturers must state how they have met AAFCO standards. The label should also list all the ingredients from largest amount to smallest.

Color, taste and texture will help maintain an interest in a specific food. Preservatives can help to maintain these factors, ensuring that the animal will continue to consume a particular food and not become ill in the process.

References

1 Case LP, Carey DP, Hirakawa DA, Daristotle L (2000) Additives and preservatives. In *Canine and Feline Nutrition* (2nd edn), pp. 180–5, St Louis, MO: Mosby.

2 Hand MS, Thatcher CD, Remillard RL, Roudebush P (2000) Preservatives, antioxidants and contaminants. Food borne illness. In MS Hand, CD Thatcher, RL Remillard *et al.* (eds), *Small Animal Clinical Nutrition* (4th edn), pp. 166–7, Marceline, MO: Walsworth Publishing.

3 Roudebush P (1993) Food additives. *JAMA* **203**: 1667–70.

4 Whitney E, Rolfes SR (2008) Consumer concerns about food and water. In *Understanding Nutrition* (11th edn), pp. 682–5, Belmont, CA: Thomson Wadsworth.

5 Zicker SC, Wedekind KJ (2010) In MS Hand, CD Thatcher, RL Remillard *et al.* (eds), *Small Animal Clinical Nutrition* (5th edn), pp. 149–55, Marceline, MO: Walsworth Publishing.

6 Dodds WJ, Donoghue S (1994) Interactions of clinical nutrition with genetics. In JM Wills, KW Simpson (eds), *Waltham Book of Clinical Nutrition in the Dog and Cat*, pp. 114–15, Tarrytown, NY: Pergamon.

7 Dzanis D (1991) Safety of ethoxyquin in dog foods. *Journal of Nutrition* **121**: S163–S164.

8 FDA Center for Veterinary Medicine: Press release. Available at: http://www.fda.gov/animalveterinary/resourcesforyou/ucm047113.htm (updated March 2010; accessed 12-4-14).

9 Crane SC, Cowell CS, Stout NP, *et al.* (2010) Commercial pet foods. In MS Hand, CD Thatcher, RL Remillard *et al.* (eds), *Small Animal Clinical Nutrition* (5th edn), p. 169, Marceline, MO: Walsworth Publishing.

10 Dzanis D (2001) Personal communication to Dr Katherine Michel (University of Pennsylvania) regarding FDA labeling requirements for antioxidants, March 21.

17   Homemade Diets

Introduction

Counseling clients on feeding is one of the most important client education services that the veterinary team can offer.[1] Even though the majority of pet owners in the United States enjoy the convenience, economy and reliability of commercially produced diet, some owners still prefer to prepare homemade diets for their pets.[2] The vast majority of dogs and cats in the United States are fed table food at some point in their lives.[3] Many pets learn of the availability of table scraps after a family meal, and are very determined to share in the leftovers. As long as the supplementation of scraps does not exceed 10% of the caloric intake, this is not usually a problem as long as the food is not toxic (i.e. onions, chocolate, grapes).[3]

The reasons that clients choose to feed a home prepared diet vary greatly, some of the more common reasons are:

- They adopt a traditional approach being among a minority of owners not using commercially prepared food.
- Induced food preference in pets by exposure to home-cooked food from kitten or puppyhood.
- Anthropomorphism: giving human food preferences to pets.
- Finicky eaters will "hold out" for tasty home-cooked treats.
- Veterinarian recommended home-prepared "elimination diets" may work better in some food-related disease, such as skin problems.
- Poor owner perception of commercially prepared foods as "unwholesome" or as unappetizing.
- Wanting to feed "what nature intended."
- Veterinary therapeutic diets may lack palatability or acceptability particularly in advanced illness.
- Wanting to be involved in the care of their pet especially older or ill animals.

- Wish to use ingredients that are fresh, wild grown, organic or natural.
- Concerned that the ingredient list is an indecipherable list of chemicals.
- They hope to construct a nutritional profile for dietary management of a disease for which no commercial food is available.
- They wish to provide food variety as a defense against malnutrition, or because of the popular idea that animals need variety.
- They wish to lower feeding costs through the use of significant quantities of table foods and leftovers.
- They wish to feed a pet according to human nutritional guidelines such as low fat or low cholesterol.
- They want to feed their pet according to their diet preferences such as vegetarian/vegan diets.[4,5]

While many pet owners consulted their veterinary team for nutrition information regarding their pet, as many as 17% of owners cited the internet as their primary source of information.[6] The concerning part of this number is the vast amount of misinformation regarding dog and cat nutrition found on the internet. Feeding unbalanced, homemade diets can lead to any number of medical complications such as osteodystrophy, osteopenia, nutritional secondary hyperparathyroidism, and pansteatitis.[6] Even when recommended by the veterinarian, as many as 90% of the homemade diets were not balanced, and were not nutritionally adequate to support the requirements for adult maintenance.[6] The most common types of imbalances seen include deficiencies of calcium, improper calcium/phosphorus rations, deficiencies of vitamins A and E, and deficiencies of potassium, copper and zinc levels.[6] When compared to AAFCO requirements for specific life stage nutrition, 55% of the veterinary recommended diets found in commonly used books had inadequate protein, with all diets being deficient in the amino acid taurine, 64% had inadequate vitamin levels, and 86% were deficient in minerals.[7]

Nutrition and Disease Management for Veterinary Technicians and Nurses, Second Edition. Ann Wortinger, Kara M. Burns
© 2015 John Wiley & Sons, Inc. Published 2015 by John Wiley & Sons, Inc.
Companion Website: www.wiley.com/go/wortinger/nutrition

Why homemade?

When clients elect to feed homemade diets, it is important to understand their reasons and motivations. In many cases it is possible to address their concerns and to recommend an appropriate commercial diet that will meet everyone's needs.[5] In those instances where a client is insistent about cooking for their pet, it is always better to provide them with a well designed homemade recipe, rather than allowing them to prepare food according to their own or a breeder's well-intentioned formulation that may have significant nutrient excesses and deficiencies.[5]

Any ingredient used in homemade diets should be fit for human consumption and preferably cooked. The quality of the nutrients depends on the source and digestibility of the ingredients.[4] One of the problems with preparing homemade diets is that many of the recipes that are available have not been adequately tested for nutrient content and availability.[2] Poor feeding management rather than faulty diets are believed to be responsible for many nutritional problems.[1] Even if a balanced diet is offered, clients will usually "adjust" the ingredients to their likes, very likely upsetting any balance that the diet did have, or will supplement with treats or snacks in excess of 10% of the caloric requirements. This practice is commonly referred to as "diet drift."[3,7]

It should be noted that the most prevalent form of malnutrition that is seen in dogs and cats today is obesity. This would be even more likely to occur when an animal is fed a homemade, highly palatable diet with unknown nutrient density (i.e. caloric concentration).

Food Preparation

Any food fed to a pet needs to be properly cooked before feeding. Cooking improves digestibility and kills bacteria and parasites that might cause disease.[8] However, cooking does not eliminate the problem caused by endotoxins released from dead bacteria such as *E.coli* and *Clostridium botulinum*.[8] These endotoxins can be found in meats previously contaminated by bacteria.[8] Nothing can be done to decontaminate a food containing endotoxins.[8] Antibiotics are also ineffective in treating a pet who has ingested these endotoxins as they are not bacteria themselves, though there are antitoxins available for some of these endotoxins but not all, nor are they commonly found in most veterinary practices.

When foods are prepared at home, safe food handling and preparation methods determine whether or not the final diet will be safe for consumption.[8] Safe handling of food by owners begins at the store and continues in the home. Safe handling prevents or minimizes hazards associated with biological (bacteria), chemical (cleaning agents) and physical (equipment) causes.[8]

According to the Centers for Disease Control (CDC) hand washing is the single most important means of preventing the spread of infection from bacteria, pathogens and viruses causing disease and food-borne illnesses.[8] Food preparation most importantly includes hand washing done before and after handling of each ingredient in the diet.[8] In addition to hand washing, counters, equipment, utensils and cutting boards should be sanitized with a dilute bleach solution.[8] Frozen foods should never be thawed at room temperature, thawing should be done in the refrigerator, the microwave or a cold water bath.[8]

All ingredients used in the diet should always be cooked thoroughly. Freezing or rinsing with cold water is not an acceptable method for destroying bacteria.[8] Once a diet is cooked, it may be stored in the refrigerator and reheated later before serving.[8]

All diets should be prepared according to the specific recipe recommended, with no substitutions, additions or omissions being done by the client or veterinarian.

Ingredient Choices

Many owners choose their pets, diet ingredients based on their own preferences, product availability or affordability.[5] Other pets are fed a variety of leftovers such as fat trimmings, vegetable skins, crusts and condiments. These diets are rarely representative of the owner's diet and are not "complete and balanced" for the pet.[5] Diet drift is commonly encountered when a client starts to substitute ingredients either based on cost or a perception of change needed by the pet. Each ingredient in a diet is important and provides specific nutrients to the diet. Inappropriate substitutions can contribute to advancement of a disease process or change the palatability of the overall diet.[6,7] Feline foods designed by clients are often deficient in fat and energy density or may contain an unpalatable fat source such as vegetable oil.[3]

Owners may also choose the ingredients based on current human nutrition trends. These include grain-free, gluten free or vegetarian/vegan diets.[6] As we know, there are several differences between canine, feline and human nutrition as well as nutrient digestion and needs. Those clients who choose to feed their pet's vegetarian/vegan diets are at greatest risk of feeding an unbalance, inadequate diet. There are a number of commercially prepared canine vegetarian diets that are complete and balanced.[5] Clients should be strongly discouraged from feeding cats vegetarian/vegan diets, cats are strict carnivores and have specific nutrient requirements that are only found in meat-based food sources, such as the amino acid taurine and the essential fatty acid arachidonic acid. Without adequate supplementation (usually available from only meat-based products) cats fed vegetarian or vegan diets are at high risk for taurine, arginine, tryptophan, lysine, arachidonic acid and vitamin A deficiency. These deficiencies are life threatening and can lead to the death of the cat.[5]

Due to inconvenience, expense or failure to understand its importance, many clients eliminate the vitamin and mineral supplements in homemade diets. This would cause a recipe that was crudely balanced to become grossly imbalanced.[5] While vitamins and minerals do not contribute calories to the diet, they are the sole source of essential nutrients required for normal, daily function of the animal.

Assess the Recipe

If possible, offer the client a nutritionally adequate recipe rather than having them either make their own, or use one from a nonveterinary source. There are a number of sources for clients to have nutritional balanced homemade diets formulated to meet their pet's needs (Table 17.1).

Homemade formulation can be checked for nutritional adequacy and adjusted using the "quick check" guidelines below:[5]

- Do all five food groups appear in the recipe?
  - Carbohydrate/fiber source
  - Protein source, preferable animal origin
  - Fat source

Table 17.1 Sources of homemade diet recipes from veterinary nutritionists

- Custom pet diets and nutrition counseling
  Phone: (865) 577–0233 or (865) 235-4356
  www.petnutritioncounsulting.com
- Pet diet evaluations
  www.PetDiets.com
  www.Balanceit.com
  http://aavn.org/site/view/58440_NutritionResources.pml (accessed 3/22/13).

  - Mineral source, primarily calcium
  - Multivitamin and trace mineral source.
- Carbohydrate source cooked and present in higher or equal quantity than the protein source?
  - Feline carbohydrate: protein 1:1 to 2:1
  - Canine carbohydrate: protein 2:1 to 3:1.
- What is the type and quantity of the primary protein source?
  - Final food should contain 25–30% cooked meat for dogs and 35–50% cooked meat for cats. Skeletal muscle meat is preferred. Liver can be used once weekly. If feeding lacto-ovo vegetarian diets, eggs are the best protein source, if feeding a vegan diet, soybeans provide the next best protein source, but has an incomplete amino acid profile.[5] For cats, organ meats have higher taurine concentrations than do muscle meats. Taurine levels can also be affected by cooking, specifically boiling leaches out available taurine rendering it unavailable to the animal.[7] Raw food diets have also been shown to have decreased taurine availability when compared to commercial and cooked diets.[7]
- Is the primary protein source lean or fatty?
  - If using a "lean" meat, an additional fat should be added either of animal, vegetable or fish source
  - 2% of the total formula weight for dogs
  - 5% of the total formula weight for cats.
- Is a source of calcium and other minerals provided?
  - Absolute calcium deficiency is most common in homemade diets
  - Milk products usually contribute inadequate amounts of calcium to diet.
- Is a source of vitamins and other nutrients provided?
  - An adult over-the-counter supplement that contains no more than 200% of the recommended

daily allowances for humans usually works well for dog and cats.

- Give $1/2-1$ tablet per day, based on pet size.
- Cats should receive additional taurine supplementation, between 200 and 500 mg/day depending on the diets calculated taurine content.
- Iodized salt should be use to meet the iodine requirement.[5]

Selecting a Diet

There are software programs available to help you formulate a balanced diet from scratch, or you can contact a member of the American College of Veterinary Nutrition (ACVN) for food recommendations and many veterinary schools also offer help with homemade recipes. In addition there are many published recipes available, just critically evaluate the source and see if any testing has been done on the recipe. References 1, 4 and 5 contain a variety of recipes as well as acceptable substitutions. The sources listed in Table 17.2 can provide or development appropriate, balanced homemade recipes. There is usually a fee for this service.

Additional Instructions

Be sure to provide specific instructions for preparation, storage and feeding of homemade foods to the pet owners. As these diets do not contain preservatives and are high in moisture, they are more susceptible to bacterial and fungal contamination when left at room temperature for prolonged periods of time.[6] Food that is not immediately fed to the pet should be stored in an airtight container in the refrigerator for no more than a few days.[6] When the food has been stored in the refrigerator, it should be warmed to body temperature before feeding to increase palatability. If using a microwave, make sure the food is mixed well before feeding to prevent the development of hot spots in the food.[6] If desired, a small amount of water can be added to the food to either increase the water intake or improve the consistency of the food. Any food that is not consumed at that meal should be discarded and not saved for the next meal.[6]

Explain the importance of each ingredient as well as the proper proportions to be used. Foods should be

Table 17.2 Veterinary schools/hospitals offering nutritional support services

Angell Animal Medical Center
  Phone consultation (617) 522-7282
Michigan State University Nutrition Support Service
  http://cvm.msu.edu/hospital/services/nutrition-support-service-1
University of Missouri, College of Veterinary
Medicine, Veterinary Medical Teaching Hospital Nutrition Consultations
  www.vmth.missouri.edu/clin_nu.htm
Ohio State University
  Phone consultations (614) 292-1221 or (614) 292-3551
Tufts Cummings School of Veterinary Medicine. Nutritional
consultations for veterinarians
  Phone: (508) 839-5395 x 84696
  VetFax: (800) 829-5690
  http://www.tufts.edu/vet
University of California, Davis, School of Veterinary Medicine
  Veterinary phone consultations (530) 752-1387
University of Tennessee
  Phone consultations (865) 974-8387
VA-MD Regional College of Veterinary Medicine
  Phone consultations: (540) 231-4621
  Fax: (540) 231-1676
  http://vetmed.vt.edu/vth/nutrition.asp
  Email: vetnutrition@vt.edu
Gulf Coast Veterinary Specialists, Houston Tx
Dr Catherine Lenox, DVM, Dipl. ACVN
  Phone: (713) 693-1144
  Email: nutrition@gcvs.com
  http://aavn.org/site/view/58440_NutritionResources.pml
  (accessed 3/22/13).

checked daily for any changes in color or odor that may indicate spoilage or deterioration.[5]

Patient Assessment and Monitoring

Dogs and cats that are fed homemade diets should be brought in to the clinic for veterinary evaluations 2–3 times per year. The physical examination should include an assessment of body condition, body weight, and if indicated, CBC chemistry and urinalysis testing.[7] This will help to identify any problems with the diet before they become too big to fix.[5]

The purpose of these exams is to evaluated the effectiveness of a diet by noting the patient's body weight, body condition and activity level. Laboratory levels such as albumin, red blood cell number and size and hemoglobin concentration are gross estimations of the animal's nutritional status. More specifically, the skin and hair should be examined closely, and an ophthalmic evaluation looking at the lens and retina should be performed. Stool quality needs to be assessed also.[5]

The diet history should be updated at every visit to determine if any changes to the diet have been done by the owner, or need to be done by the veterinarian.[7] Often what appear to be simple substitutions on the client's part can result in significant changes in the nutrition distribution in the diet.[7] A list of Board-certified veterinary nutritionists can be located through the American College of Veterinary Nutrition (ACVN) at www.acvn.org.

References

1 Strombeck DA (1999) Introduction. In *Home-prepared Dog and Cat Diets, a Healthful Alternative*, pp. 3–19, Ames, IA: Iowa State Press.

2 Case LP, Carey DP, Hirakawa DA, Daristotle L (2000) Types of pet foods. In *Canine and Feline Nutrition* (2nd edn), p. 196, St Louis, MO: Mosby.

3 Remillard RL, Crane SW (2010) Making pet foods at home. In MS Hand, CD Thatcher, RL Remillard *et al.* (eds), *Small Animal Clinical Nutrition* (5th edn), pp. 207–19, Marceline, MO: Walsworth Publishing, Mark Morris Institute.

4 Kelly NC (1996) Food types and evaluation. In N Kelly, J Wills (eds), *Manual of Companion Animal Nutrition and Feeding*, pp. 38–41, Ames, IA: Iowa State Press.

5 Remillard RL, Paragon B-M, Crane SW, *et al.* (2000) Making pet foods at home In MS Hand, CD Thatcher, RL Remillard *et al.* (eds), *Small Animal Clinical Nutrition* (4th edn), pp. 163–79, Marceline, MO: Walsworth Publishing.

6 Schenck P (2010) Homemade diets. In *Home-prepared Dog and Cat Diets* (2nd edn), pp. 5–13, Ames, IA: Wiley-Blackwell.

7 Delaney S, Fascetti A (2012) Commercial and home-prepared diets. In S Delaney, A Fascetti (eds), *Applied Veterinary Clinical Nutrition*, pp. 98–105, Ames, IA: Wiley-Blackwell.

8 Strombeck DA (1999) Food safety and preparation. In *Home-prepared Dog and Cat Diets, A Healthful Alternative*, pp. 43–61, Ames, IA: Iowa State Press.

Feeding Management of Dogs and Cats

18 Feeding Regimens for Dogs and Cats

Introduction

To understand normal feeding behaviors in domestic dogs and cats you first need to understand where these behaviors developed from, and how they differ from those still found in their wild counterparts.

Feeding behaviors include searching, hunting and caching of prey, as well as postprandial grooming and sleeping.[1] An obvious difference between domestic dogs and cats and their wild ancestors is the amount of energy expended in obtaining a meal.[2] Wild ancestors of domestic dogs and cats expended considerable amounts of energy locating and capturing a meal, and their success was not guaranteed. They, for the most part, did not have a reliable and consistent source of food.[2] In an effort to maintain access to food, additional energy was expended in territorial behaviors.[1] Our domestic pets are usually provided with a consistent source of nutritious and palatable foods, and expend only the effort required for begging to obtain this.[2]

Dogs

Wolves, our modern day dogs' wild ancestor, hunt in packs, using cooperative behavior to prey on large animals that otherwise would be unavailable to an animal hunting on its own.[2] This cooperative behavior allows for larger amounts of food to be obtained, but also dictates the type of feeding behavior seen, that of gorging themselves immediately after a kill and then not eating for extended periods of time.[2] Food is consumed rapidly, and in a predetermined order within the pack. Any food that is left over is hoarded or cached for consumption later, when food is not so readily available.[2]

These gorging and hoarding behaviors can be seen in some of our domestic dogs today. This can lead to choking and swallowing of large amounts of air during eating (aerophagia).[2] Dogs may also eat more rapidly, and consume more food if fed in a group situation rather than alone.[3] Changing the feeding situation can help to curb the gorging behavior if this is occurring in a pack situation, removing the dog from the pack and feeding them by themselves may decrease the desire to gorge and overeat. If the dog is consuming the food too quickly, sometimes changing the type of food being fed can help as well as changing how that food is offered. It is much easier to eat large amounts of canned food out of a bowl, than it is to eat large amounts of dry food fed off of a flat tray.[2] There are also special bowls that have a raised center that makes the dog work harder to obtain individual kibbles from around the side. This decreases the ability to consume large amounts of food in a short period of time (Figure 18.1).

Conversely, the presence of another dog may stimulate the appetite of a poor eater so they consume more food than if fed alone.[2] Dominance may also play a part

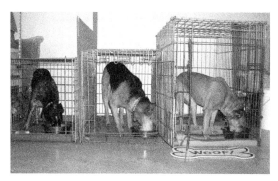

Figure 18.1 Dogs being group fed using the portion controlled method. (Courtesy Heidi Reuss-Lamky LVT, VTS (Anesthesia, Surgery).)

Nutrition and Disease Management for Veterinary Technicians and Nurses, Second Edition. Ann Wortinger, Kara M. Burns
© 2015 John Wiley & Sons, Inc. Published 2015 by John Wiley & Sons, Inc.
Companion Website: www.wiley.com/go/wortinger/nutrition

on the amount of food consumed within a group, with the dominate dog eating more than their share and the subordinate dog not getting enough food to eat. Separating the dogs at meal time may help, as well as designating feeding location or bowls for each dog.[2]

Domestic dogs still hoard choice food items, as can be seen with buried bones in the yard and treats hidden in furniture and under beds.[2] Unlike their wild ancestors, domestic dogs often forget about these hidden items, leading to quite a collection in various places within the house and yard.[3]

If we look to the wolf for our domestic dogs feeding schedule, large meals fed infrequently would seem to be the natural way to feed.[2] However, when domestic dogs are given free-choice access to food, they tend to eat small meals frequently throughout the day.[1,2] This pattern is similar to that seen with cats, with the exception that dogs tend to only eat during the day.[2] Our domestic dogs can readily adapt to a number of feeding regimes, the primary ones being portion-controlled feeding, time-controlled-feeding and free-choice or ad libitum feeding.[2]

It has been shown that dogs can learn food preferences for novel flavors from other dogs in the house.[4] They also learn to follow human pointing gestures during feeding, and have been known to select a smaller portion of a food over another larger portion at the pointing direction of the owner.[4] Given that the vast majority of dogs live in multi-dog households, the presence of another dog during feeding and directions from the owner can have a significant influence on individual eating behaviors.

Cats

As much as domestic cats look like their wild ancestors the tiger and lion, they are actually descendant from the much smaller African wildcat, *Felis libyca*. This distinction is important because the larger cats eat larger prey less frequently, while the smaller African wildcat consumes multiple small meals throughout the day. The primary prey for *F. libyca* is small rodents that are similar in size to our common field mouse.[4] This leads to a more ad libitum type of feeding schedule for the smaller cats.[1] There is no convincing evidence that the smaller cats engage in cooperative hunting behaviors, even when living in large groups (Figure 18.2).[1]

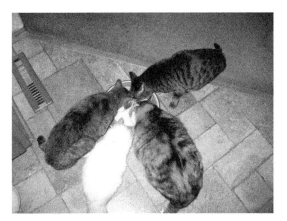

Figure 18.2 Cats being group fed using ad lib feeding.

Because these cats hunt alone and consume small meals frequently, they tend to consume their meals slowly and are uninhibited by the presence of other animals.[2,3] This same type of behavior can readily be seen with our own domestic cats. If fed free choice, they will nibble at their food throughout the day and night. It is not unusual for a cat to eat between 9 and 16 meals per day, with each meal having a calorie content of about 23 kcal. The average caloric value of a typical field mouse is ~30 kcal/animal.[4] If a 10 lb cat needs ~235 kcal/day, which would be ~8 mice/day to meet their caloric requirements. That is assuming that the mice are all adults and in good nutritional status prior to being caught and eaten.

Like the dog, the cat is able to adapt to a number of different feeding regimes, though time-controlled feeding with cats doesn't work as well as with dogs due to their nibbling behavior and desire for small meals frequently.[2] The method of feeding used is often dependent on the owner's preference rather than the ingrained preference of an individual species.[3]

What to Feed

As listed in previous chapters the food choices for owners include dry, semi-moist, moist and homemade diets. Most owners prefer the convenience, cost-effectiveness and reliability of feeding commercial foods. If the choice is made to feed a homemade diet, care must be exercised to ensure that the diet is complete and balanced, and that all ingredients and the final product are safe to consume, provide all the essential nutrients, and are stored properly.[2] Surveys have shown that more than 90% of owners feed commercial foods to their pets.[2]

One of the most important considerations when deciding what is feed is the life stage of the pet.[2] Nutrient and energy needs will differ according to an animal's age, activity level, reproductive status and health.[2] Specific diets have been developed by commercial pet food manufacturers to address the needs of pets during different ages, physiologic states and disease conditions.[2,4]

When evaluating a diet to be fed, some other important considerations for all life stages are:

- Does the food provide all the essential nutrients in adequate amounts and proper balance to meet the lifestyle and life stage needs?
- Does the food supply sufficient energy to maintain ideal body condition and weight as well as support optimal tissue growth?
- Is the food palatable enough to ensure that the animal will willingly consume it over an extended period when fed as the primary diet?
- Does extended use support proper gastrointestinal function and consistently results in the production of regular, firm, well formed stools?
- With extended use is the animal subjectively healthy with good coat quality, healthy skin condition, proper body physique and muscle tone and does it have sufficient energy to function as desired?[2]

While many of these qualities are subjective and can only be assessed over an extended period of time, some of these can be found in the product reference guides supplied by the pet food manufacturers. Have feeding trials been done on this food, what is the life stage rating, what is the metabolizable energy of the diet and what is the nutrient density of the diet? Many clients do not connect the quality of the diet being fed to their pet to the condition of the skin and coat, the stool quality or the lack of endurance when exercising.

If pet owners are reluctant to follow your dietary recommendations, use the list from above to compare the diet they are currently feeding with what you are recommending. Point out the significance of each point, and how the current food compares to the desired food. Referencing a Pet Food Library that you have prepared can help you with having copies of individual food labels available as well as additional nutritional information from the manufacturer.

Feeding Regimens

The three primary feeding choices available for dogs and cats are free-choice or ad libitum, time-controlled feeding and portion-controlled or measured feeding.[2]

The method used will be determined by the owner's daily schedule, the number of animals being fed, the type of food being fed and the acceptability of the method to the pet or pets.[2]

Free Choice Feeding

Free-choice feeding is having a surplus of food available at all times. This enables the pet or pets to consume as much food as desired at any time of the day.[2] This feeding method relies on the animal's ability to self-regulate food intake so that only the actual energy and nutrient needs are met, and no excess energy is consumed.[2] Dry food is the best choice for this method as it will not spoil or dry out as easily as other products. This does not mean that by feeding dry food, the dishes do not need to be cleaned or the food refreshed daily though.[2]

When compared to the other methods, free-choice feeding requires the least amount of work and knowledge by the owner.[2] The food and water supply is only replenished once daily (or less often) and it is not necessary for the owner to determine the pet's exact daily energy requirements.[2] When dogs are fed free-choice, they tend to consume frequent small meals throughout the day. This feeding pattern has the advantage of greater meal-induced energy loss through digestion when compared to dogs eating larger meals, less frequently.[2] However, this increased energy loss is usually more than compensated for by increased energy intake by most dogs (Figure 18.3).

Free-choice feeding can be a helpful way to feed those animals that are "poor doers" or have higher energy expenditure and do not or cannot eat sufficient calories to support themselves when fed time-controlled meals.[3] This allows them to eat multiple small meals throughout the day, increasing their overall energy intake. This method can also be helpful for animals that work at a very high energy level such as hunting dogs, service dogs and search and rescue dogs, by allowing them to replenish their energy reserves throughout the day.[2]

Free-choice feeding can be a disadvantage if animals are having problems with anorexia or over consumption

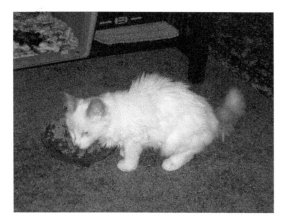

Figure 18.3 Ad lib feeding of a special needs kitten in a multi-cat household to ensure adequate food intake.

as these problems may go undetected for an extended period of time as the owners are not feeding and monitoring the intake daily.[2] If these problems are related to a medical condition, valuable treatment time may be lost until the animal is sick enough for the owner to notice a change in the condition, where if the animal was meal or portion fed, the problem with increased or decreased intake would be evident to the owner within a short period of time.[2]

Obesity is a common problem with animals that are fed free choice food. With a highly palatable diet, and a sedentary lifestyle the normal regulatory mechanisms used to control food intake are easily overridden.[2] In young growing animals this over consumption of energy has been shown to cause an accelerated growth rate and increased fat deposition within the body, further contributing to obesity later in life.[2] This increased growth rate has also been linked to the development of degenerative joint diseases as the animal matures, as well as decreased overall life expectancy.[3]

Time-controlled Feeding

Time-controlled feeding involves controlling the amounts of time that the animal is given access to the food, but they can eat as much as they want or can within this period of time.[2] Time-controlled may also pertain to portion controlled feeding where the food is only given as a specific volume for a controlled period of time. If this volume of food is not consumed within this

time period, it is removed until the next feeding.[4] This method also relies on the animal's ability to regulate its own energy intake. At mealtime, a surplus amount of food is supplied and the animal is allowed to eat for a predetermined period of time.

For most dogs and cats that are not physiologically stressed, 15–20 minutes is sufficient time to meet their energy requirements.[2] This is usually done in either one or two meals daily. While most animals can eat a sufficient amount of food when fed once daily, twice daily is healthier and more satisfying for the animal.[2] Twice daily feeding will also help to reduce hunger between meals and decrease food-associated behaviors such as begging and stealing food.[2]

Some animals do not adapt well to time-controlled feedings. Some may not consume a sufficient quantity within the time period allotted, while other will gorge themselves throughout the entire period of time leading to overeating and obesity. Time-controlled feedings may actually encourage gluttonous behavior because animals quickly learn that they have to "beat-the-clock."[2]

Picky eaters or those who are intimidated by the presence of other animals during meal time may not be able to consume enough calories to meet their energy requirements. There are also those who will only pick at their food, but hold out for table food and scraps from the owners, more frequent meals, thus defeating the purpose of time-controlled meals.[4]

Portion-controlled Feedings

Portion-controlled feedings are the preferred method in most situations.[2] By feeding a predetermined amount of food once, twice or more often daily the owner is given the greatest amount of control over the pet's diet. Portion-controlled feedings also allow the owners to monitor the food intake more closely and notice any changes in intake or behavior quickly.[2] This method provides the most control over growth rate and weight, and can be adjusted as needed to maintain the desired effect.[2] By doing this, conditions related to overweight, underweight or inappropriate growth can be corrected at an early stage (Figure 18.4).[2]

Portion-controlled feeding also demands the most amount of knowledge and effort by the owner. Guidelines for feeding amounts are provided on the bags or containers of food; these can be used as a starting

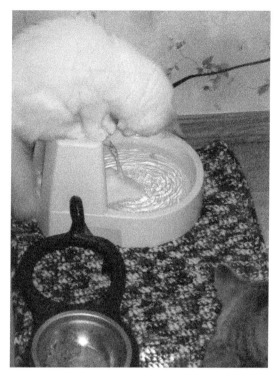

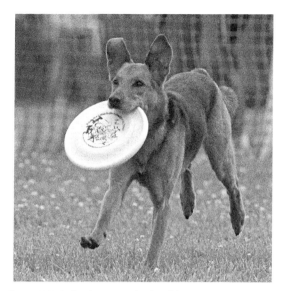

Figure 18.5 Active dog competing in Frisbee tournament. (Courtesy Heidi Reuss-Lamky LVT, VTS (Anesthesia, Surgery).)

Figure 18.4 Portion-controlled feeding of the same special needs cat as an adult. He often got distracted by the waterer.

point to determine the amount of food to be fed to the animal.[2] The Daily Energy Requirements (DER) can also be calculated using the pets' weight, activity level and the energy density of the food. The manufacturer can be contacted to determine the energy density of the food, since this is usually not provided on the product label. Internet sites maintained by the manufacturer will often contain the energy density of the food, as well as the nutrient distribution. When in doubt always contact the manufacturer for the correct information (Figure 18.5).

Guidelines for expectations need to be provided to owners as to desired outcomes for using portion-controlled feedings. We need to ensure that adequate food is being fed to meet the animal's energy requirements, as well as providing all the necessary nutrients in the correct portions. This is a good time to introduce the concept of Body Condition Scoring, and give clients a lesson on how to conduct these at home, as well as the desired number to achieve. It is also important to ensure that you and the clients are talking

about the same unit of measure when determining feeding volumes. A standard 8 oz measuring cup does not provide the same volume of food as the standard 7/11 Big Gulp cup, but both constitute a "cup."

The time-commitment for portion-controlled feeding is usually not a problem for most owners unless a large number of animals are being fed at any one time. The easiest method is to coordinate the pets' meal time with the owners' meal time; this would also have the added benefit of decreasing begging at the table because they're eating their own food.[2]

The amount of food being fed can be adjusted based on the individual animal's activity level, growth rate, body condition and any life style changes. Any treats being fed will need to be figured into the total caloric allotment for each animal. There are no free calories, and portion controlled feeding do not work if treats and snacks are not also controlled. This also allows the owner to monitor food intake more closely and make any adjustments as needed before significant changes have occurred in the animal's body condition (Figure 18.6).

There are a number of timed feeders on the market that are designed to help with portion-controlled feeding that require less effort by the owner. They usually provide a specific amount of food delivered using a timer set by the owner. This method can also help those animals

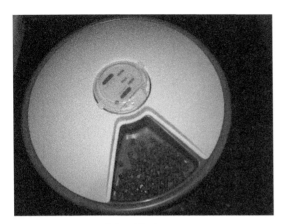

Figure 18.6 Automated timed feeder.

who have extreme begging behavior by removing the owner from the feeding process. These timed feeders can be set for multiple feedings per day, and are also helpful for those owners who have unreliable schedules and are not always at home at the designated meal time.

References

1 Voith VL (1994) Feeding behaviors. In JM Wills, KW Simpson (eds), *The Waltham Book of Clinical Nutrition of the Dog and Cat*, pp. 119–27, Tarrytown, NY: Elsevier.

2 Case LP, Carey DP, Hirakawa DA, Daristotle L (2000) Feeding regimens in dogs and cats. In *Canine and Feline Nutrition* (2nd edn), pp. 217–24, St Louis, MO: Mosby.

3 Case L (1999 Feeding management throughout the life cycle. In *The Dog, Its Behavior, Nutrition and Health*, pp 311–28, Ames, IA: Iowa State Press.

4 Case LP, Daristotle L, Hayek MG, Raaasch MF (2011) Feeding regimens in dogs and cats. In *Canine and Feline Nutrition* (3nd edn), pp. 191–7, Maryland Heights, MO: Mosby.

5 Case L (2003) Feeding management throughout the life cycle. In *The Cat, Its Behavior, Nutrition and Health*, pp. 329–40, Ames, IA: Iowa State Press.

19 Body Condition Scoring

Introduction

With humans, body condition and percent of body fat can be assessed using body mass indexing (BMI). For the majority of humans, this method is a helpful way of determining body condition and if the person is under weight, ideal, or overweight/obese. Unfortunately for us, our patients' sizes are too wide and their body types too diverse to make this system usable for veterinary medicine.

In an attempt to determine the ideal weight for our patients, a number of systems have been developed. The use of weight/height charts are impractical especially for dogs not only because of their different body types, but also the difficulty in obtaining the information on a moving, happy animal.[1] Zoometric methods, similar to anthropometric methods used in humans have been developed, but are more useful in a research setting as they are difficult to use on a daily basis on pets. Morphometric methods have also been developed, but require acquiring a number of measurements and plugging these into a complex formula to determine percent body fat. Due to the difficulty in obtaining these measurements, and the complexity of the formula, errors are common making the use of this method impractical.[1] In animals, the subcutaneous fat adheres more to muscle than to skin, making skin-fold thickness a questionable means for determining body fat in cats and dogs.[2]

Body condition scoring (BCS) is a subjective (not objective) assessment of an animal's body fat and to a lesser extent protein stores.[3] The scoring system takes into account the animal's frame size independent of its weight. BCS involves both visual assessment and physical assessment through palpation to assess body fat over the rib, abdomen, lumbar area and tail base.[1]

There are two main scoring systems, the 5-point scale and the 9-point scale. Both systems use defined criteria to help make the subjective process of body evaluation more objective, but all subjectivity can not be removed when assigning a score to an animal. For this reason, it is important that the same person try to assign the score each time the animal is evaluated. The 5-point scale scores the animals to the nearest half score, and a 9-point scale scores to the nearest whole score.[3]

Studies have shown that body fat increases 5–7% for each whole increment increase using a 9-point scale with mid-range scoring dogs (4/9–5/9) having 15–20% of their body mass as fat.[2] For cats, a mid-range score would be consistent with a body fat percentage of 25–30%.[1] On a 5-point scale the change of body fat for each increment change is ~10–15%.[1] When trying to detect small changes in body fat, the use of BCS scores would probably not be your best choice, but for monitoring and routine care it is quick, easy and painless. Body condition scores are ideally used with body weight measurement, not in place of weighing the animal at every visit.

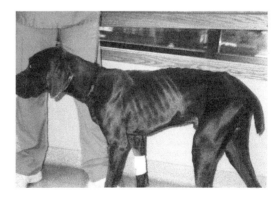

Figure 19.1 BCS 1/5 with obvious muscle wasting and loss of fat layer.

Nutrition and Disease Management for Veterinary Technicians and Nurses, Second Edition. Ann Wortinger, Kara M. Burns
© 2015 John Wiley & Sons, Inc. Published 2015 by John Wiley & Sons, Inc.
Companion Website: www.wiley.com/go/wortinger/nutrition

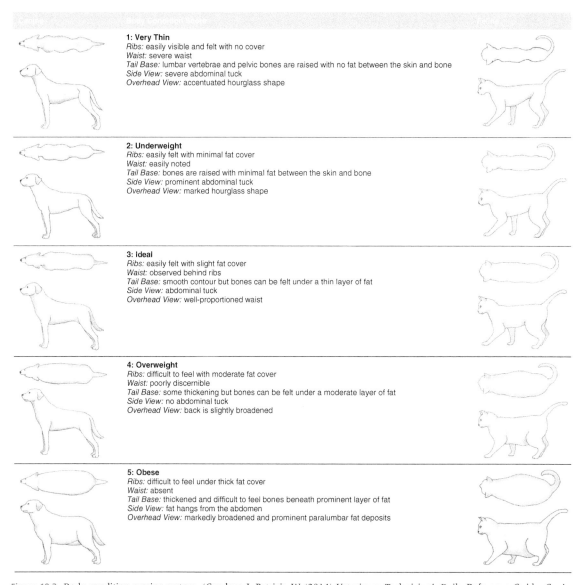

1: Very Thin
Ribs: easily visible and felt with no cover
Waist: severe waist
Tail Base: lumbar vertebrae and pelvic bones are raised with no fat between the skin and bone
Side View: severe abdominal tuck
Overhead View: accentuated hourglass shape

2: Underweight
Ribs: easily felt with minimal fat cover
Waist: easily noted
Tail Base: bones are raised with minimal fat between the skin and bone
Side View: prominent abdominal tuck
Overhead View: marked hourglass shape

3: Ideal
Ribs: easily felt with slight fat cover
Waist: observed behind ribs
Tail Base: smooth contour but bones can be felt under a thin layer of fat
Side View: abdominal tuck
Overhead View: well-proportioned waist

4: Overweight
Ribs: difficult to feel with moderate fat cover
Waist: poorly discernible
Tail Base: some thickening but bones can be felt under a moderate layer of fat
Side View: no abdominal tuck
Overhead View: back is slightly broadened

5: Obese
Ribs: difficult to feel under thick fat cover
Waist: absent
Tail Base: thickened and difficult to feel bones beneath prominent layer of fat
Side View: fat hangs from the abdomen
Overhead View: markedly broadened and prominent paralumbar fat deposits

Figure 19.2 Body condition scoring system. (Candyce J, Patricia W (2014) Veterinary Technician's Daily Reference Guide: Canine and Feline (3rd edn), John Wiley & Sons, Inc.)

Body Condition Score Uses

A body condition score (BCS) should be recorded with the weight each time an animal is examined. Body weight alone does not indicate how appropriate the weight is for that individual animal. The BCS puts in perspective what an Figure 19.1 and Figure 19.2 individual animal should weigh.[3]

In general, dogs and cats with an optimal body condition have:

• Normal body contours and silhouettes.
• Boney prominences that are easily palpated but not seen or felt above the skin surface.
• Intra-abdominal fat that is insufficient to obscure or interfere with abdominal palpation.

Table 19.1 Five-point body condition score[4]

BCS	What you see:	What you feel:
1/5 Emaciated	Obvious ribs, pelvic bones and spine, no body fat or muscle mass	Bones with little covering of muscle
2/5 Thin	Ribs and pelvic bones, but less prominent; tips of spine, an "hourglass" waist (looking from above), a tucked up abdomen (looking from side).	Ribs and other bones with no palpable fat, but some muscle is present.
3/5 Moderate	Less prominent hourglass and abdominal tuck	Ribs without excess fat covering.
4/5 Stout	General fleshy appearance, hourglass and abdominal tuck hard to see	Ribs, with difficulty
5/5 Obese	Sagging abdomen, large deposits of fat over chest, abdomen and pelvis	Nothing, except general flesh

Table 19.2 Nine-point body condition score[5]

BCS	What you see:	What you feel:
1/9 Emaciated	Obvious ribs, pelvic bones and spine, no body fat or muscle mass	Bones with little covering of muscle
2/9	Obvious ribs, pelvic bones and spine, minimal body fat, minimal loss of muscle mass	Bones with some covering of muscle
3/9 Thin	Ribs and pelvic bones, but less prominent; tips of spine, an "hourglass" waist (looking from above), a tucked up abdomen (looking from side).	Ribs and other bones with no palpable fat, but more muscle is present.
4/9 Ideal	Minimal fat covering, waist easily seen from above, abdominal tuck evident	Ribs easily palpated, muscle mass present
5/9	Less prominent hourglass and abdominal tuck	Ribs without excess fat covering.
6/9 Heavy	Slight fat covering, waist evident when viewed from above, but not prominent, abdominal tuck apparent	Ribs palpable with slight excess fat covering
7/9	General fleshy appearance, hourglass and abdominal tuck hard to see	Ribs, with difficulty, noticeable fat deposits over lumbar and at base of tail.
8/9	Heavy fat deposits over lumbar area and at base of tail, waist absent, no abdominal tuck evident, obvious abdominal distension	Ribs not palpable under heavy fat cover, obvious fat deposits over lumbar and at base of tail, abdominal palpation difficult
9/9 Obese	Sagging abdomen, large deposits of fat over chest, abdomen and pelvis	Nothing, except general flesh

Normal BCSs are 3/5 or 4–5/9; when scores are below 2/5 or 3/9 or above 4/5 or 7/9 then action should be taken to bring the animal into a more normal BCS (Table 19.1, Figure 19.2, Table 19.2 and Figures 19.3).[3]

Studies have shown that people are more likely to underestimate their own pet's BCS. This may be due to daily exposures making the clients more accepting of any increases that may have occurred, or acceptance of a heavier body condition as normal.[1] We as a veterinary health care team are often willing to ignore, and not bring to the owners attention increases in body condition. Whether this is due to failure to appreciate the problems that being overweight or obese can pose to the animal, or an unwillingness to engage the owner in a discussion on obesity management is undetermined. In a large survey of veterinary practices in the United States, ~ 28% of the dogs and cats were scored as overweight or obese, but only 2% had this problem recorded as an issue on the medical record.[1]

Best practice would dictate that the weight be recorded at every visit to the client, a BCS be done at

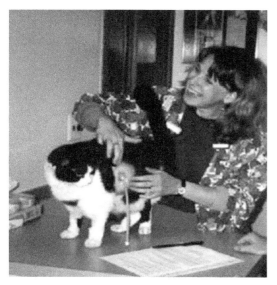

Figure 19.3 Discussing BCS scoring during a hepatic lipidosis discharge. BCS instruction allows the owner to continue to monitor the cat's condition in between recheck visits.

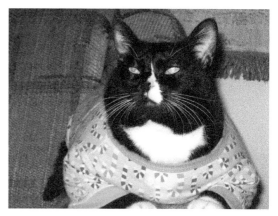

Figure 19.4 This cat developed diabetes after years of obesity.

every physical exam and a discussion be done with the client regarding any abnormalities at every visit.[1] Sometimes this can seem like we are talking to a brick wall when discussing overweight and obesity issues with clients, but our job is to advocate for the pet. Our knowledge of obesity related issues continues to grow at least as fast as the obesity problem in our patients. We also need to remember to encourage those owners with pets within a normal range to continue with the excellent work.

Just because an animal scores a 5/5 or a 9/9, does not mean that this is the maximum size or weight that this animal can attain. In fact animals can be scored as a 5/5+ or 9/9+ if morbid obesity is present. There is no "maximum" amount of body fat compatible with life (Figure 19.4).[3]

Using BCS is an effective means of monitoring an animal's condition as well as its weight, and is something that can be easily learned by most pet owners and done at home. By teaching clients how to do this, our assessment should come as less of a surprise to them, and make them involved in maintaining a healthy weight in their dogs and cats. This should be instituted early on in the client/patient/veterinary team relationship so that we can prevent obesity and all of the associated problems.

References

1 Delaney S, Fascetti A (2012) Nutritional management of body weight. In S Delaney, A Fascetti (eds), *Applied Veterinary Clinical Nutrition*, pp. 111–15, Ames, IA: Wiley-Blackwell.
2 Burkholder WJ (2000) Precision and practicality of methods assessing body composition of dogs and cats. In *Nutrition Forum Proceedings*, pp. 1–9, St Louis, MO, Ralston Purina Co.
3 Burkholder WJ, Toll PW (2000) Obesity. In MS Hand, CD Thatcher, RL Remillard *et al.* (eds), *Small Animal Clinical Nutrition*, (4th edn), pp. 405–6, Marceline, MO: Walsworth Publishing.
4 Case LP, Carey DP, Hirakawa DA, Daristotle L (2000) Adult maintenance. In Canine and Feline Nutrition, (2nd edn), pp. 256–7, St Louis, MO: Mosby.
5 Nestlé Purina Body Condition Score card.

20 Pregnancy and Lactation in Dogs

Introduction

In general, gestation for dogs averages 63 days (+/- 2 days) and can be divided into 21-day trimesters.[1] Nutrition for the bitch during gestation and lactation should take place long before she is bred or the litter is whelped. Before breeding, both the sire and the dam should be in excellent physical condition, moderate body condition and well exercised. They should both have complete physical exams done by a veterinarian, be current on all preventative health programs such as vaccinations, heartworm medications and intestinal dewormers and be tested for the presence of brucellosis and herpes virus.[1,2] If this is a pure bred litter, both parents should also be screened for any congenital problems such as hip dysplasia, elbow dysplasia or retinal problems, as well as shown to adhere to established breed standards.[1]

If the bitch is underweight, she may not be able to consume enough food during the pregnancy to provide for both her physical needs as well as the needs of her developing puppies. Lack of proper nutrition in the bitch can result in decreased conception rates, decreased birth weight, increased neonatal mortality and perform poorly during lactation.[1,3] Puppies born to underweight bitches have been shown to have decreased birth weights, have increased incidence of experiencing hypoglycemia and show lower survival rates.[3]

A bitch that is overweight at the time of breeding may experience lower ovulation rates, have smaller litters and perform poorly during lactation.[3] They are predisposed to the development of very large puppies and resultant dystocia due to fetal maternal disproportion, which puts the life of both the bitch and puppies at risk. It is recommended that overweight bitches lose weight before breeding to optimize fertility and decrease the risk of developing dystocia.[4]

What to Feed

If the breeding pair is in good physical and nutritional condition, no special foods need to be fed prior to, or during the breeding. Feeding a complete and balance, highly digestible diet that has undergone feeding trials for pregnancy and lactation would be recommended.[1,2,4] It is not unusual for the bitch to have a slightly depressed appetite during estrus; this can be due to hormonal changes as well as nervousness.[1,4] The diet should be changed if needed early in her reproductive cycle to allow her to fully adjust to the new food prior to breeding and to help prevent any abrupt change in diets during gestation or lactation.[1]

Gestation is a unique situation in which nutritional requirements increase markedly over a relatively short period of time.[4] The bitch's energy requirements do not increase substantially until the last third of gestation.[3] The average bitch will gain approximately 15–25% of their pre-pregnancy weight during gestation.[3] Actual energy requirements for gestation peak anywhere between 30% and 60% of the pre-breeding requirements. This variation is dependent on the size of the litter and the activity level of the bitch.[3] These increased energy requirements continue to increase after whelping and into lactation reaching their highest levels approximately 3–5 weeks after whelping.[3] It is suggested to increase the amount of food fed to the bitch by 15% each week from the fifth week of gestation until parturition. Following this regimen would mean that by whelping, the bitch should be eating 60% more food than when she was mated.[5] As the pregnancy advances, it is reasonable to decrease the size of the meals and offer them more frequently. This allows a bitch with a large litter, and little free abdominal space to still meet her energy requirements.[5] During lactation, most dogs can be fed ad lib or small meals frequently to allow them

Nutrition and Disease Management for Veterinary Technicians and Nurses, Second Edition. Ann Wortinger, Kara M. Burns
© 2015 John Wiley & Sons, Inc. Published 2015 by John Wiley & Sons, Inc.
Companion Website: www.wiley.com/go/wortinger/nutrition

to meet their energy requirements while producing adequate milk for the puppies.[3] The exception to this would be a bitch that experiences fetal loss and is only left with 1–2 puppies to care for – they will not experience increased energy requirements at the same level as a bitch with a larger litter.[3]

As lactation progresses, the bitch will gradually start weaning the puppies. The amount of calories offered can be reduced correspondingly. Not only does this help prevent the development of obesity in the bitch, but will also help to reduce the amount of milk that she is producing. Once weaning has been completed, usually by 6–8 weeks, the bitch should be back to the amount of calories that she was consuming prior to breeding.[3]

The Puppies

Although the puppies are developing rapidly, they are very small until the last third of the 63-day gestation.[1] They have little impact on the bitches weight and nutritional needs until after the 5th week of pregnancy. After the fifth week, fetal size and weight increase rapidly for the remaining 3–4 weeks of gestation. In the dog, greater than 75% of the weight and at least half of the fetal length are attained between the 40th and 55th day of gestation.[1]

Lactation

Lactation presents the biggest test of nutritional adequacy of any feeding regimen.[5] The bitch must eat, digest, absorb and use large amounts of nutrients to produce sufficient milk of adequate quality to support the growth and development of several puppies.[5] Not only does she need to meet the entire energy requirements for the rapidly growing puppies, but she must also be able to meet all of her energy and nutrient requirements. The amount of energy needed to meet these multiple requirements is dependent on the normal energy intake of the bitch, and the size and age of the litter.[5] A 5 lb Maltese with 2 puppies would require must less energy per pound than would a 15 lb Beagle with 6 puppies.[5] The bitch does not require additional vitamin or mineral supplements if a balance diet suitable for gestation and lactation is being fed.[5]

Table 20.1 Recommended nutrient levels during canine pregnancy and lactation

Nutrient	Recommended levels in food
Protein	25–35% ME
Fat	20% ME higher (if needed)
Carbohydrates (soluble)	23% ME
Calcium	1–1.7% ME
Phosphorus	0.7–1.3% ME
Calcium:phosphorus ration (6)	1.1:1–2:1

After whelping, the bitch's energy requirement steadily increases and peaks between three and five weeks post-partum to a level 2–4 times higher than Daily Energy Requirements (DER) for nonlactating adults.[4] The energy requirements return to normal levels about 8 weeks post-partum.[4] If the energy density of the food is too low, the bitch may not be able to physically consume enough food to meet both her and the puppies' energy requirements, if this happens her milk production will decrease, she will lose weight and may display signs of severe exhaustion.[4] This is most pronounced in giant-breed dogs with large litters (Table 20.1).[4]

Nutrients

Water is of utmost importance during lactation. Inadequate water intake leads to a significant decrease in the quantity of milk produced. Water is needed to produce the milk as well as for thermoregulation.[6] Water requirements are roughly equivalent to the energy requirements in kcals.[6] Fresh, cool water should always be readily available to the lactating bitch, allowing her to determine optimal water intake.[1]

Protein

Protein requirements for mating are the same as for maintenance for young adult dogs, and do not increase substantially for the first 2 trimesters of pregnancy. When entering the third trimester, protein requirements increase from 40% to 70% above maintenance as the puppies do their most growth.[6] At this point, the food should contain ~ 4 grams of digestible protein/100 kcal of metabolizable energy. The recommended crude protein allowance for foods fed during gestation and lactation ranges from 20% DM (NRC, 2006) to 22% DM (AAFCO, 2007). Because very few proteins are 100% digestible, the recommended dietary amounts of proteins found in diets fed during gestation and lactation would be between 25% and 35% DM.[6]

Fats and Fatty Acids

Fats provide increased energy when compared to proteins or carbohydrates as well as providing essential fatty acids and aiding in absorption of the fat soluble vitamins.[6] Increased fat intake has also been shown to improve food efficiency during lactation.[6] Increased fat intake by the bitch may increase the fat content of the milk. As puppies have very low energy reserves, this can increase the energy available through the milk.[6] The minimum recommended level of fat found in food for late gestation on into lactation is 8.0% DM (AAFCO, 2007) and 8.5% DM (NRC, 2006). Remembering that the NRC and AAFCO recommendations are minimums, and we are aiming for optimal performance, the recommended levels for bitches with fewer than 4 puppies would be at least 20% DM crude fat. For giant breeds dogs, the recommendation would also be 20% DM crude fat and higher levels may be needed to meet energy requirements for those dogs with larger litters.[6]

The omega 3 (n-3) and omega 6 (n-6) fatty acids have received a lot of attention lately as they relate to pregnancy and lactation. The diet should ideally be supplement with both fatty acids in a ratio of 5 parts n-3: 1 part n-6 up to 10 parts n-3: 1 part n-6.[7] The n-3 docosahexaenoic acid (DHA) is essential for normal neurologic and retinal development in puppies. Adult animals have a limited ability to synthesize DHA from alpha-linolenic acid; the best way to ensure that the developing fetuses have enough DHA for optimal development is through supplementation of the bitche's diet.[7]

Carbohydrates

While the body does not have a "requirement" for carbohydrates, feeding carbohydrate-free diets to pregnant bitches may result in weight loss, decreased food intake, reduced birth weight in the puppies and

decreased neonatal survival with a possible increased risk of stillbirth.[6]

With more than 50% of the energy required for fetal-development being supplied by glucose, bitches have an increased requirement for glucose during the last trimester of pregnancy. While glucose can be supplied by gluconeogenic amino acids, this is an expensive way to supply glucose. When using fats for energy production, the risk of ketosis increases during late pregnancy.[6] A diet providing approximately 20% of the energy from soluble carbohydrates (i.e. starches and glycogen) is sufficient to prevent the negative effects of a carbohydrate-free diet.[6] Foods fed during lactation should contain at least 23% DM from digestible carbohydrates.[6]

Calcium and Phosphorus

For most breeds of dogs, calcium and phosphorus requirements are the same for the first 2 trimester of pregnancy as they are for adult maintenance (Ca:P ratio 1:1 to 1.5:1).[6] Due to rapid fetal skeletal growth during the final weeks of pregnancy, the requirements for calcium and phosphorus increase by 60%.[6] The NRC recommends a minimum recommended allowance for calcium in foods intended for late gestation and peak pregnancy is 0.8% DM. AAFCOs recommendations are 1.0% DM.[6] Excessive calcium intake during late pregnancy may decrease parathyroid gland activity and predispose the bitch to developing eclampsia during lactation.[6] Because of this, we need to find a balance between meeting minimum levels of calcium without over supplementing. The recommended calcium level is 1–1.7% DM, phosphorus levels of 0.7–1.3% DM with a calcium-phosphorus ratio of 1.1:1 to 2:1.[6] These levels apply to large and giant breed dogs as well. Calcium supplementation is not recommended during gestation or lactation if the appropriately balanced commercial diet is being fed.[6]

Digestibility

During late gestation, the actual caloric requirements for the bitch and fetuses may exceed what she is able to consume. This occurs most often if the food is poorly digestible. Digestibility is determined through the use of

Table 20.2 Sample calculation of bitch and puppy feeding requirements

Example

60 lb Labrador (pre-pregnancy weight) with 7 puppies
60 lb = 27.3 kg
RER= (30 × wt kg) + 70
RER = (30 × 27.3 kg) + 70 = 889
Lactation = RER × 1.9 = 1689 kcal/day
25% for each puppy = 422.25 kcal/puppy
7 puppies = 2955.75 kcal/day
Bitch + puppies = 1689 + 2955.75 = 4644.75
Commercial dry puppy food = 375 kcal/cup
4644.75 kcals/ 375 kcal/cup = 12.4 cups/day
Feed 12.4 cups/day

If we increase the energy content to 454 kcal/cup,
4644.75 kcal/ 454 kcal/cup = 10.2 cups/day
Feeding amount could be decrease to 10.2 cups and still meet energy requirements.

feeding trials to measure the energy found in the food and the amount of energy actually available to the animal through digestion. The higher the digestibility the more energy is available to the bitch. While there is no requirement for digestibility, a food having an energy density of 4 kcals ME/gram or higher will have more fat and less fiber increasing overall digestibility.[6]

When determining energy requirements, as a rough estimate, daily energy requirements (DER) for a lactating bitch would be 1.9 X RER. Each puppy would account for an additional 25% for DER for each puppy (Table 20.2).

References

1 Case LP, Carey DP, Hirakawa DA, Daristotle L (2000) Pregnancy and lactation. In *Canine and Feline Nutrition* (2nd edn), pp. 225–32, St Louis, MO: Mosby.
2 Buffington CA, Holloway C, Abood SK (2004) *Normal dogs. In Manual of Veterinary Dietetics*, pp. 9–11, St Louis, MO: Saunders.
3 Delaney S, Fascetti A (2012) Feeding the healthy dog and cat. In S Delaney, A Fascetti (eds), *Applied Veterinary Clinical Nutrition*, pp. 82–3, Ames, IA: Wiley-Blackwell.
4 Debraekeleer J, Gross KL, Zicker SC (2000) Normal dogs. In MS Hand, CD Thatcher, RL Remillard, P Roudebush (eds), *Small Animal Clinical Nutrition* (4th edn), pp. 232–41, Marceline, MO: Walsworth Publishing.
5 LeGrand-Defretin V, Munday HS (1995) Feeding dogs and cats for life. In I Burger (ed.), *The Waltham Book of Companion Animal Nutrition*, pp. 57–9, Tarrytown, NY: Elsevier.
6 Debraekeleer J, Gross KL, Zicker SC (2010) Feeding reproducing dogs. In MS Hand, CD Thatcher, RL Remillard *et al.* (eds), *Small Animal Clinical Nutrition* (5th edn), pp. 281–90, Marceline, MO: Walsworth Publishing.
7 Case LP, Daristotle L, Hayek MG, Raasch MF (2011) Pregnancy and lactation. In *Canine and Feline Nutrition* (3rd edn), pp. 199–206, St Louis, MO: Mosby.

21 Pregnancy and Lactation in Cats

Introduction

As with dogs, any cat being considered for breeding should be in excellent physical condition, moderate body condition and well exercised. Both the queen and tom should have complete physical exams by a veterinarian, be current on all preventative health programs such as vaccinations, heartworm medications and intestinal dewormers and be tested for the presence of feline leukemia virus and feline immunodeficiency virus.[1,2] If this is a pure bred litter, both parents should also be screened for any congenital problems as well as shown to adhere to established breed standards.[1] If the queen is significantly underweight (BCS <2/5 or 3/9) or overweight (BCS > 4/5 or 6/9) she should not be bred until she is closer to her ideal body weight and condition.[3]

Queens that are underweight or in poor body condition may fail to conceive, abort or bear small underweight kittens. They may also have markedly reduced lactation. Obesity in cats can lead to large kittens resulting in increased incidence of dystocia.[3,4]

First Heat Cycle

Domestic cats generally have their first heat cycles between 6 to 9 months of age. This does not mean that they are physically ready to have a litter of kittens. Before 10–12 months of age, queens are still growing and if they become pregnant must support not only their own continued growth but also that of their kittens.[4] The best age for breeding is between 1.5 years and 7 years of age. Queens older than 7 years should not be bred due to reproductive complications, irregular estrous cycles and reduced litter size.[4]

What to Feed

Unlike most species, weight gain in a queen increases linearly from conception to parturition. This weight gain in early pregnancy is not associated with significant growth of reproductive tissues or fetal growth, but appears to be stored in energy deposits (presumably as fat) to support lactation.[1,4] Energy intake parallels the linear pattern of weight gain. The amount of weight gain is also independent of the number of fetuses being carried.[3] This stored energy can account for up to 60% of the weight gained during the pregnancy and is gradually lost during lactation.[1] Energy requirements increase to 90–100 kcal/kg of body weight/day.[3] The average weight gain should be about 40% of the pre-mating weight.[4]

The queen should be fed a diet that is intended for reproduction throughout gestation and lactation.[1,4] The amount of food should be gradually increased, beginning at the second week of gestation and continuing until parturition. At the end of gestation, the queen should be consuming about 25–50% more food than during her normal maintenance needs.[1] Due to the high energy demands during pregnancy and lactation, free choice or ad lib feeding is recommended to allow the queen to meet her increased energy demands.[3]

After parturition, approximately 40% of the weight gained during pregnancy is lost. By the time the kittens are weaned (7–8 weeks post parturition) the queen should be back to her pre-breeding weight.[3]

Once the kittens are weaned, the queen can be returned to her regular maintenance diet with a goal to maintain optimal BCS (Table 21.1).[3]

The Kittens

Kittens should exhibit steady weight gain, have good muscle tone and suckle vigorously. Young kittens are

Nutrition and Disease Management for Veterinary Technicians and Nurses, Second Edition. Ann Wortinger, Kara M. Burns
© 2015 John Wiley & Sons, Inc. Published 2015 by John Wiley & Sons, Inc.
Companion Website: www.wiley.com/go/wortinger/nutrition

Table 21.1 Recommended nutrient levels during feline pregnancy and lactation[1]

Nutrient	Recommended levels in food
Protein	32% ME
Fat	Minimum 20% ME
Omega 3: Omega 6 FA ratio	5:1 – 10:1

quiet between feedings.[4] Kittens that are restless and cry excessively may not be receiving enough milk due to poor lactation. Gastric distension is not a good indicator of adequate nursing. Excessive swallowing of air during nursing can give the appearance of gastric fullness, despite inadequate milk intake.[4] Kitten mortality reportedly varies from 9% to 63%, depending on the source of the cats and the cattery.[4] Several genetic, husbandry and nutritional factors can contribute to high mortality. If kitten death or cannibalism by the queen is high, all three areas should be investigated.[4]

Lactation

Lactation presents the biggest test of nutritional adequacy of any feeding regimen.[5] The queen must eat, digest, absorb and use large amounts of nutrients to produce sufficient milk of adequate quality to support the growth and development of several kittens.[5] Not only does she need to meet the entire energy requirements for the rapidly growing kittens, but she must also be able to meet all of her energy and nutrient requirements. The amount of energy needed to meet these multiple requirements is dependent on the normal energy intake of the queen and the size and age of the litter.[5]

Lactation is considered to be the most physically demanding life stage with regards to energy and nutrient requirements.[3] When lactating, energy needs for the queen increase with a peak at 7 weeks post parturition, though peak lactation amounts is reached at 3 weeks post parturition.[3] This discrepancy can be explained by looking at the calories consumed by the queen for maintenance and lactation, and including the calories consumed by the kittens from both lactation but also oral intake of the queen's food.[3]

Depending on litter size, the queen should be eating 2 – 3 times her maintenance energy requirements during lactation.[1] A general guideline is to feed 1.5 times DER during the first week of lactation, 2 times DER during the second week, and 2.5 – 3 times DER during the fourth week of lactation.[1] If the energy density of the food is too low, the queen may not be able to physically consume enough food to meet both her and the kittens' energy requirements. If this happens her milk production will decrease, she will lose weight and may display signs of severe exhaustion.[4]

Milk production depends on litter size and stage of lactation.[4] Peak lactation occurs between 3 and 4 weeks post-partum.[4] Continuous weight gain by the kitten is the best indicator of adequate milk production by the queen.[4]

Nutrients

Protein

Feeding a diet that meets the minimum AAFCO and NRC requirements is essential for optimal production and growth during gestation and on into lactation. Due to the carnivorous nature of cats, attention also needs to be paid to the type of protein that the queen is consuming. Taurine, an essential amino acid for cats, can only be found in animal-based protein sources. When insufficient taurine is in the diet, both conception rate and neonate birth weights are decreased.[6]

Fat

Litter size can be positively influenced by the fat level found in the queen's diet. This fat should include the essential fatty acids (EFAs) as well as arachidonic acid. Arachidonic acid is an EFA for cats, and can only be found in fats obtained from animal sources.[6]

The omega 3 (n-3) and omega 6 (n-6) fatty acids have received a lot of attention lately as they relate to pregnancy and lactation. The diet should ideally be supplement with both fatty acids in a ratio of 5 parts n-3: 1 part n-6 up to 10 parts n-3: 1 part n-6.[6] The n-3 docosahexaenoic acid (DHA) is essential for normal neurologic and retinal development in kittens. Adult animals have a limited ability to synthesize DHA from alpha-linolenic acid; the best way to ensure that the developing fetuses have enough DHA for optimal development is through supplementation of the queen's diet.[6]

Water is the most important nutrient the queen consumes during lactation. Because milk has an estimated 78% water content, inadequate water intake leads to a significant decrease in the quantity of milk produced.[6]

As lactation increases post-parturition, the queen's water requirements will increase significantly.[6] Fresh, cool water should always be readily available to the lactating queen.[1]

References

1 Case LP, Carey DP, Hirakawa DA, Daristotle L (2000) Pregnancy and Lactation. In *Canine and Feline Nutrition* (2nd edn), pp. 225–32, St Louis, MO: Mosby.

2 Buffington CA, Holloway C, Abood SK (2004) Normal dogs. In *Manual of Veterinary Dietetics*, pp. 9–11, St Louis, MO: Saunders.

3 Delaney S, Fascetti A (2012) Feeding the healthy dog and cat. In S Delaney, A Fascetti (eds), *Applied Veterinary Clinical Nutrition*, pp. 81–2, Ames, IA: Wiley-Blackwell.

4 Kirk CL, Debraekeleer J, Armstrong PJ (2000) Normal cats. In MS Hand, CD Thatcher, RL Remillard, P Roudebush (eds) *Small Animal Clinical Nutrition* (4th edn), pp. 320–8, Marceline, MO: Walsworth Publishing.

5 LeGrand-Defretin V, Munday HS (1995) Feeding dogs and cats for life. In I Burger (ed.), *The Waltham Book of Companion Animal Nutrition*, pp. 57–9, Tarrytown, NY: Elsevier.

6 Case LP, Daristotle L, Hayek MG, Raasch MF (2011) Pregnancy and lactation. In *Canine and Feline Nutrition* 3rd edn, pp. 199–206, St Louis, MO: Mosby.

22 Neonatal Puppies and Kittens

Introduction

The neonatal period of a dog's or cat's life is considered to be the first 2 week of their life.[1] The first week of this period is the most critical for its survival. Newborn puppies and kittens are physiologically immature, with low percentages of body fat, 1–2% compared to 12–35% in adults. This immaturity is termed altricial, which means that they are born immature and are therefore completely dependent on their mother for survival.[1] If they are orphaned, then that care will depend on their foster parents until they mature enough to start caring for themselves.

Nutrition

The first nutritional concern for newborns is that they receive colostrum immediately after birth. Colostrum is milk produced by the mother during the first 24–72 hours after parturition. Colostrum provides nutrients, water, growth factors, digestive enzymes and maternal immunoglobulins (antibodies).[2] Most of the immunoglobluins and other factors transmitted through the colostrum are in the form of large proteins. Once they are absorbed across the intestinal barrier, they confer passive immunity to the neonate.[1] The ability of the neonate to absorb these large proteins across the intestinal barrier is lost after the first 24–72 hours. Continuation of colostrum after this period provides no additional immunity to the neonate. It is important to remember the neonate can only receive protection from diseases the mother has either been vaccinated for or has contracted and developed natural immunity to. This passive immunity will help to protect the neonate until into the weaning period and is considered gone by ~16 weeks of age.[1]

All of the components of colostrum are critical to the survival of the newborn. The main difference between colostrum and milk is in the water content and nutrient composition.[2] The water content of colostrum is lower than that of milk, which accounts for its sticky, concentrated appearance when compared with regular milk. The water content found in the milk will gradually increase from day 1 to day 3.[2] Lactose concentrations found in colostrum are also lower than that found in milk with protein and fat levels being higher. Energy content found in milk also increases throughout lactation.[2] Due to their immaturity, neonates do not develop adequate glycogen reserves until after the first few days of nursing.[3] This lack of glycogen reserves means that they need to nurse or be fed frequently, sometimes as often as every 2 hours for the first week or so of life.

Maintenance of body temperature is the second most important concern for newborns. Neonatal puppy and kittens are unable to thermoregulate and must be kept in an environment that is 85–90°F during the first week of life, and 80–85°F during the second week.[3] If the neonates are not kept warm enough and develop hypothermia, they will be unable to eat, and if tube fed will be unable to digest the food. This failure to eat may result in rejection by the bitch or queen.[3] The best source of warmth is the mother. After 6 days the neonates are able to shiver, but are still very susceptible to chilling. Keeping the environment warm and free of drafts is of utmost importance during the first few weeks of life.[4]

Orphaned neonates have the same requirements as do neonates that have a mother; they still need adequate nutrition and warmth. Obviously the best course for the young puppy or kitten would be to have a foster mother; if this is not available they can be hand-raised. If they are hand-raised, not only do they need to be fed, but they also have to have their urination and defecation

Nutrition and Disease Management for Veterinary Technicians and Nurses, Second Edition. Ann Wortinger, Kara M. Burns
© 2015 John Wiley & Sons, Inc. Published 2015 by John Wiley & Sons, Inc.
Companion Website: www.wiley.com/go/wortinger/nutrition

Table 22.1 Nutrient composition of various milks[2]

Nutrient	Queen's milk	Bitch's milk	Cow's milk	Goat's milk
Moisture (g/100 g)	79	77.3	87.7	7.0
Crude protein (g/100 g)	7.5	7.5	3.3	3.6
Crude fat (g/100 g)	8.5	9.5	3.6	4.1
Lactose (g/100 g)	4.0	3.3	4.7	4.0
Calcium (mg/100g)	180	240	119	133
ME (kcal/100 g)	121	146	64	69

stimulated. The mother would do this through licking of the anogenital area. Since the foster parent is unlikely to consider this option, using a dry dish rag or cotton ball can provide the same stimulation. If using a damp cloth, make sure that the area is thoroughly dry after defection/urination or chapping can occur in this very delicate area. This will need to be continued until the puppy or kittens are between 16 and 21 days old.[5]

Milk from other species is inadequate substitutes for mothers' milk. The protein, fat and calcium levels found in goat and cows milk are too low for either puppies or kittens.[5] The ratio of casein:whey in the milk is also different for each species. Casein is the solid protein found in milk, while whey is the liquid protein found in milk. The amount of casein found in milk can affect protein digestion, mineral utilization and the milk's amino acid composition. The ratio for cats is 60:40, while dogs are 70:30.[1] Queen's milk would also be inadequate for puppies because of inadequate lactose and calcium levels. Bitch's milk contains almost twice as much protein compared to cow's milk. It also provides branched chain amino acids and high levels of arginine and lysine (Table 22.1).[5]

Surveys indicate that a high percentage of deaths before weaning are due to a relatively small number of causes: infectious diseases, congenital defects and malnutrition.[3] Infectious diseases are more of a concern with neonates who did not received adequate colostrum from their mothers, and are therefore deficient in passive immunity. The cause of malnutrition is usually from death of or neglect from the mother, lactation failure or a litter that is too large for the milk supply.[3]

If the puppy or kitten is raised by its mother, they should be allowed free access to her. They should be monitored to ensure that they are receiving adequate nutrition, and have received colostrum during the first 24 hours of life.[5] During the first few weeks of life they

should nurse at least 4–6 times per day. In healthy puppies and kittens, the mothers' milk supports normal growth until approximately 4 weeks of age.[4] Supplemental feedings should only be necessary with unusually large litters or with maternal rejection.[4] After 4 weeks of age, milk alone does not provide adequate calories or nutrients for continued normal development.[4]

Milk Replacers

Commercially available milk replacers can be used to supply or supplement the nutritional needs of neonates. Most milk replacers are based on cow or goat's milk and modified to more resemble the nutrient profile for bitch and queens milk.[6]

While there are "homemade" recipes for milk replacers for puppies and kittens, most of these recipes were developed through trial and error, and their actual nutrient content is unknown.[4] If fed straight cow's milk, neonate puppies develop severe diarrhea. Cow's milk contains nearly three times the lactose found in bitch's milk.[4] Cow's milk also contains an excessive proportion of casein for neonatal puppies and kittens and supplies insufficient calories for both.[4]

Commercial milk replacers are the preferred source of nutrition for orphans or as supplemental feeding to those neonates who are not receiving enough nutrition from their mother.[4] A product that has been tested for the specific purpose of raising neonatal puppies or kittens should be selected. Even though the nutrient content and bioavailability is guaranteed, commercial formulas vary in their ability to provide adequate nutrition and calories.[4] Most commercial replacement formulas have a nutrient density of ~1 kcal/ml, though dilution with water will reduce that.[7] Recommendations for feeding vary from 13 to 18 ml/100 grams of body weight, using a formula with ~1 kcal/ml.[7] This amount will be gradually increased as the neonate gains weight. Frequent reassessment of the feeding plan should be done looking at overall health, appearance, activity level, hydration status, and weight gain of the orphans. For kittens the expected weight gain would be ~18–20 grams/day. For puppies, due to the larger variation in size is ~1 gram of weight gain for every 2–5 grams of milk consumed during the first 5 weeks of life.[7] Chronic whimpering or vocalization may be an indication of discomfort or hunger, and would warrant a reassessment of the feeding plan.[7]

The American Association of Feed Control Officials (AAFCO) does not provide detailed guidelines for testing milk replacers. Obtaining the manufacturers' information related to nutrient composition, nutritional integrity and feeding efficacy is helpful in selecting the best replacement.[4] It is important to remember, even the best milk replacer can not provide the neonate with the antibodies found in colostrum, therefore extra care must be taken to maintain a clean environment and prevent transmission of disease.[4] Feeding materials such as bottles, nipples and tubes should be cleaned and disinfected between feedings. The milk replacer itself should be made fresh or refrigerated between feedings to decrease the incidence of bacterial contamination. Only the volume of milk replacer that will be consumed within a 24-hour period should be made up. Any milk replacer that is not used at that feeding should be stored in the refrigerator.[8]

Weaning

Weaning is a gradual process with two phases. The first phase begins when the neonate begins to eat solid food between 3–4 weeks of age.[2,4] This can be encouraged by mixing a commercial food specifically made and tested for all life stages, or a thick gruel made by mixing a small amount of warm water with the mother's food which has also been made and tested for all life stages including lactation.[1,7] Cow's milk should not be used to make the gruel as the lactose level is too high and may contribute to diarrhea.[1] This semi-solid food should be provided in a shallow dish, with the puppies or kittens allowed free access to the fresh food several times per day.[2,4] The food should be removed after 20–30 minutes to discourage bacterial growth in the food. A homemade weaning formula should not be fed, as the nutrient content would

be unknown, leading to nutrient, vitamin and mineral imbalances and the caloric density is unknown.[1]

Initially the intake of food will be minimal, but by 5–6 weeks of age the deciduous teeth will have begun to erupt enabling the puppies and kittens to chew and eat dry food.[2,4] As the food intake increases in the neonates, the mothers' milk production will decrease. By 6 weeks of age, the second stage of weaning can begin with the puppies and kittens obtaining their full nutrition from their food and not from their mother (nutritional weaning).[2,4] Even though some mothers will continue to nurse their young past this time, very little milk is being produced with little nutrition being obtained. It is believed that the psychological and emotional benefits of suckling may be as important as the nutritional benefits in animals that are older than 5 weeks of age.[4] For this reason, complete weaning (behavioral weaning) should not be done until puppies and kittens are at least 7–8 weeks of age.[4]

References

1 Case LP, Daristotle L, Hayek MG, Raasch MF (2010) Nutritional care of neonatal puppies and kittens. In *Canine and Feline Nutrition* (3nd edn), pp. 209–17, St Louis, MO: Mosby.

2 Kirk CL, Debraekeleer J, Armstrong PJ (2000) Normal cats. In MS Hand, CD Thatcher, RL Remillard, P Roudebush (eds), *Small Animal Clinical Nutrition* (4th edn), pp. 331–2, Marceline, MO: Walsworth Publishing.

3 Buffington CA, Holloway C, Abood SK (2004) Normal dogs. In *Manual of Veterinary Dietetics*, pp. 11–12, St Louis, MO: Saunders.

4 Case LP, Carey DP, Hirakawa DA, Daristotle L (2000) Nutritional care of neonatal puppies and kittens. In *Canine and Feline Nutrition* (2nd edn), pp. 233–43, St Louis, MO: Mosby.

5 Gross KL, Debraekeleer J, Zicker SC (2000) Normal dogs. In Hand MS, Thatcher CD, Remillard RI, Roudebush P (eds), *Small Animal Clinical Nutrition* (4th edn), pp. 244–7, Marceline, MO: Walsworth Publishing.

6 LeGrand-Defretin V, Munday HS (1995) Feeding dogs and cats for life. In I Burger (ed.), *The Waltham Book of Companion Animal Nutrition*, pp. 61–5, Tarrytown, NY: Elsevier.

7 Delaney S, Fascetti A (2012) Feeding the healthy dog and cat. In S Delaney, A Fascetti (eds), *Applied Veterinary Clinical Nutrition*, p. 83, Ames, IA: Wiley-Blackwell.

8 Gross KL, Becvarova I, Debraekeleer J (2010) Feeding nursing and orphaned kittens from birth to weaning. In MS Hand, CD Thatcher, RL Remillard *et al.* (eds), *Small Animal Clinical Nutrition* (5th edn), pp. 415–27, Marceline, MO: Walsworth Publishing.

23　Growth in Dogs

Introduction

The dog is unique among other mammals in that it has the widest range of normal adult body weight within any single species, ranging in size from adult Yorkshire Terriers and Chihuahuas weighing only 3 lb (1.4 kg) to adult Great Danes and Mastiffs that can top 200 lb (90 kg).[1] Because of this wide range in sizes, growth in the early stages of life is very rapid and, in general most breeds of dog will reach 50% of their adult weight between 5–6 months old.[1] Different breeds will continue to mature at different rates with some of the larger breeds not reaching maturity until almost 2 years of age. Initial weight gain should be between 2 and 4 gram/day/kg of anticipated adult weight for the first 5 months of life.[2] While this can be helpful in pure bred dogs where anticipate adult weight can at least be guessed, for mixed breed dogs where the adult size of both parents may not even be known – this doesn't provide much helpful information.

After nursing, post-weaning growth is the most nutritionally demanding period in a dog's life. With large and giant breed dogs, the length and speed of their growth poses an even higher nutritional demand. First we will address normal growth, and then how this differs with the large and giant breeds. Obviously what works nutritionally for a Chihuahua, won't necessarily work for an Irish Wolfhound.

Normal Growth

The most rapid period of growth is seen during the first 6 months of life. With this comes an increased requirement for all nutrients, with energy and calcium being of special concern.[3] Most small breed dogs will have reached their adult size by 8–12 months, medium breed dogs by 12–18 months and large and giant breed dogs not reaching their mature size until 18–24 months of age.[4] By maturity, most dogs will have increased their birth weight by 40–50 times.[4]

Diet restriction, and thus energy restriction, has been shown to affect the life span of dogs, with the primary research being done on Labrador Retrievers over the span of 15 years. All dogs were housed in the same conditions, received the same level of care and were fed the same food; the only difference between the two groups was in the amount of food consumed. One group of 24 dogs was designated the control group and was fed 62.1 kcal of ME/kg of estimated ideal body weight, the remaining 24 dogs were fed 25% less than their pair-mate. The group fed the larger amount had a body condition score of 6–7/9, with the restricted group having body condition scores of 4–5/9, with 1 being emaciated and 9 being severely obese. The group that received the larger amount of food, on average died 2 years younger than their pair-mates, developed osteoarthritis 1.1 years sooner and developed chronic health conditions 6 months sooner.[5] The only difference between these two groups was the amount of food fed. Following body condition scoring, none of the group fed the larger amounts was obese, and none of the restricted fed dogs was emaciated; these were all "average" sized Labradors.

This group of Labradors was fed controlled amounts from the time they entered the study at 6 weeks of age until they either died or were euthanized.[5] Because of the rapid growth that is seen in dogs during the first 12–18 months, this restriction can become very important when we are looking at the development of orthopedic problems later in life. While these problems occur later in life, they do not develop later in life, but while the dog is going through this rapid growth phase.

Even though calcium is essential for bone growth, the actual requirements in puppies is quite low. The American Association of Feed Control Officials (AAFCO)

Nutrition and Disease Management for Veterinary Technicians and Nurses, Second Edition. Ann Wortinger, Kara M. Burns
© 2015 John Wiley & Sons, Inc. Published 2015 by John Wiley & Sons, Inc.
Companion Website: www.wiley.com/go/wortinger/nutrition

Nutrient Profiles recommend that dog foods formulated for growth contain a minimum of 1% calcium on a dry-matter basis.[4] In general, calcium absorption from the food is dependent on requirements and calcium intake.[3]

What to Feed

The protein requirements for growing puppies is higher than that for adult dogs, this is because not only does the puppy have normal maintenance needs, but it also needs protein to build new tissue associated with growth.[4] Since puppies eat higher amounts of energy the total amount of protein eaten is naturally higher. Foods fed to growing puppies should contain slightly higher levels of protein than those fed for adult maintenance. Most importantly, this protein should be of high quality and highly digestible.[4] The minimum level of protein found in puppy diets should be 22% of the ME, with optimal levels between 25% and 29%. The type of protein included in the diet should be of high quality to ensure that all of the essential amino acids are being delivered to the body for use in growth and development.[4] This does not mean that only muscle meats provide adequate protein of high digestibility.

Because of the quantity of food needed to meet energy requirements, energy density is very important for growing puppies. If they are fed a poor quality food with low energy density and low digestibility, they need to consume large quantities to meet their energy requirements.[3] This intake of large volumes of food can increase the incidence of flatulence, vomiting, diarrhea, fecal volume and the development of a "pot-bellied" appearance.[3] When feeding poor quality food, even an inexpensive food can cost more to feed than a higher quality food, more expensive food, since so much of it will not be utilized by the body and will instead end up as feces.

While puppies do have higher requirements for energy and other essential nutrients than do adults, they also tend to have less digestive capacity, smaller mouths and smaller and fewer teeth with which to eat their food. This is especially true for small and toy breeds of dogs.[4] These differences limit the amount of food that the puppy can consume and digest within a meal or a given amount of time.[4]

It is equally important to not over-feed growing dogs; not only can this lead to an accelerated growth rate due to excess energy consumption, but also causes a build-up of adipose tissue that can contribute to obesity later in life.[4] Many well-meaning owners supplement an otherwise balanced diet, causing nutrient excessive that would not have existed before. It is not advised to supplement a balanced diet. If the owner feels that a supplement is needed, maybe the diet should be changed instead to a better quality diet.

Feeding Regimens

When a new puppy is initially brought home, the diet should not be changed from what had been fed previously, unless the food was of a very poor quality. Moving to a new home and leaving the bitch and litter mates is quite stressful for a young dog.[4] A new diet can be introduced 2–3 days after the move home, although it is best to do this transition slowly over 5–7 days. The easiest way to do this is to mix the food in quarters, so for Day 1 give 3/4 of the old diet mixed with 1/4 of the new diet, Day 2 and 3 give 1/2 of the old diet mixed with 1/2 of the new diet, Day 4 and 5 give 1/4 of the old diet with 3/4 of the new diet and on Day 6 the transition is complete.[3] If the initial food is of poor quality, switching over all at once is acceptable, though some diarrhea may also be expected.

Free-choice and time-restricted feedings are not recommended for puppies. Free-choice feedings may increase the amount of body fat, predisposing the dog to obesity later in life and cause skeletal deformities at a young age. Studies using time-restricted feedings have shown that the puppies increase body weight, have more body fat and increase bone mineralization faster than puppies fed free-choice.[3] During periods of rapid growth it is better to do measured feedings 2–4 times per day. The amount fed should be based on the growth rate of the dog, and the BCS. The feeding guides listed on the package can be used as a starting point. Because the feeding directions on the package are designed to provide enough calories for all dogs on a specific diet, the amounts given tend to overestimate the actual volume needed. Amounts should be adjusted to maintain an ideal BCS.[2] Puppies should be lean, not skinny and not roly-poly throughout their growth phase.

Large and Giant breed Puppies

Nutrient excesses, rapid growth rates and excessive weight gain appear to be important factors contributing to the incidence of skeletal disorders in growing large and giant breed dogs.[6] While we continue to select for increased size for many of our larger dogs, size itself is not detrimental to the dog, but management practices that allow growth rates to be maximized can cause the negative consequences that we see in these dogs.[7] It has been estimated that more than 20% of orthopedic diseases in dogs are due to dietary origins, with more than 22% of these showing up in dogs under 1 year of age.[8]

It is well documented that the incidence of skeletal disease, including osteochondrosis, hypertrophic osteodystrophy and hip dysplasia, is markedly increased in the growing large breed dog if management practices are such that this maximal genetic potential for rate of growth is realized.[7] The primary management practice affecting growth rate and ultimately skeletal disease is nutritional support.[7]

The primary nutritional considerations implicated in skeletal disease development in growing large breed dogs are dietary concentrations of protein, energy and calcium.[7] To ensure a slower growth rate, energy intake needs to be managed through measured feedings and monitoring BCS to maintain a lean body weight. A minimum of 2 meals should be fed daily, while 3–4 meals may be more appropriate for some dogs.[2] Slight underfeeding of energy during growth will slow the overall rate, but has not been shown to negatively impact the final adult size of the dog.[8]

Hip Dysplasia (CHD)

Hip dysplasia is a common, heritable developmental orthopedic disease. Studies have shown that dysplastic dogs are born with normal hips, but develop hip dysplasia as a result of growth disparity during their first 6 months of life.[8] Abnormal development of the hip joint results due to disparity between the strength of the soft tissues supporting the joint and the increasing biomechanical forces associated with weight gain. This causes the coxofemoral joint to not "fit" properly; this subluxation causes remodeling of the joint including a shallowing of the acetabulum (hip socket in the pelvis), a flattening of the femoral head and eventually osteoarthritis.[6,7] Hip dysplasia can affect any breed but is more prevalent in large breed dogs, and is generally accepted as polygenic in its inheritance.[6,7] This means that the disease is not caused by one gene but by a combination of multiple genes and outside factors, and predisposition is genetic.

A controlled study conducted on Labrador Retrievers showed that significantly less hip joint laxity and a lower incidence of hip dysplasia was seen in the group of dogs receiving 25% less food than their pair-mates. The food restricted group grew at a slower rate than those receiving 25% more food; this is believed to be the reason for the significant decrease in hip dysplasia.[5,6] In the food restricted group, 16 of 24 dogs developed osteoarthritis with the mean age of onset of 13.3 years, for the unrestricted group 19 of 24 dogs developed osteoarthritis with the mean age of onset being 10.3 years.[5]

Diet will not cure hip dysplasia once it has developed, but it can affect the phenotypic expression if growth rates are managed in at risk puppies by optimizing the development of the hip joints during early growth.[8]

Osteochondrosis (OCD)

Osteochondrosis is a focal area of disruption in the endochondral ossification and is characterized by impaired maturation of chondrocytes and delayed cartilage mineralization.[6,9] If this disturbance occurs in articular cartilage (that cartilage lining moving joints) then OCD may develop.[8] The most commonly affected joints are the shoulder, elbow, hock and stifle. Acute pain and swelling is seen in the affected areas with stiffness and lameness aggravated by exercise often results.[6]

It is believed that over-nutrition as the result of too much energy being taken in, or a food enriched with calcium, whether from ad lib feeding, over-calculation of measured feeding or addition of supplements, helps to stimulate skeletal growth, bone remodeling and weight gain in breeds already having a genetic potential for rapid growth.[8,9] This combination of rapid growth and remodeling weakens the subchondral region in its support of the cartilage surface.[9] The increasing body weight exerts excessive biomechanical forces on the cartilage and leads to secondary disturbances in chondrocyte nutrition, metabolism, function and viability.[9] Acute inflammatory joint disease begins when the subchondral bone is exposed to synovial fluid. Inflammatory mediators and cartilage fragments are released into the joint and perpetuate the cycle of degenerative joint disease.[9] In a rapidly growing puppy, over-nutrition can result in a mismatch between body weight and skeletal growth which can lead to overloading of the skeletal structures.[9]

Dietary modifications at an early stage can positively influence the spontaneous resolution of disturbed endochondral ossification. Dietary modifications will not normalize cases of OCD in which severe of complete detachment of the cartilage in the joint has already occurred.[8]

What to Feed

Over-nutrition to achieve maximal growth rate causes excessive bodyweight which overloads the young skeleton and may contribute to the development of skeletal disorders.[6] Since fats contain over twice the caloric density of protein and carbohydrates, a diet lower in fat is recommended for large and giant breed puppies.[6]

A BCS of 2–3/5, or 4/9 should be maintained throughout puppy hood. Limiting energy intake to maintain these physical parameters will not affect the dog's final adult size, but it will reduce food intake, fecal output, obesity and the risk of skeletal disease.[9]

Protein has not been shown to have any negative consequences on calcium metabolism or skeletal development in the dog.[9] A minimum level of protein in the diet depends on digestibility, amino acid profile and bioavailability and should at minimum meet the AAFCO recommendations for growth.[9]

The absolute level of calcium rather than a calcium/phosphorus imbalance is responsible for negatively influencing skeletal development.[9] Young, large breed dogs fed a diet high in calcium have a significant increase in incidence of developmental skeletal disease.[9] Large breed puppies should not be switched to an adult maintenance diet too early, because of the difference in energy density between a puppy and adult diet; the puppy would actually consume more calcium in an adult diet because it would need to eat more to meet its energy needs.[9] Under no circumstances should these puppies receive calcium supplements.[9]

Feedings Regimens

A combination of time-restricted and measured feedings are recommended for large and giant breed puppies.[9] Because of their steep growth curve, measured feedings may not be able to keep up with their energy requirements, and frequent body weight checks and caloric recalculations would be necessary to provide the proper amount of food. When combined with time-restricted feedings offered 2–3 times/day, enough energy can be provided for growth, but not too much as would be seen with ad lib feeding.[9] Frequent assessment of BCS will help to determine the proper amount of food to offer the puppy.

Table 23.1 Nutrient profiles[10]

Small breed puppy food dry
Caloric distribution (% ME)

Protein	29%
Fat	46%
Carbohydrate	25%
Calories	485 kcal/cup

Large breed puppy food dry
Caloric distribution (% ME)

Protein	25%
Fat	36%
Carbohydrate	39%
Calories	362 kcal/cup

Table 23.1 (Continued)

Adult maintenance food dry

Caloric distribution (% ME)

Protein	24%
Fat	38%
Carbohydrate	38%
Calories	405 kcal/cup

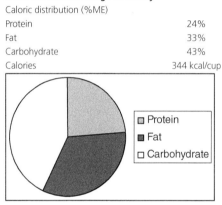

Adult maintenance large breed dry

Caloric distribution (%ME)

Protein	24%
Fat	33%
Carbohydrate	43%
Calories	344 kcal/cup

If puppies are fed based on energy requirements, activity levels and body condition, growth diets do not increase the risk of developmental bone disease in large and giant breed dogs.[9] It is not only important to feed the appropriate diet, but to feed the diet appropriately! (Table 23.1).[9]

References

1 LeGrand-Defretin V, Munday HS (1995) Feeding dogs and cats for life. In I Burger (ed.), *The Waltham Book of Companion Animal Nutrition*, pp. 63–4, Tarrytown, NY: Elsevier.

2 Delaney S, Fascetti A (2012) Feeding the healthy dog and cat. In S Delaney, A Fascetti (eds), *Applied Veterinary Clinical Nutrition*. Delaney, p. 84, Ames, IA: Wiley-Blackwell.

3 Gross KL, Debraekeleer J, Zicker SC (2000) Normal dogs. In MS Hand, CD Thatcher, RL Remillard, P Roudebush (eds), *Small Animal Clinical Nutrition* (4th edn), pp. 247–50, Marceline, MO: Walsworth Publishing.

4 Case LP, Carey DP, Hirakawa DA, Daristotle L (2000) Growth. In *Canine and Feline Nutrition* (2nd edn), pp. 245–54, St Louis, MO: Mosby.

5 Kealy RD, Lawler DF, Ballam JM *et al.* (2002) Effects of diet restriction on life span and age related changes in dogs, *JAVMA*, **220**(9), May 1: 1315–20.

6 Kuhlman G, Biourge V (1997) Nutrition of the large and giant breed dog with emphasis on skeletal development, *Veterinary Clinical Nutrition* **4**(3): 89–95.

7 Lepine AJ, Reinhart GA (1998) Feeding the growing large breed dog. In *Clinical Nutrition Symposium XXIII Congress of the World Small Animal Veterinary Association*. Buenos Aires, Argentina, October 6, pp. 12–16.

8 Hazewinkel H, Mott J (2006) Main nutritional imbalances implicated in osteoarticular diseases. In Pibot P; Biourge V; Elliott D (eds), *Encyclopedia of Canine Clinical Nutrition*, pp. 348–79. Aimargues, France: Aniwa SAS.

9 Richardson DC (1999) Developmental orthopedics: Nutritional influences in the dog. In SJ Ettinger, EC Feldman (eds), *Textbook of Veterinary Internal Medicine, Diseases of the Dog and Cat* (4th edn), pp. 252–8, Philadelphia, PA: Saunders.

10 Eukanuba Veterinary Diets, Product Reference Guide 2003, pp. 69–71.

24 Growth in Cats

Introduction

Unlike dogs, cats do not have a wide variety of sizes or shapes and they do not have as rapid of a growth phase. But like dogs, they should be fed to achieve normal growth and development.[1] Nutrient and energy needs during this phase of life exceed those for any other period, except lactation, with the most rapid growth occurring during the first 3–6 months of life.[2]

Normal Growth

As young animals, kittens have a small physical capacity for food. Because of this it is recommended to feed energy dense foods, and to feed them frequently.[3] The ultimate goal of feeding kittens is to ensure a healthy adult cat. The objective being to optimize growth, minimize risk factors for disease and achieve optimal health.[4] Energy requirements are highest at about 10 weeks of age and after this point the energy requirements per unit of body weight gradually decreases, although they remain relatively high for at least the first 6 months of life.[3] Most cats will achieve skeletal maturity at about 10 months of age even though all growth plates may not have closed by this time.[4] Additional weight gain may occur after 12 months of age, and represents a phase of maturation and muscle development.[4] In kittens, excessive growth rates do not cause the same orthopedic problems that we see associated with rapid growth in dogs.[5] However, deposition of excessive fat cells (adipocytes) during this phase of growth may predispose the cat to obesity throughout its life. Once a fat cell has been formed it will remain with the animal throughout the rest of its life, and will continue to secrete hormones that encourage fat deposition.

Growing kittens have high energy requirements to meet the needs of rapid growth, thermoregulation and maintenance.[4] Feeding an energy dense food allows for smaller volumes to be consumed to satisfy caloric needs.[4] However, growing cats with BCS of 4/5 or 6/9 should be fed foods with lower energy density to prevent obesity. The prevalence of obesity increase after 1 year of age, and over-nutrition is more of a problem in most kittens than under-nutrition.[4] Kittens should be fed a diet that meets the nutrient and energy requirements for growth or all life stages.[5]

There is no evidence that the age of neutering alters the rate of growth. Unfortunately, energy requirements do decline with neutering, increasing the risk of obesity if energy intake is not adjusted.[4] As neutering is typically performed between 6 and 12 months of age, as the caloric requirements are decreasing as the animal matures, there is also a corresponding decrease in caloric requirements secondary to the neutering procedure.[5]

Obesity should be prevented in young cats as this increases the number of fat cells capable of storing fat as the cat enters adulthood. Neutering reduces energy requirements by 24–33% regardless of age of neutering.[4] The food intake or caloric requirements should be adjusted immediately after neutering, and including this information on surgical discharge instructions would be helpful to the owners. Kittens and juvenile cats that were previously fed ad lib should be transitioned to measured feeding to help prevent weight gain. Also changing the food from energy dense, growth diets to low fat, lower energy dense food can help to prevent weight gain after neutering.[5] Total energy intake can be decreased as much as 25% after neutering.

What to Feed

The requirement for protein is already relatively high for the adult cat; it is even higher for growing kittens

---

Nutrition and Disease Management for Veterinary Technicians and Nurses, Second Edition. Ann Wortinger, Kara M. Burns
© 2015 John Wiley & Sons, Inc. Published 2015 by John Wiley & Sons, Inc.
Companion Website: www.wiley.com/go/wortinger/nutrition

by about 10%.[3] At least 19% of the protein should be from an animal source to ensure adequate amounts of the sulfur-containing amino acids (i.e. taurine, cysteine, methionine), which are required in larger amounts in kittens than in other species.[4] Taurine has a well-documented role in reproduction and growth, and all foods for growing kittens should contain adequate amounts.[4] Rapid tissue formation associated with growth accounts for much of the increased protein needs for young cats.[2] The actual percentage of protein found in the diet is not as important as the balance between protein and energy found in the food.[2] The AAFCO recommends a minimum protein level of 26% ME, with optimal levels being as high as 29% ME.[2,4]

Dietary fats provide energy, fat-soluble vitamins and essential fatty acids to growing cats. Kittens can tolerate foods with a wide variety of fat contents, but when given a choice they will usually go with the food with the higher fat content. Optimal growth rates are also achieved with diet containing higher levels of fats.[6]

The essential fatty acids linoleic acid and arachidonic acid are required by all cats, especially those that are still growing. Increasing evidence has shown the importance of the omega 3 fatty acids, DHA (docosahexaenoic acid) and EPA (eicosapentaenoic acid) in growth. DHA is made in the body from alpha-linolenic acid and is required for normal neural, retinal and auditory development in kittens.[6] Conversion of alpha-linolenic acid to DHA is inefficient and affected by age, therefore supplementing amounts in the food is recommended to ensure adequate intake.[2]

Deficiencies in energy, protein, essential fatty acids, certain vitamins and minerals have been shown to negatively affect a growing cat's immune system decreasing their immune response and defense.[2] Adequate levels of antioxidants included in the food help support the immune system and have the potential to enhance the immune response. The most widely used nutrients that have antioxidant activity include vitamin E, beta-carotene (provitamin A), lutein (another carotenoid antioxidant), vitamin C, flavonoids, zinc and selenium.[2]

Carbohydrates are not required in the food used for growing kittens as long as sufficient gluconeogenic amino acids are available.[4] Cats can readily digest carbohydrates, though feeding a diet high in poorly digestible carbohydrates may result in flatulence, bloating and diarrhea.[4] This can often be seen in kittens fed cow's milk after weaning. Cow's milk has higher levels of lactose than does cat's milk, and after weaning a kitten's level of lactase, the enzyme that breaks down lactose declines.[4] This leads to incomplete digestion of the lactose, causing digestive upset in the cat.

The palatability of the food should be good enough to ensure adequate energy intake, with a digestibility of at least 80%, and protein digestibility of at least 85%.[4] A high-quality commercial kitten food that has been shown to be adequate for growth through AAFCO feeding trials is recommended.[1] Supplementation of this diet is not recommended and should not be necessary.[1]

Table 24.1 Nutrient profiles[7]

Kitten food dry
Caloric distribution (% ME)

Protein	31%
Fat	48%
Carbohydrate	21%
Calories	568 kcal/cup

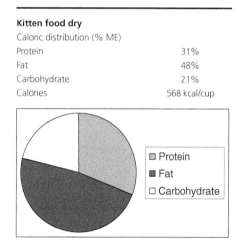

Cat adult maintenance dry
Caloric distribution (% ME)

Protein	30%
Fat	46%
Carbohydrate	24%
Calories	536 kcal/cup

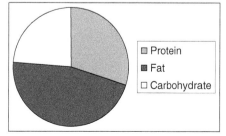

It is better to change to a food specifically formulated for kittens than to try balancing an inappropriate food.[4] A balanced kitten food can be fed until kittens reach adulthood at approximately 10–12 months of age, though feeding amounts should be adjusted to maintain an ideal BCS.[4] If a young adult cat is showing signs of obesity, they can be switched to a balanced adult diet by 6 months of age.[3]

Feeding Regimens

Free choice feeding is often preferred with kittens because it reduces the risk of underfeeding and reduces the marked gastric distension that sometimes accompanies rapid meal feeding in kittens.[4] This feeding method may not be a good option if older cats are in the house, as they may push the kitten away from the food and eat it all themselves. Measured feedings can be used in a mixed age household if 2–3 meals per day are offered and everyone is fed in separate areas to allow the kitten to eat unharassed.

A good option with a kitten in a house of older cats is to either separate the kitten at meal times, or to make an area that is accessible to the kitten but not to the older cats and place the food there. This can be as easy using a plastic or cardboard box, turning it upside down and cutting a size-appropriate hole in the box. Place the box where it can not be tipped over, and put the food inside out of reach of the older cats.

Body condition scores should continue to be done, and food intake adjusted to maintain at 3/5 or 4–5/9 BCS throughout kittenhood and into adulthood. Obesity is much easier to prevent than to treat (Table 24.1).

References

1 Case LP, Carey DP, Hirakawa DA, Daristotle L (2000) Growth. In *Canine and Feline Nutrition* (2nd edn), p. 245, St Louis, MO: Mosby.
2 Case LP, Daristotle L, Hayek MG, Raasch MF (2011) Growth. In *Canine and Feline Nutrition* (3rd edn), pp. 221–33, St Louis, MO: Mosby.
3 LeGrand-Defretin V, Munday HS (1995) Feeding dogs and cats for life. In I Burger (ed.), *The Waltham Book of Companion Animal Nutrition*, pp. 64–5, Tarrytown, NY: Elsevier.
4 Kirk CL, Debraekeleer J, Armstrong PJ (2000) Normal cats. In MS Hand, CD Thatcher, RL Remillard, P Roudebush (eds), *Small Animal Clinical Nutrition* (4th edn), Marceline, MO: Walsworth Publishing.
5 Delaney S, Fascetti A (2012) Feeding the healthy dog and cat. In S Delaney, A Fascetti (eds), *Applied Veterinary Clinical Nutrition*. Delaney, p. 84, Ames, IA: Wiley-Blackwell.
6 Gross KL, Becvarova I, Debraekeleer J (2010) Feeding growing kittens: Postweaning to adulthood. In MS Hand, CD Thatcher, RL Remillard *et al.* (eds), *Small Animal Clinical Nutrition* (5th edn), pp. 429–34, Marceline, MO: Walsworth Publishing.
7 Eukanuba Veterinary Diets, Product Reference Guide 2003, p. 77.

25 Adult Maintenance in Dogs

Introduction

Dogs that have reached mature adult size and are not pregnant, lactating or working strenuously are defined as being in a state of maintenance.[1] Depending on breed, these are usually dogs between 1 and 7 years of age. Some breeds mature more slowly, and do not reach their full mature size until 18–24 months of age, while others are full grown by 10 months of age.[1,2]

Most companion dogs live indoors in a temperate environment. They are usually not pregnant or lactating, not involved in regular work or excessive exercise and are not subject to extremes of temperature.[3] For an animal in maintenance the diet must:

- provide the correct amount, balance and availability of nutrients to sustain physical and mental health and activity;
- promote peak condition and therefore reduce the dog's susceptibility to disease;
- be sufficiently nutrient dense to allow the animal to meet it nutrient requirements by eating an amount within the limits set by appetite;
- be sufficiently palatable to ensure an adequate intake.[3]

Requirements

The ultimate goal of any maintenance diet is to minimize risk factors for disease, and achieve optimal health. Maintenance of ideal BCS has been shown to increase the quality and quantity of life in dogs.[4] It is much easier to keep an animal lean than to work on weight loss after they have become overweight or obese. Once a fat cell has formed, it will never go away, even when emptied due to dieting. It will also try very hard to maintain the stored contents, making weight loss even more of a challenge.

Healthy adult dogs have relatively small nutrient requirements when compared to those in the reproductive stages of life. They may be maintained for years on a wide range of diets with little apparent consequences.[5] The probability of a diet related problem should be lower for dogs fed properly formulated commercial diets due to the AAFCO testing required. Dogs that are fed homemade diets or those that haven't undergone AAFCO certification would pose significantly higher risks for diet related problems. Just because an adverse consequence has not been seen in a single animal does not mean that a diet provides superior nutrition.[5] Remember AAFCO requirements provide the minimal levels to sustain a dog; you cannot feed minimal foods and expect optimal results.

The guidelines printed on pet food labels provide an estimate of the amount of food to feed an average adult dog that is living indoors and provided with moderate amounts of exercise.[1] These estimates may not take into consideration whether the animal is neutered or intact, if they engage in 2 walks a day, or are confined to the yard and go on no walks. These amounts are guidelines at best, and adjustments would need to be made based on each individual animal. An estimate of the amount to feed can also be calculated using the dog's ideal body weight, with adjustments in intake being made based on changes in BCS. An animal housed outside of these conditions may require more of less food than recommended. Label guidelines are also based on the food being the only source of nutrition for the dog; this means that no treats, snacks or table food are being fed. The addition of these foods can significantly change the amount of food that the dog actually requires. Current recommendations are that additional sources of nutrition (i.e. snacks) not compose more than 10% of the entire caloric intake.[2]

A wide variety of foods are not necessary for most dogs, picky eaters are made by the owner not by the

Nutrition and Disease Management for Veterinary Technicians and Nurses, Second Edition. Ann Wortinger, Kara M. Burns
© 2015 John Wiley & Sons, Inc. Published 2015 by John Wiley & Sons, Inc.
Companion Website: www.wiley.com/go/wortinger/nutrition

breeder. Most dogs are best managed on a diet of balanced dog food with a constant supply of fresh, clean water.[1] Frequent changes in the diet can result in gastrointestinal tract upset with resulting diarrhea or vomiting. The cause for these GI upsets can usually be traced back to lack of digestive enzymes to meet the diet formula. The body does not have unlimited amounts of enzymes in place at all times. If will usually take 5–7 days for the enzyme production to be adjusted to meet the new diet's requirements.

Sometimes these changes can be seen when feeding a lower quality commercial brand of food, which utilizes a variable feed formula as opposed to a fixed feed formula. With a variable feed formula, the ingredient amounts and types can vary from batch to batch based on market conditions or product availability. As long as the product conforms to the minimums and maximums listed on the guaranteed analysis, the manufacturers can do this. With a fixed feed formula, the ingredients do not change but remain constant from batch to batch. Unfortunately, this information is not listed on the label, and can only be obtained by contacting the manufacturer.

Owners should be encouraged to weigh their dog every month or so, with adjustments in intake based on any changes seen. Dogs who are nutritionally well managed are alert, have ideal BCS (3/5, 4–5/9) with a stable, normal body weight, a healthy coat and able to maintain an active lifestyle. Stools should be firm, well-formed and a medium to dark brown in color.[2,4]

Stress

Stress can affect the caloric intake of a dog in a number of ways. It is not uncommon for working or boarding dogs to refuse to eat for no apparent reason. Conversely, a dog's appetite may improve with the addition of another dog to the household. If one dog is more dominant and allowed to control access to the food dish, weight loss may be seen in one dog, with weight gain seen in the other.[2]

Environmental stress can also change energy requirements. In a hot environment increased water intake can be seen to help with cooling. In colder environments, dogs kept outdoors, even within shelters, need increased energy intake to maintain their body temperatures.[2] If a

change is seen in appetite or BCS, look at possible stressors within the dog's environment.

Obesity

Studies indicate that up to 60% of dogs within the United States seen by veterinarians were overweight or obese (BCS 4–5/5, 7–9/9).[6] By definition, obesity is the accumulation of an excessive amount of body fat.[4] Excess body weight is by far the most prominent form of malnutrition seen in companion animals.

Risk factors associated with obesity include:
• middle age;
• neuter status;
• low activity;
• high-fat, high calorie foods.

Obesity occurs twice as often in neutered dogs than in intact dogs. Neutering does not appear to have a marked impact on resting energy expenditure of female dogs; however it can significantly increase food intake.[2] This may be due to a reduction of the appetite-suppressing hormone estrogen.[2] A decrease in physical activity is also assumed to occur in many dogs after neutering and may play a more important role in weight gain for male dogs due to decreased roaming activity.[2]

Obesity has been linked to increased incidence of diabetes mellitus, lameness and degenerative joint disease, and skin disease. By preventing the occurrence of these diseases, we can in turn increase the quality and quantity of life our dogs can have.[4]

It is much easier to prevent an obese animal than it is to treat obesity once it has occurred. Following BCS in puppyhood to get an adult in the normal to lean range is the best way to prevent obesity later in life. True obesity is the direct result of consumption of too much energy without a corresponding increase in activity level (Table 25.1).

Table 25.1 Influence of age on daily energy requirements (DER) for dogs[7]

Age in years	DER adjustment
1–2	1.7–2.0 × RER
3–7	1.14–1.9 × RER
>7	1.1–1.7 × RER

Table 25.2 Calculating daily energy requirements (DER)

1 Determine ideal maintenance body weight in kilograms.
2 Determine RER using this number.
3 Determine DER by multiplying RER by the estimated adjustment factor based on age and activity.
4 Determine the caloric density of the food.
5 Take the DER divide it by the caloric density to determine volume to feed/day.
6 Divide this volume by the desired number of feedings/day.

Example: Zeus is a 5-year-old beagle who weighs 25 lb, with an ideal BCS of 3/5. His owner wants to switch his food and needs help with determining the volume to feed. Zeus is a house beagle, who has access to the outdoors, but doesn't go on many walks. The new food has a caloric density of 254 kcal/cup.

1 25 lb/ 2.2 = 11.36 kg
2 RER = (wt in kg × 30) + 70 (or whichever formula you prefer)
   (11.36 × 30) + 70 = 411 kcal/day
3 411 kcal/day × 1.4 (low activity level for age) = 575 kcal/day
4 254 kcal/cup
5 575/254 = 2.25 cups/day
6 3 meals/day = 2.25/ 3 = 0.75 cup/meal

What to Feed

While owners are directly responsible for selecting what food is fed to their dogs, recommendations should be made by and sought from the veterinary team. Ad lib or free choice feeding has been associated with obesity, but may be of benefit for those shy animals who may not have unlimited access to the food dish due to the presence of a more dominate animal or activity levels within the house disrupting feeding time.

Measured and timed feeding will help to control the volume of food a dog consumes, but unless the appropriate amount is determined, the animal can easily become over or under weight. Working with clients to determine the ideal food for that dog as well as an appropriate amount to feed and feeding method to use is part of our jobs. A good starting point when doing energy calculation is to determine RER at desired body weight. DER is calculated by taking 1.0–1.6 × RER to determine estimated caloric intake. The caloric density of the food will need to be used to calculate the desired volume to feed. This can be found either from the product reference guide, an internet search or by contacting the manufacturer.[7] Regular contact with clients with BCS and weight checks of dogs can help to control food related weight issues ensuring we can keep them healthy and happy for as long as possible (Table 25.2).

References

1 Case LP, Carey DP, Hirakawa DA, Daristotle L (2000) Adult maintenance. In *Canine and Feline Nutrition* (2nd edn), pp. 255–6, St Louis, MO: Mosby.
2 Gross KL, Debraekeleer J, Zicker SC (2000) Normal dogs. In MS Hand, CD Thatcher, RL Remillard, P Roudebush (eds), *Small Animal Clinical Nutrition* (4th edn), pp. 219–29, Marceline, MO: Walsworth Publishing.
3 JM Wills (1996) Adult maintenance. In *Manual of Companion Animal Nutrition and Feeding*, pp. 44–6, Ames, IA: Iowa State University Press.
4 Delaney S, Fascetti A (2012) Feeding the healthy dog and cat. In S Delaney, A Fascetti (eds), *Applied Veterinary Clinical Nutrition*. p. 85, Ames, IA: Wiley-Blackwell.
5 Buffington CA, Holloway C, Abood SK (204) Normal dogs. In *Manual of Veterinary Dietetics*, pp. 15–18, St Louis, MO: Saunders Burkholder.
6 Burkholder WJ, Toll PW (2000) Obesity. In MS Hand, CD Thatcher, RL Remillard, P Roudebush (eds), *Small Animal Clinical Nutrition* (4th edn), pp. 401–9, Marceline, MO: Walsworth Publishing.
7 Debraekeleer J, Gross KL, Zicker S (2010) Feeding young adult dogs: Before middle age. In MS Hand, CD Thatcher, RL Remillard *et al.* (eds), *Small Animal Clinical Nutrition* (5th edn), p. 260, Marceline, MO: Walsworth Publishing.

26 Adult Maintenance in Cats

Introduction

Cats that reached mature adult size and are not pregnant, lactating or working strenuously are defined as being in a state of maintenance.[1] Cats generally reach adult size between 10–12 months of age, and reach their full mature weight by 18 months. Adult maintenance is usually the time from 12 month to 8 years.[2]

Most companion cats live indoors in temperate environments. They are usually not pregnant or lactating, not involved in regular work or excessive exercise and are not subject to extremes of temperature.[3] For an animal in maintenance the diet must:

- provide the correct amount; balance and availability of nutrients to sustain physical and mental health and activity;
- promote peak condition and therefore reduce its susceptibility to disease;
- be sufficiently nutrient dense to allow the animal to meet it nutrient requirements by eating an amount within the limits set by appetite;
- be sufficiently palatable to ensure an adequate intake.[3]

Requirements

The ultimate goal of any maintenance diet is to minimize risk factors for disease, and achieve optimal health and longevity of life. Healthy adult cats have relatively small nutrient requirements when compared to those in the reproductive stages of life. They may be maintained for years on a wide range of diets with little apparent consequences.[4] The probability of a diet related problem should be lower for cats fed properly formulated commercial diets due to the AAFCO testing required. Cats that are fed homemade diets or those that are fed diets that haven't undergone AAFCO certification would pose significantly higher risks for diet related problems. Just because an adverse consequence has not been seen in a single animal does not mean that a diet provides superior nutrition.[4] Remember that AAFCO requirements provide minimal levels of nutrients. You cannot feed a minimal diet and expect optimal results.

It has been shown that for dogs, maintaining a lean BCS throughout their lives increases the quality and quantity of their lives. We could safely surmise that these conditions would also benefit cats by avoiding conditions that contribute to early mortality such as diabetes mellitus, lameness, cardiac disease and skin diseases.[5]

The guidelines printed on pet food labels provide an estimate of the amount of food to feed an average adult cat that is living indoors and provided with moderate amounts of exercise.[1] An estimate of the amount to feed can also be calculated using the cat's ideal body weight, with adjustments in intake being made based on changes in BCS. An animal housed outside of these conditions may require more or less food than recommended. Label guidelines are also based on the food being the only source of nutrition for the cat; this means that no treats, snacks or table food are being fed. The addition of these foods can significantly change the amount of food that the cat actually requires. Current recommendations are that additional sources of nutrition not compose more than 10% of the entire caloric intake.[2]

A wide variety of foods are not necessary for most cats, picky eaters are not born but made by the owner. Most cats are best managed on a diet of balanced cat food with a constant supply of fresh, clean water.[1] Frequent changes in the diet can result in gastrointestinal tract

Nutrition and Disease Management for Veterinary Technicians and Nurses, Second Edition. Ann Wortinger, Kara M. Burns
© 2015 John Wiley & Sons, Inc. Published 2015 by John Wiley & Sons, Inc.
Companion Website: www.wiley.com/go/wortinger/nutrition

upset with resulting diarrhea or vomiting. The cause for these GI upsets can usually be traced back to lack of digestive enzymes to meet the diet formula. The body does not have unlimited amounts of enzymes in place at all times. It will usually take 5–7 days for the enzyme production to be adjusted to meet the new diet requirements.

Sometimes these changes can be seen when feeding a lower quality commercial brand of food that utilizes a variable feed formula as opposed to a fixed feed formula. With a variable feed formula, the contents can vary from batch to batch based on market conditions or product availability. As long as the product conforms to the minimums and maximums listed on the guaranteed analysis, the manufacturers can do this. With a fixed feed formula, the ingredients do not change but remain constant from batch to batch. Unfortunately, this information is not listed on the label, and can only be obtained by contacting the manufacturer.

Neutering reduces the daily energy requirements by 24–33% compared to intact animals.[2] This decrease does not appear to be affected by age of neutering. The reduction in energy requirements are most likely due to a reduction in basal metabolic rate, since obvious changes in behavior and activity are usually not seen after neutering especially in young cats.[2]

By nature, cats do not usually participate in heavy work or endurance-like activities, thus the variation in energy requirements between active and sedentary cats is small when compared to dogs.[2] Even considering this, a twofold increase can be seen between sedentary and active cats' energy requirements (DER = RER x 2). Food intake should be adjusted according to activity level to maintain a BCS of 3/5, 4–5/9.

Sedentary, inactive, caged or older cats often have energy requirements very near or even below the average resting energy requirement. (DER = RER × 1 or less) Cats with unlimited activity may have energy needs 10–15% above normal.[2] Very active or "high-strung" cats may have markedly higher energy expenditures than normal cats, as much as 30% higher than average.[2]

Although different breeds of cats may have varying nutritional requirements, this variation is less pronounced than that seen with dog breeds.[2] Some of the more active breeds, such as Abyssinians and Siamese, may have higher energy requirements, while others such as Persians or Rag dolls tend to be very tranquil and expend little energy above maintenance.[2] Disposition tends to affect energy requirements more than does breed.

Cats that are provided proper nutrition are healthy and alert, have ideal body condition and stable weight, and have a clean, glossy hair coat. The owners should ideally evaluate BCS every 2 weeks, and daily monitor daily food and water intake and observe the cat's interest in food and its appetite. Stools should be evaluated regularly for changes in frequency or character, with normal stools being firm, well-formed and medium to dark brown in color.[2]

Canned versus Dry Food

One of our most prevalent controversies in feeding cats currently involves the discussion on whether canned or dry food diets are better for the cat. We know that cats evolved eating a meat-based diet, and in fact, due to their classification of obligate carnivores require meat in their diets to meet their essential nutrient requirements.[6] We also know that cats produce amylase as a pancreatic enzyme and are able to digest and utilize carbohydrates for energy.[5]

In the wild (which our current companions are not in) cats consumed few carbohydrates, other than those already consumed by their preferred prey.[6] Small rodents such as moles, voles and field mice make up 40% or more of a feral domestic cats diet, supplemented with young wild rabbits and hares, birds, reptiles, frogs and insects making up the remaining portion of the diet.[7] The average mouse contains approximately 30 kcals of metabolizable energy. For an active (DER = RER × 1.7–2.0), 12 lb cat, this would be an average caloric intake of 370–440 kcals/day. This would be approximately 12–15 mice/day (Table 26.1).[7] Since cats eat 10–20 small meals a day, this works out well for most cats in the wild. How do we translate these behaviors and physiologic needs into a process that works for humans?

Proponents of canned food diets cite the documented increase in water consumption that occurs when feeding a canned food diet. With canned food diets having about 80% moisture as opposed to 8–10% found in dry food diet. This increase in water intake may be helpful in prevention of urinary tract problems and may decrease

Table 26.1 Nutrient levels found in a rat carcass[7]

Nutrient	Rat carcass
Moisture %	63.6
Protein %	55
Fat %	38.1
Carbohydrate %	1.2

food intake and help prevent obesity due to the dilution of calories with water.[5]

One other advantage cited for feeding canned food diets is the nutrient profile typically found in these diets. They tend to be higher protein, lower carbohydrate diets that more accurately reflect the nutrient profile found in their wild prey. A typical mouse only contains 3–5% carbohydrates.[7] Canned food diets can have as few carbohydrates as 0%, but may also contain as much as that found in dry food diets. This would really depend on the ingredients, and one cannot automatically assume that all canned food diets contain a low-carbohydrate nutrient profile. One reason commonly given for reluctance to feed canned food diets exclusively to companion cats is the cost. With a typical 3.5 oz can containing approximately 90–100 kcals, a normal 10 lb cat would need to be fed 2.5–3.0 cans day. With the cost of each can ranging from $1 to $2/can, and most cats living in multi-cat households, this can become quite expensive very quickly.

Proponents of dry food diets cite the dental health benefits and the ability to feed a schedule more typical of their natural diet (10–20 small meals daily). Due to their processing methods, dry food diets can range from 10% to 50% carbohydrates based on metabolizable energy content.[7] Again the assumption cannot be made that all dry diets have the same nutrient composition, and that all dry food diets are inherently high in carbohydrate levels. The cost of feeding a dry food diet is significantly less expensive for owners, and is easier to feed with our busy schedules. After all, who has time to feed their cat's 10–20 small meals daily?

Cats are very sensitive to the physical form, odor and taste of their foods. Mouth feel (oral tactile sensation) is important to normal feeding behavior in cats.[7] Cats also develop fixed taste preferences early in life, and may be very reluctant to eat a food that doesn't "feel right" to them regardless of how yummy it may taste.[7] Because of this, the recommendation to owners is to feed young cats a variety of foods to increase their exposure before these fixed taste preferences are fully developed.

In general, cats prefer solid, moist foods and do not like foods that have a powdery, sticky or greasy texture. If fed a moist diet, they prefer it to be near or at normal body temperature.[7] Even with all this information we have regarding feeding and eating preferences for cats, owners will often cite a cat who will willingly eat fruits and vegetables. After all, cats are individuals too (Table 26.2).

Obesity

By definition, obesity is the accumulation of an excessive amount of body fat.[6] Excess body weight is by far the most prominent form of malnutrition seen in companion animals.

Studies indicate that up to 60% of cats within the United States seen by veterinarians were overweight or

Table 26.2 Calculating daily energy requirements (DER)

- Determine ideal maintenance body weight in kilograms.
- Determine RER using this number.
- Determine DER by multiplying RER by the estimated adjustment factor based on age and activity.
- Determine the caloric density of the food.
- Take the DER divide it by the caloric density to determine volume to feed/day.
- Divide this volume by the desired number of feedings/day.

Example:
Stryder is a 5 year old DSH who weighs 12 lb, with an ideal BCS of 3/5. His owner wants to switch his food and needs help with determining the volume to feed. Stryder is a house cat, who has access to a screened-in porch, but doesn't go outdoors. The new food has a caloric density of 479 kcal/cup.

- 12 lb/2.2 = 5.45 kg
- RER = (wt in kg x 40) (or whichever formula you prefer) (5.45 x 40)= 218 kcal/day
- 218 kcal/day x 1.3 (low activity level for age) = 284 kcal/day
- 479 kcal/cup
- 284/479 = 0.6 cups/day
- 3 meals/day = 0.6/ 3 = 0.2 cup/meal

obese (BCS 4–5/5, 7–9/9).[5,7] The highest prevalence being seen in the middle-aged cats (7–8 years old) with ~50% of this group being overweight or obese (BCS 4–5/5. 7–9/9)

Risk factors associated with obesity include:

* middle age;
* neuter status;
* low activity;
* high-fat, high calorie foods.[2]

Neutered cats have resting energy requirement 20–25% less than intact cats of similar age. In practical terms, this means that a neutered cat would require only 75–80% of the food required by an intact cat to maintain optimal body condition.[2,7]

It is much easier to prevent an obese animal than it is to treat obesity once it has occurred. Following BCS in kitten hood to get an adult in the normal to lean range is the best way to prevent obesity later in life. True obesity is the direct result of consumption of too much energy with insufficient energy expenditure.

References

1 Case LP, Carey DP, Hirakawa DA, Daristotle L (2000) Adult maintenance. In *Canine and Feline Nutrition* (2nd edn), pp. 255–6, St Louis, MO: Mosby.

2 Gross KL, Debraekeleer J, Zicker SC (2000) Normal cats. In MS Hand, CD Thatcher, RL Remillard, P Roudebush (eds), *Small Animal Clinical Nutrition* (4th edn), pp. 306–14, Marceline, MO: Walsworth Publishing.

3 Wills JM (1996) Adult maintenance. In N Kelly, J Wills (eds), *Manual of Companion Animal Nutrition and Feeding*, pp. 44–6, Ames, IA: Iowa State University Press.

4 Buffington CA, Holloway C, Abood SK (2004) Normal dogs. In *Manual of Veterinary Dietetics*, pp. 30–1, St Louis, MO: Saunders.

5 Delaney S, Fascetti A (2012) Feeding the healthy dog and cat. In S Delaney, A Fascetti (eds), *Applied Veterinary Clinical Nutrition*. Delaney, p. 85, Ames, IA: Wiley-Blackwell.

6 Pierson L (2013) *Feeding Your Cat: Know the Basics of Feline Nutrition*. http://www.catinfo.org (updated November 2013; accessed 12/01/2014).

7 Armstrong PJ, Gross KL, Becvarova I, Debraekeleer J (2010) Introduction to feeding normal cats. In MS Hand, CD Thatcher, RL Remillard *et al.* (eds), *Small Animal Clinical Nutrition* (5th edn), p. 362, Marceline, MO: Walsworth Publishing.

27 Feeding the Healthy Geriatric Dog and Cat

Introduction

Continued improvements in control of infection and nutrition in recent years has resulted in a gradual increase in the average lifespan of the companion cat and dog. The maximum lifespan of any given species has remained relatively fixed; the average lifespan within a given population can be affected by genetics, health care and nutrition.[1] It is estimated that more than 40% of the dogs and 30% of the cats in the United States are at least 6 years old, and approximately 30% of these animals are older than 11 years.[1] While we are seeing more and more older animals, it is important to remember that old age is not a disease, and if they are otherwise healthy, old age alone will not kill any animal.[2]

The average lifespan of the dog is about 13 years, with a maximal life span of 27 years. Small breeds of dogs tend to live longer than do large and giant breeds.[1]

Aging has been defined as "a complex biologic process resulting in progressive reduction of an individual's ability to maintain homeostasis under physiologic and external environmental stresses thereby decreasing the individuals viability and increasing its vulnerability to disease, and eventually death."[2] While old age is difficult to define, the aging process can vary tremendously from one individual to another. Cats appear to age more slowly than do dogs, and do not show breed differences in aging or longevity.[1] The average life span of the domestic cat is 14 years, with a maximal life span as high as 25–35 years. Healthy cats are considered to be geriatric when they are between 10–12 years old (Table 27.1).[1]

Table 27.1 Onset of old age[2,3]

Category	Body weight in pounds	Age of onset
Small	Under 20 lb	11.5 years
Medium	20–50 lb	10 years
Large	50–90 lb	8.8–9 years
Giant	Greater than 90 lb	7.5 years
Cats		12 years

Table 27.2 Most common causes of mortality in cats[9]

Cause of death	Percentage of occurrence
Cancer	35%
Kidney disease	24.9%
Heart disease	10.7%
Diabetes mellitus	7.6%

There are breed and size differences at which dogs are considered to be geriatric. We know that larger breeds tend to age more quickly than do smaller breeds, and mixed breed dogs tend to live longer than pure breeds of a similar size.[2] According to Fascetti and Delany, a survey of veterinarians revealed that clinicians believe the term "geriatric" is appropriately applied to small dogs (<20 lb) at 11.5 years of age, medium dogs (21–50 lb) at 10 years old, large breeds dogs (51–90 lb) at 9 years of age, and giant breed dogs (>90 lb) at 7.5 years old.[2] Other experts suggest that "old age" is when an animal has completed approximately 75–80% of its expected life span, or 5–7 years old (Table 27.2).[2]

Nutrition and Disease Management for Veterinary Technicians and Nurses, Second Edition. Ann Wortinger, Kara M. Burns
© 2015 John Wiley & Sons, Inc. Published 2015 by John Wiley & Sons, Inc.
Companion Website: www.wiley.com/go/wortinger/nutrition

Feeding Requirements

Though old age is not a disease, there are biologic effects of aging on the body. These include a gradual decline in the functional capacity of organs which begins shortly after the animal has reached maturity.[1] These changes occur in tissue structure and composition, rate of metabolism, cardiovascular and pulmonary function, renal and gastrointestinal tract excretion, special senses, skin, and reproductive system, virtually all functional and structural systems of the body.[3]

Different systems age at different rates and the degree of compromise that must occur before the onset of clinical signs also depends on many factors.[1] It is not unusual for more than one chronic disease to be present in a single geriatric dog or cat.[1] Because of this variability, each older animal should be assessed as an individual, using functional changes in body systems rather than chronological age to assess old age changes.[1]

In dogs and cats, the three leading causes of nonaccidental death are cancer, kidney disease and heart disease.[4]

The objectives for nutritional management of old dogs and cats are:

- enhancing the quality of life;
- delaying the onset of aging;
- extending life expectancy;
- slowing or preventing progression of disease;
- eliminating or relieving clinical signs of disease;
- maintaining optimal body condition.[3−5]

Metabolism

Dogs and cats metabolism naturally slows as they age, causing a reduction in their resting and maintenance energy requirements. This decline is due primarily to the loss of lean body mass, even without subsequent loss of body weight.[1] There also tends to be a decrease in activity level as animals age, decreasing their energy output, and also decreasing their muscular activity.[3] The degree at which these changes occur appear to be breed and size related in dogs. In cats, maintenance energy requirements remain fairly constant throughout their lives.[2] Recent studies have documented a decrease energy requirement in mature adult cats, but an increase energy requirement when these cats reached 10–12 years of age. These changes were not linear, but

continued to rise between 12–15 years of age. It has also been reported that loss of lean body mass, body fat and bone mass put an older cat at increased risk of early death, with significant changes occurring within the last year of life.[2]

The minimum nutrient requirements for older animals are probably similar to those of young to middle-aged animals.[6] Because of this, nutritional recommendations for these animals are based on risk factor management, using information obtained on other species, and good sense.[6] To date the only nutritional modification known to slow aging and increase life span is reduction in caloric intake over the life of the animal with the goal of maintaining a lean BCS.[5,6] Reducing caloric intake by 20–30% of normal while meeting essential nutrient needs reduces the aging process, cancer incidence, occurrence of renal disease and immune-mediated disease.[5,6] This means that animals should be maintained with a BCS of 3/5 or 4/9, significantly lower than what we normally see in our companion animals.

Digestion

There is little to no evidence that healthy older animals are less able to digest their food than younger animals.[3] Though changes in the digestive tract may contribute to inadequate food intake, decreased appetite, and systemic disease.[2] Structural changes in the canine digestive tract are not evident during aging and atrophy and fibrosis of the intestinal villi are seldom seen.[2] Despite histologic changes seen in older dogs, there does not appear to be any apparent loss in nutrient digestibility.[2]

Similar changes have not been well studied in cats, though several studies have demonstrated reductions in protein, fat and carbohydrate digestibility in older cats. A study conducted by Carolyn Cupp *et al.* was able to demonstrate that significant increases were seen in average life span in cats fed a diet supplemented with increased levels of antioxidants, prebiotic fibers and a blend of oils over those cats not receiving the supplemented foods.[7]

The nutrient requirements for elderly dogs and cats are the same as for their younger counterparts. There may be changes in the volume consumed to maintain their body weight as well as some adjustments needed in the way these nutrients are provided in the diet.[2]

There is no evidence that "geriatric diets" are necessary if the animal is healthy and eating a sufficient amount of a good quality diet to maintain body weight and body mass.[8]

Many geriatric diets are reduced in fat and caloric density to help prevent weight gain as activity level reduces with age. While this may be of benefit to many animals, there are some that have a difficult time maintaining their weight either due to decreased caloric intake or to decreased appetite secondary to various disease processes.[2] It would be prudent to switch these animals to a higher calorie diet, be it a kitten, puppy or recovery diet or in the case of dogs, a performance diet to enable them to meet their caloric requirements.[2]

Protein

There are no actual protein reserves in the body. All protein found in the body, with the exception of a small amount of amino acids found within each cell, is functional and plays a role in maintenance of that body. When reductions in protein reserves are seen, that is a decrease in the actual functional proteins found in the body. Due to the lack of actual protein reserves in older animal's avoidance of negative nitrogen balance is important as this indicates an additional loss of functional tissue within the body.[3] These "reserves" are used by the body to help combat stress and disease.[2]

Dietary protein should not be reduced in apparently healthy older dogs and cats. Adequate protein and energy intake are needed to sustain lean body mass, protein synthesis, and immune function.[5] An additional benefit to maintaining moderate protein concentration in foods for older animals is an increase in palatability, which may help maintain an adequate caloric intake.[5]

Evidence exists that feeding reduced protein diets to animals already showing signs of renal failure will result in an improvement in clinical signs. But there is no evidence to suggest that feeding reduced protein diets to otherwise healthy animals provides any renal protection or prevents development of chronic kidney disease.[2]

In animals with chronic kidney disease, a reduction in dietary protein may be needed to help decrease the serum/plasma urea nitrogen (BUN/SUN). The kidneys are responsible for excretion of the end products of protein catabolism, with impaired function these end products can accumulate in the blood stream and cause problems for the animal through development of uremia.[3,5] Feeding of a protein source with high biologic value will help to decrease the accumulation of these by-products. The higher the biologic value, the greater the efficiency of the protein in replenishing or maintaining tissue protein and the less, in proportion to intake, is excreted in the urine as urea.[3] A reduction of protein intake without evidence of chronic renal failure has not been shown to prevent the occurrence of renal failure and may actually cause more problems such as decreased lean body mass and decreased body weight due to decreased energy intake and increased protein catabolism or body tissues to meet the animals' protein requirements.[1,2]

Healthy older animals should receive sufficient protein to adequately meet their protein needs and avoid protein-calorie malnutrition.[5] With decreased energy intake, if these older animals are feed a diet that meets the minimum protein requirements for adult animals, they may actually be in a protein deficient (protein-calorie malnutrition).[1] Therefore older animals should be fed diets with a percentage of calories from protein slightly higher than the minimum recommended for adult maintenance.[1]

Fat

Fats provide energy, essential fatty acids, and act as a carrier for fat-soluble vitamins and improve the palatability of foods.[3] Because of their high energy density (8.5 kcal/gram), the most effective way to affect caloric intake is to modify the fat content of a diet. Although weight loss can be seen in some older animals, obesity by far is the most common problem. It has been theorized that the increase in the percentage of body fat that occurs with aging is partially due to an increased inability of the body to metabolize lipids.[1] There is also evidence that aging is associated with a gradual decline in the ability to desaturate the essential fatty acids (EFAs).[1]

Supplementing foods with antioxidants to support immune function has become commercially popular. The implication is that the supplements will slow down the aging process and reduce the likelihood of disease development.[2] We do know that certain of these supplements, such as the omega-3 fatty acids, and beta-carotene have been shown to improve the immune response in young animals, but few studies have actually been done on older animals to evaluate their response to these supplements.[2] The exception to this would be the previously mentioned study done by Dr Cupp, where using older cats, they evaluated the effects of antioxidants vitamin E and beta-carotene, and a blend of omega-3 and omega-6 fatty acids on overall life spans of cats.[7] The positive effects were statistically significant between the control and the ones fed the enhanced diet.

Certain diseases associated with obesity are also commonly seen in older animals, primarily diabetes mellitus, hypertension and heart disease as well as pancreatitis and arthritis.[3,5] The risk of death also increases significantly in older obese animals.[3,5]

Moderate to low levels of fat in the diet is indicated to reduce the risk of obesity, or treat obesity that already exists.[5] These very same animals may also have impaired fat digestion, and fat metabolism. Fats included in foods for older animals should be highly digestible and contain high levels of essential fatty acids (EFAs). Foods with lower fat levels are recommended for those animals that are obese or obese-prone, while foods with higher fat levels should be fed to thin animals (BCS < 3/5, 4/9).[2]

Fiber

Dietary fiber can promote gastrointestinal health by aiding normal motility and providing fuel for colonocytes through the production of the fatty acid butyrate. Not all dietary fibers act the same way in the intestines, some are highly digestible and can cause diarrhea (i.e. lactulose), some allow the colonic bacteria to make butyrate (i.e. beet pulp) and some are nondigestible and act as bulking agents (i.e. cellulose).[3,5]

Many older animals have problems with constipation; this can be treated in one of two ways: by increasing the bulk of the stool to increase frequency of defecation, or by feeding a low fiber food to increase digestibility and decrease stool volume and therefore colonic distention.[1,5] In refractory cases, lactulose may be added to the diet to increase the amount of water pulled into the colon, keeping the stool moister and making it easier to defecate. As it is difficult to tell which method will work best for any individual animal, all three methods may need to be tried.

Conclusion

Many older animals become very particular about their eating habits. There may be a decreased willingness to eat new foods, and it may be necessary for the owners to provide especially strong smelling or highly-palatable foods.[1] The animals may also develop very fixed food preferences; if possible owners should accommodate these provided the food provides adequate nutrition to the animal to ensure continued food intake and help prevent loss of lean body mass and weight.[1]

If a chronic disease is present that requires specific nutrient alterations such as diabetes, renal disease, arthritis or obesity, the animal should be fed a diet that is appropriate for the management of that disorder. If multiple diseases are present, feed for the most life-threatening disease.[1]

Proper care of teeth and gums is especially important as animal's age; if their mouths hurt or are a source of bacteria, this can negatively affect their overall health. As animals age, there is also a decrease in the amount of saliva that is produced, which can contribute to a decrease in food intake.[2] If owners are unable or unwilling to provide at home dental care, yearly to bi-yearly oral health care should be done through the veterinarian.[1]

Exercise is also important in the older animal to help maintain muscle tone, enhance circulation, improve gastrointestinal motility and prevent excess weight gain. The level and intensity of the exercise should be adjusted to an individual animal's physical and medical condition.[1] Keeping an animal active will help to preserve lean body mass, engage the brain to maintain mental acuity and prevent the development of obesity (Table 27.3).

Table 27.3 Practical feeding tips for geriatric dogs and cats[1]

- Provide regular geriatric health exams at least twice yearly.
- Avoid sudden changes in daily routine or diet.
- Feed a diet that contains high-quality protein formulated for adult animals.
- Use measured feedings to help prevent obesity and maintain ideal body weight.
- Provide a moderate amount of regular exercise.
- Maintain proper dental health with home care and regular dental cleanings.
- If needed, provide a therapeutic diet to help manage or treat a disease.

References

1 Case LP, Carey DP, Hirakawa DA, Daristotle L (2000) Geriatrics. In *Canine and Feline Nutrition* (2nd edn), pp. 275–86, St Louis, MO: Mosby.

2 Delaney S, Fascetti A (2012) Feeding the healthy dog and cat. In S Delaney, A Fascetti (eds), *Applied Veterinary Clinical Nutrition*, pp. 85–6, Ames, IA: Wiley-Blackwell.

3 Anderson RS (1996) Feeding older pets. In N Kelly, J Wills (eds), *Manual of Companion Animal Nutrition and Feeding*, pp. 93–8, Ames, IA: Iowa State University Press.

4 Gross KL, Debraekeleer J, Zicker SC (2000) Normal dogs. In MS Hand, CD Thatcher, RL Remillard, P Roudebush (eds), *Small Animal Clinical Nutrition* (4th edn), pp. 229–32, Marceline MO: Walsworth Publishing.

5 Gross KL, Debraekeleer J, Zicker, Steven C (2000) Normal cats. In MS Hand, CD Thatcher, RL Remillard, P Roudebush (eds), *Small Animal Clinical Nutrition* (4th edn), pp. 314–20, Marceline, MO: Walsworth Publishing.

6 Kealy RD, Lawler DF, Ballam JM *et al.* (2002) Effects of diet restriction on life span and age related changes in dogs, *JAVMA* **220**(9), May 1: 1315–20.

7 Cupp C, Jean-Phillipe C, Kerr W, *et al.* (2006) Effect of nutritional interventions on longevity of senior cats, *International Journal of Applied Research in Veterinary Medicine* **4**(1): 34–50.

8 Buffington CA, Holloway C, Abood SK (2004) Normal dogs. In *Manual of Veterinary Dietetics*, pp. 21–3, St Louis, MO: Saunders.

9 Gross KL, Becvarova I, Debraekeleer J (2010) Feeding mature adult cats: Middle aged and older. In MS Hand, CD Thatcher, RL Remillard *et al.* (eds), *Small Animal Clinical Nutrition* (5th edn), p. 394, Marceline, MO: Walsworth Publishing.

28 Performance and Dogs

Introduction

People have spent much time and energy over the years molding dogs into various shapes to suit our needs; *The Illustrated Encyclopedia of Dog Breeds* lists 91 hound breeds, 43 working breeds, 44 herding breeds, 49 gun dogs and 31 terrier breeds.[1,2] Due to our changing lifestyle, many of these breeds are no longer needed for what they were bred. These breeds still contain the genetic make-up for their original activities; this means that many of our companions have much more energy than is needed for a couch potato, leading to the development of many behavioral problems if they are not given an appropriate outlet for all this energy.

Working dogs are still found in many areas though. The federal, local and state governments employ dogs in areas of national defense, customs service drug reinforcement and border patrol. Dogs are trained as service animals for the deaf and blind as well as the physically and mentally disabled. They are also still used for hunting, racing, endurance sled pulling and other athletic competitions. Canine agility competitions, Frisbee competitions, and herding competitions are found in many parts of our country. These provide a wonderful opportunity for human and dog to work together again as they were originally trained without having to maintain a herd of sheep (Figure 28.1)!

Just like people who are athletes, training and nutrition can play a major role in the canine athletes' success. But nutrition cannot overcome deficits in genetics and training. Matching nutrition to exercise type allows a canine athlete to perform to its genetic potential and level of training.[1] In general, all working dogs have increased energy requirements over those of an adult dog during time of normal activity.[3] The type of work being done and the intensity of work may require modifications in the nutrient composition of the food and the feeding schedule.[3] Individual variations

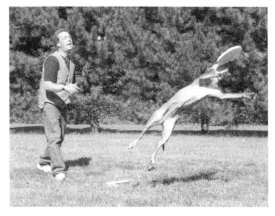

Figure 28.1 An owner and his dog competing in a Frisbee competition. (Courtesy of Heidi Reuss-Lamky LVT, VTS (Anesthesia, Surgery).)

in energy requirements exist and calculation of ME requirement based on DER provides no more than an estimate of their true requirements.[4] Let the animal dictate if they are receiving enough energy for their activity level, and adjust intake as required to meet these needs.

An ideal BCS for performance dogs has not been determined, but studies have shown that dogs live longer and perform better when they are fed less food, and weigh slightly less than is typically seen as "normal."[4] Racing greyhounds trained to run a 500 m race were on average 0.7 kn/h faster if they weighed 6% less and were fed 15% less food than when they were fed free choice.[4] These dogs had a BCS of 3.5/9 when fed the lesser amount of food, and when fed free choice had a BCS of 3.75/9.[4]

Most of our performance dogs typically are "weekend athletes," for optimal performance their training should match the intensity, duration and frequency of the desired level of performance.[2] It is unrealistic to expect

Nutrition and Disease Management for Veterinary Technicians and Nurses, Second Edition. Ann Wortinger, Kara M. Burns
© 2015 John Wiley & Sons, Inc. Published 2015 by John Wiley & Sons, Inc.
Companion Website: www.wiley.com/go/wortinger/nutrition

a dog that has not done any work since last season to go out the first day of duck season and work for 6–8 hours.

The work performed by most intermediate athletes (hunting dogs, field trials, Frisbee trials, agility, service work, police work, search and rescue, livestock management and exercise with people) resembles that done by endurance athletes (sled pulling), but is of shorter duration. The muscle-fiber type profile of intermediate athletes should resemble that of an endurance athlete over that of a sprint athlete (sight hounds).[3] In general, endurance athletes have an increased number of well-developed slow-twitch fiber muscles; athletes involved in high speed sprinting have increased numbers of fast-twitch muscles.[3] Slow-twitch muscles have a higher capacity for aerobic metabolism, meaning that they primarily use fat in the form of free fatty acids for energy. Fast-twitch muscles can use both aerobic and anaerobic pathways in that they can use both carbohydrates in the form of glycogen and glucose for immediate energy and fat for longer term energy use.[1,3]

Exercise requires transfer of chemical energy into physical work. ATP (adenosine triphosphate) is the sole source of energy for muscle contraction.[1] ATP is formed from metabolic fuels stored in muscle (endogenous) and from other body stores (exogenous). The energy is converted to ATP using either aerobic pathways using oxygen, or anaerobic pathways that can work without oxygen.[1] The proportion of each pathway used is determined by duration and intensity of exercise, conditioning and nutritional status of the animal.[1]

Training and conditioning results in adaptive physiological changes, which facilitate efficient delivery of oxygen and other nutrients to the working muscles. Some of these changes include increased blood volume, increased red blood cell mass, increased capillary density, increased mitochondrial volume, increased bone mass, muscle hypertrophy, increased activity level and increased total mass of metabolic enzymes.[2,3]

Fats

Fats, on average provide 8.5 kcal of ME per gram of dry matter. Carbohydrates provide 3.5 kcal of ME per gram of dry matter. The easiest and quickest way to increase the energy density of a food is to increase the fat content in the diet.

The two primary fuels used by the body for working muscles are muscle glycogen and free fatty acids. An intermediate athlete would receive ~70–90% of their energy from fat metabolism, and only a small amount from carbohydrate metabolism.[3] Dogs rely more heavily on free fatty acids for energy generation at all exercise levels than do people.[1] Feeding a higher fat diet to endurance and intermediate trained athletes prepares the muscles to efficiently mobilize and use free fatty acids for energy. It also exerts a glycogen sparing effect that can help prolong glycogen use during work.[3] By increasing dietary fat concentration you can increase the energy intake and encourage stressed dogs to increase food intake due to the increased palatability of fat in the diet.[1] Increased dietary fat levels may also enhance free fatty acid availability.[1] As the duration of the event performed by the dog increases, so should the dietary fat intake. Fatigue and dehydration may decrease appetite, making intake of adequate amounts of energy even more challenging.[2]

Carbohydrate

Provided sufficient gluconeogenic precursors are available in the diet, no dietary requirements for carbohydrates exist for dogs except during gestation and neonatal development.[1] Gluconeogenesis (formation of glucose from noncarbohydrate sources) is done by the liver and kidneys using glycerol, lactate and glucogenic amino acids.[1] Stored fat in adipose tissue supplies glycerol for glucose production by breaking down triglycerides and fatty acids for oxidation to supply energy, whereas muscle catabolism releases glucogenic amino acids, lactic acid and pyruvate for glucose production by the liver.[1]

Since digestible carbohydrates contain only 3.5 kcal of ME per gram of dry matter, adding additional carbohydrates to a diet will not increase the caloric density and will not provide additional energy.[2] Dogs at rest obtain energy equally from the oxidation (aerobic metabolism) of fat and glucose. When trained dogs begin to walk and run, glucose oxidation increases only slightly, with most of the increased energy obtained from oxidation of fat.[2] As the intensity of exercise increases, the supply of oxygen becomes limited, and lactic acid is produced. The increased levels of lactic acid further decrease the use of fat for energy.[2]

Even though fat provides more energy than carbohydrates do, the inclusion of carbohydrates in performance diets has been shown to decrease the incidence of "stress diarrhea" in endurance athletes. With sprinting athletes, onset of fatigue can be delayed with the inclusion of carbohydrates, who are working at or above their anaerobic threshold.[2] Despite this fact, carbohydrate loading of canine athletes is probably not as beneficial for dogs, as would a continuous diet of foods with higher fat levels. The exception to this would be sprinting greyhounds. Since they do not have dramatically increased energy needs (small bursts of energy for less than 60 seconds), and rely primarily on glycogen for energy and seldom get to the point of utilizing free fatty acids, and would not appreciate the value of a higher-fat diet other than for provision of additional energy in the diet.[2]

Carbohydrates fed to athletes should be highly digestible to decrease fecal bulk in the colon. Excessive amounts of undigested carbohydrates reaching the colon can also increase water loss through the stool; increase colonic gas production and increase overall fecal bulk and therefore add unneeded weight.[1] Adding moderately fermentable fibers may provide some benefit for racing dogs, especially those fed raw food diets. Rapid fermentation of these fibers to oligosaccharides may decrease colonic pH and inhibit clostridial growth.[2]

Protein

Endurance training results in increased protein needs through increased protein synthesis (anabolism-the building up of muscle), protein degradation (catabolism-the breaking down of muscle) and gluconeogenesis.[1,3] Catabolism is only a small portion of the overall protein needs; the primary use is anabolism.[3] Increased tissue mass associated with training must be supplied by increased protein in the diet.[3] Amino acids are used in the formation of new muscle and repair damage to muscle and connective tissue during intensive conditioning; exercise increases the amino acid catabolism.[1] Dogs initially use glycogen as a source of glucose during submaximal exercise, but gluconeogenesis from protein increases after about 30 minutes.[4] Because of this, dogs running for longer than 30 minutes require more

protein in their diets than do dogs that only do short bursts of activity, such as Greyhounds.[4]

Amino acids provide ~5–15% of the energy used during exercise; most of this energy comes from the branched-chain amino acids (leucine, isoleucine and valine). All of these are essential amino acids and cannot be synthesized from other amino acids; they must be included in the diet.

The "biologic value" of a protein is an indicator of the amount of essential amino acids found in that product. Egg has the highest biologic value, followed closely by casein and whey both milk based proteins. Muscle and organ meat-based proteins have the next highest level of essential amino acids, and are also highly digestible and bioavailable.[1,2]

Excessive protein intake may predispose an athlete to increased amino acid catabolism. Amino acids are not stored as proteins in the body but are deaminated (broken down) to ketoacids. These ketoacids are either oxidized for energy or converted to fatty acids and/or glucose and stored as adipose tissue (fat) or glycogen.[1] The diet fed should supply adequate calories as fat and carbohydrate so that the protein fed can be used primarily for tissue synthesis and not for energy.[3] During long periods of exercise DER may increase 2–3 times over RER, while protein requirements only increase slightly.[2]

Water

Water is used as a solvent for biological solutes; it acts as a transport medium for nutrients, wastes and heat, absorbs physical shock and lubricates various internal and external surfaces.[2] Heat is the primary byproduct of muscle contraction and the respiratory tract through panting is responsible for dissipation of this heat.[1]

Because evaporative heat loss is the primary way dogs dissipate heat, ensuring adequate hydration is crucial for the maintenance of normal body temperature.[1] Depending on the type of work done and environmental conditions, water losses can increase by 10–20 times normal during exercise.[3] Even mild dehydration can lead to decreased performance, decreased strength and hyperthermia.[3] Water should be offered in small amounts frequently throughout the exercise period. If an insufficient amount is consumed, the dog might benefit by having water added to its food.[1]

While dogs require unlimited and frequent supplies of water, before, during and after exercise, they do not require additional electrolytes including sodium or additional vitamins.[4] As dogs do not sweat, they do not lose electrolytes during exercise as do humans. Sports drinks designed for humans are not recommended for dogs and could actually decrease performance.[4] Any salt consumed in the drinking water will have to be excreted in the urine, increasing the rate of water loss and may exacerbate dehydration.[4]

Supplements

Many breeders, exhibitors and trainers believe stressed dogs must also receive supplements of certain vitamins and minerals. There is no evidence to suggest that working dogs have increased requirements of these nutrients.[3] If a diet is nutritionally balanced and the dog is consuming enough to meet its energy requirements during work, then additional supplements should not be necessary.[1]

Requirements for antioxidant vitamins such as vitamin E increase as the level of fat in the diet increases, especially poly unsaturated fatty acids (PUFAs).[4] We have not been able to determine if exercising dogs require more antioxidants than do sedentary dogs. But antioxidant requirements for moderately active dogs may be less than for sedentary dogs. It is better to exercise the dogs more frequently, than to increase the antioxidants in the diet over recommended levels.[4] Oxidative stress can be decreased to a degree through adequate pre-exercise training.[2]

The addition of glucosamine/chondroitin may be of benefit for dogs with existing osteoarthritis, but there is no evidence that the inclusion of these supplements in the diet prevents the occurrence of osteoarthritis.[4]

Diet Requirements

A diet needs to be highly digestible to limit the total volume of food consumed at each meal. Some maintenance diets may supply enough energy if consumed in large enough quantities, but may become bulk limiting and thereby limits performance in hard working dogs (too much stool production due to low digestibility).[3] By increasing digestibility, you can reduce fecal bulk and

therefore unnecessary weight, decrease fecal water loss and may decrease the incidence of "stress diarrhea."[2]

An ideal diet would provide increased levels of high quality protein to meet anabolic requirements and enough nonprotein energy nutrients (fats and carbohydrates) to meet energy requirements. By doing this, the diet provides sufficient calories with fat to limit the use of amino acids for energy leaving them available for muscle repair and replacement.[3] Dogs doing short-duration, maximal intensity exercise, may benefit from a lower fat, higher carbohydrate diet to increase available glycogen stores for immediate use.[2]

The food needs to be calorically dense and palatable, highly digestible and practical, so that the dog can physically consume enough to meet their caloric requirements.[1] The price of the food, the form it is available in, storage conditions required and number of animals being fed also needs to be taken into account. What may be practical for 1 dog may be impractical for a kennel of 15 dogs.[1]

Most intermediate athletes are fed commercial diets, while many elite sprint and endurance athletes are fed homemade diets or a mixture of commercial diets with additional ingredients added in.[2] It is important to compare the nutritional content of the current food to the key nutritional factors (protein, fats, carbohydrates) to determine the adequacy of food for that dog. If the current food contains appropriate levels to meet that dog's needs, than it can continue to be fed. If discrepancies are found, a more balance diet would be recommended.[2] Determining the nutrient content for homemade and supplemented diets is difficult at best, and digestibility can only be determined using feeding trials. Consulting a veterinary nutritionist to formulate a homemade diet would be recommended to ensure nutritional adequacy for those clients who don't want to feed commercially available balanced diets.

Energy Considerations

Daily energy requirements (DER) can be highly variable and are directly related to the amount of work being done and the condition and training of the dog. Ambient temperature, psychological stress and geography are all environmental factors that may influence nutritional needs of the canine athlete.[1] Of these ambient temperature can exert the greatest effect; with increased environmental temperature you get increased work and increased water loss. Lower environmental temperature increases energy expenditure for thermogenesis; this may be as much as a 50% increase over DER.[1,3]

Stress in the form of intense physical exertion, weather extremes and psychological strain may negatively affect food intake, and an adequate amount of energy may not be available for the work required.[1,3] Geographical factors such as elevation above sea level and changing elevations throughout a course as well as working in sand or tall grass may increase the workload and therefore energy expenditure.[1]

Dogs require time to adapt to diet changes, when these changes are dramatic as with significant increases in fat or protein content, gastrointestinal and metabolic adaptations need to occur. GI adjustments can happen over the course of a couple of days, whereas metabolic adjustments can take longer. Allowing adequate amounts of time for the body to adjust to a diet change is important to optimize the desired result. This can be especially important for seasonal athletes such as hunting dogs.[2] These dogs may be fed a maintenance diet during non-hunting season, with transition to a performance diet during hunting season. This should not be done opening weekend!

Diet Calculations

The amount of energy required depends on the total work done: intensity × duration × frequency. DER (daily energy requirements) is ~1.6 × RER (resting energy requirements) for the average canine athlete. Sprinters may require 1.6–2 × RER and endurance or other high-end athletes may require 2–5 × RER.

Resting energy requirements can either be figured using $(70 \times \text{body weight in kilograms})^{0.75}$, or $70 + (30 \times \text{body weight in kilograms})$. From there you can calculate the DER. Maintenance is typically 1.0–1.6 × RER depending on activity.

Feeding Plan

Look at where the dog is housed (inside/outdoors), medications or supplements they may be taking, dietary history; amount fed, type of food fed and timing of meals in relation to exercise/training and the nutrient profile

of the diet, exercise and training history (amount of exercise done, frequency and performance of exercise).[1]

Compare the current diet's key nutritional factors to the recommended levels; determine the amount to be fed and the timing of the meals. Estimate energy expenditure using body condition scoring and exercise level.

Timing of meals is important to allow the most availability of nutrients to the athlete. A recommended feeding schedule would be: 1 meal at least 4 hours before

Table 28.1 Comparison of nutrient content for various commercial canine performance foods[1]

Food	Caloric density (kcal)	ME protein	ME fat	ME carbohydrate
Diamond Performance Dog Food, dry	448/cup	28%	45%	27%
Eagle Pack Power pack, dry	439/cup	28%	44%	28%
Hill's Science Diet High Energy, dry	560/cup	23%	50%	26%
Iams Eukanuba Premium Performance, dry	431/cup	27%	48%	28%
Nutro Natural Choice High Endurance, dry	339/cup	27%	41%	32%
Purina Pro Plan Performance, dry	430/cup	28%	42%	30%

Table 28.2 Sample calculation for calories/100 grams of food

Total calories in 100 grams of food
Protein = 3.5 kcal/gram × grams in food
Fat = 8.5 kcal/gram × grams in food
Carbohydrate = 3.5 kcal/gram × grams in food
Total calories/100 gram = protein calorie + fat calorie + carbohydrate calorie

Percentage of ME contributed by each nutrient (caloric distribution)
Protein = (protein calories/100 gram ÷ by total calories/100 gram) × 100 = % ME
Fat = (fat calories/100 gram ÷ by total calories/100 gram) × 100 = % ME
Carbohydrate = (carbohydrate calories/100 gram ÷ by total calories) × 100 = % ME

exercise, l meal within 2 hours after exercise and if necessary, due to the duration of exercise, small amounts during exercise. The largest meal should be given post exercise after the dog has calmed down.[4] Eating a meal directs blood to the intestinal tract for digestion, if fed soon before exercise or fed a large meal during exercise this could compromise both performance and digestion.[4] It is also very important to allow access to plenty of fresh clean water to prevent dehydration.[1]

For optimal performance and long term health, exercising dogs should not be fed free-choice but rather should receive measured feeding based on the volume of food required to maintain their desired level of activity and BCS.[4]

Reassess your plan based on body condition scoring, weight, hydration and performance. Adjust as needed to get the results that you want from your canine athlete (Table 28.1).

Adapted from a table in *Small Animal Clinical Nutrition 4th Edition*, this list represents products with the largest market share and for which published information is available. Values are expressed on percentage of metabolizable energy.[1]

To express nutrients as a percentage of metabolizable energy, see Table 28.2.

Comparing products using ME gives a better idea of caloric distribution, and allows you to accurately compare canned and dry diets. This does not take into account digestibility. It is also important when comparing foods to see if feeding trials have been done on the product and look at digestibility, if given. If you chose a food that has not had feeding trials done by the manufacturer, then you are doing the feeding trials for them (Table 28.3).

Table 28.3 Recommended caloric distribution for canine athletes[3]

Calories from protein: 30–35% ME
Calories from fat: 50–65% ME
Calories from carbohydrate: 10–15% ME

References

1 Toll PW, Reynolds AJ (2000) The canine athlete. In MS Hand, CD Thatcher, RL Remillard, P Roudebush (eds), *Small Animal Clinical Nutrition* (4th edn), pp. 261–83, Marceline, MO: Walsworth Publishing.

2 Toll P, Gillette R, Hand M (2010) Feeding working and sporting dogs. In MS Hand, CD Thatcher, RL Remillard *et al.* (eds), *Small Animal Clinical Nutrition* (5th edn), pp. 321–52, Marceline, MO: Walsworth Publishing.

3 Case LC, Carey DP, Hirakawa DA, Daistotle L (2000) Performance and stress. In *Canine and Feline Nutrition* (2nd edn), pp. 259–73, St Louis, MO: Mosby Publishing.

4 Hill R (2012) Nutritional and energy requirements for performance. In S Delaney, A Fascetti (eds), *Applied Veterinary Clinical Nutrition*, pp. 47–55, Ames, IA: Wiley-Blackwell.

29 Nutritional Requirements of Cats

Introduction

In their natural environment, cats are an obligate carnivore, meaning that their nutritional needs can only be met by eating a diet that consists of animal-based proteins (i.e. mice, birds). How have our efforts to domesticate cats been affected by this dietary requirement?

Strictly speaking, cats and dogs are members of the order *Carnivora* and are therefore classified as carnivores. From a dietary perspective, dogs are omnivores and cats and other members of the suborder *Feloidea* are strict carnivores. Domesticated cats (*Felis catus*) have evolved unique anatomic, physiologic, metabolic and behavioral adaptations consistent with eating a strictly carnivorous diet.[1,2]

By recognizing and addressing these special nutritional requirements for cats we can help to ensure they have the best chance at a long, healthy life. As veterinary nutrition evolves, we will continue to update our information regarding feline nutrition.

Feeding Behaviors

The evolutionary history of the cat indicates that it has eaten a purely carnivorous diet throughout its entire development.[2] Feeding behaviors that have evolved to fit this lifestyle include searching, hunting and caching of prey as well as postprandial behaviors such as grooming and sleeping.[3] Feral or outdoor cats feeding primarily on mice, voles and insects tend to live solitary lives when food is scarce and spread over a large area, but when food is plentiful and concentrated as with households, dumps, and farms, cats can be found living in large groups.[3]

Cats typically eat 10–20 small meals throughout the day and night. This eating pattern probably reflects the relationship between cats and their prey. Small rodents make up ~40% or more of the feral domestic cat's diets, with small rabbits, insect, frogs and birds making up the remainder. The average mouse provides ~30 kilocalories or an estimated 8% of a feral cat's daily energy requirements (DER). Repeated cycles of hunting throughout the day and night are required to provide sufficient food for the average cat.[1,2] House cats typically continue this pattern by eating 10–20 small meal throughout the day and night with each meal having a caloric content of ~23 kilocalories, very close to the caloric value of one small mouse.[1,2]

For thousands of years the primary economic value of cats has been their hunting skills.[3] Until recently, there has been little or no selective breeding done to alter their behavior or looks. The predatory drive is so strong in cats that they will stop eating to make a kill. This behavior allows for multiple kills, which optimizes food availability.[1] From their viewpoint, the dead meal isn't going anywhere, and they have no assurance that another prey will show up within the next 2–3 hours when they are due for their next meal. Many owners will feed outdoor cats thinking that this will decrease their hunting, especially of small song birds. Unfortunately, supplemental feeding may reduce the time spent hunting, but otherwise will not alter hunting behavior.[1]

Cats are very sensitive to the physical form, odor and taste of foods. They consume live prey beginning at the head, this head first consumption is dictated by the direction of hair growth on the prey.[1] Food temperature also influences acceptance by cats. They do not readily accept food served at either temperature extreme, but prefer food near body temperature (~38°C, 101.5°F) as

Nutrition and Disease Management for Veterinary Technicians and Nurses, Second Edition. Ann Wortinger, Kara M. Burns
© 2015 John Wiley & Sons, Inc. Published 2015 by John Wiley & Sons, Inc.
Companion Website: www.wiley.com/go/wortinger/nutrition

would be found with freshly killed prey.[1,3] House cats accustomed to a specific texture or type of food may refuse foods with different textures. An individual cat's preferences are often influenced by early experiences (good or bad). Many cats will choose a new food over a diet that is currently being fed. The reverse is true in new or stressful situations, such as illness or hospitalization, where cats tend to refuse novel foods. This can be important when trying to switch foods or forms of food fed.[1]

Anatomic Adaptations

Cats have adapted physiologically to the life of a hunter. Their visual acuity is greater than that of dogs. In addition, their sense of hearing is well developed- their ears are upright, face forward and have 20 associated muscles to help them precisely locate sound. Their highly sensitive facial whiskers and widely dispersed tactile hairs are thought to help them hunt in dim light and to protect their eyes.[1] Sharp and dagger-like, their retractable claws are ideal for capturing and securing prey, yet they are easily retracted to decrease noise when stalking.[1]

The scissor-like carnassial teeth are ideal for delivering the cervical bite used to sever the spinal cord and immobilize or kill prey.[1] Cats are able to taste foods as early as 5 days before they are born, with continued improvement in their taste sensitivity as they age. They are able to taste 4 of the 5 main flavor classes: acid > bitter > salty > sweet. Cats do not have active sweet receptors in their tongues, and do not appear to taste or appreciate sweet tastes, and they lack receptors to savory or umami tastes.[4] Cats have the receptors to detect sweet tastes, but they appear to have been switched off and have instead become a pseudogene. When synthetic sweeteners such as saccharine or cylamates are used to flavor medications, cats detect a bitter, not a sweet taste.[4] An important fact to keep in mind when administering liquid human medications that use sweeteners to cover up the taste of the medication.

Their stomachs are smaller than dogs and simpler in structure. Because cats do not consume large meals, the stomach is less important as a storage reservoir.[1]

Intestinal length, as determined by the ratio of intestine to body length, is markedly shorter in cats than in omnivores and herbivores. The ratio for cats is 4:1, meaning that the intestinal length is 4 times longer than the length of the cat, for dogs this is 6:1

and for pigs 14:1.[1] Cats do have greater villus height in their intestinal lining improving their absorptive capacity over that of dogs, so that overall they are only ~10% less efficient in digestion especially with complex starches or fibers even with their shorter intestinal length.[1] The bacterial populations found in the feline small intestine are higher than those found in dogs and other omnivores.[5] These additional bacteria may be needed to increase digestive process due to their shorter intestinal length. The bacteria may also be beneficial in protein and fat digestion.[5]

Physiologic Adaptations

Cats are not able to adapt to varying levels of carbohydrates in their diets due to various changes in the digestive and absorptive functions of intestine. Salivary amylase, the enzyme used to initiate digestion of dietary starches, is absent in cats, and intestinal amylase appears to be exclusively derived from the pancreas. These enzymes were not necessary in a prey based diet with minimal starch content.[1] The level of pancreatic amylase is only 5% of that found in dogs. The sugar transporter in the intestine is nonadaptive to changes in dietary carbohydrate levels. Disaccharide activity (i.e. the brush border enzymes responsible for sugar digestion) is also nonadaptive and only ~40% that found in dogs.[1,6] These changes evolved because cats had little natural carbohydrate intake and it was not necessary to have systems intact that were of little use to the animal.

Despite these adaptive changes, cats are still able to use carbohydrates in their diets, with a sugar digestibility of ~94% with a few exceptions. Lactose digestion declines sharply in kittens after 7 weeks of age. This is due to a decrease in intestinal lactase activity that is typical in mammals. Most adult cats can consume small amounts of milk without problems, but larger amounts (>1.3 gram/kilogram of body weight) can lead to signs of bloating, diarrhea and gas.[1]

High amounts of dietary carbohydrate levels can negatively impact diet digestibility. With high levels of dietary carbohydrates, decreases in protein digestibility are seen due to a combination of factors including reduced fecal pH caused by incomplete carbohydrate digestion, and increased microbial fermentation in the colon with increased production of organic acids.[1,6] Cats have a vestigial cecum and short colon, which limits their ability to use poorly digestible starches and fiber for energy through bacterial fermentation in the large bowel.[1]

Metabolic Adaptations

Energy

The liver of most animals has two active enzyme systems for converting glucose to glucose-6-phosphate (the first step to forming glycogen-the storage form of glucose within the cells); hexokinase and glucokinase.[7] The glucokinase system is used primarily when a large load of glucose is received by the liver as would be seen with a high carbohydrate meal. Cats have very low liver glucokinase activity and therefore limited ability to metabolize large amounts of simple carbohydrates by this route. Blood glucose levels in carnivores are more consistent with less postprandial fluctuations because glucose is released in small continuous boluses over a longer period of time as a result of gluconeogenic catabolism of proteins.[1] If sufficient protein is not included in the diet (exogenous source), body muscle and organ tissue will be used to meet the cat's protein requirements (endogenous source). If fed according to their nutritional requirements, cats did not need to handle large carbohydrate loads and therefore only use the hexokinase system for glucose metabolism.

Cats can often be seen eating grass, or grazing on house plants. This is a natural phenomenon which makes vomiting easier helping with the expulsion of hairballs.[4] This is not a dietary requirement, but rather a behavior. As cats can become quite destructive if allowed unlimited access to house plants, and many house plants pose a poisoning hazard to cats when consumed this behavior should be discouraged by owners.[4] Plants can either be placed in areas inaccessible to the cat, sprayed with hot pepper spray or other noxious tasting sprays to make them taste bad or using a water sprayer to convey to the cat that this behavior is unacceptable.[4]

Water

Domestic cats are thought to have descended from the small African wildcat (*Felis silvestris libyca*), a cat naturally found in the deserts of Africa. Due to their limited water availability *F. libyca* evolved to conserve water by concentrating their urine to reduce water

loss.[4] Because of this ancient relationship, cats today maintain this adaptation to a dryer environment. Cats seem to be less sensitive to the stimulus of thirst, and are able to survive on less water than can dogs.[1,2,7] Average water requirements for cats vary from 55 to 70 ml/kg/day. This requirement is related to the dry matter intake in the diet.

With this decreased response to thirst, cats may ignore minor levels of dehydration (up to 4% body weight). They are able to compensate for this reduced water intake by forming highly concentrated urine.[7] Cats adjust their water intake based on the dry matter content of their diet rather than the moisture content. They consume 1.5–2 ml of water/g of dry matter. This 2:1 ratio of water to dry matter is similar to that of their typical prey.[1,6,7]

Practically, this means that cats consuming a dry food diet will consume substantially more water through drinking, compared to cats eating a canned food diet.[1,7] For us, if increased water turnover is necessary as with FLUTD or formation of urinary calculi, feeding a canned food diet can increase water intake without any additional work by the client or cat.

Protein

Protein metabolism in cats is unique; this is apparent because of their unusually high maintenance requirement for protein in the diet as compared to dogs or other omnivores. Cats have both a higher basal requirement for protein and an increased requirement for essential amino acids.[7] Cats depend on protein not only for structural and synthetic purposes but also for energy. They will continue to use protein in the form of gluconeogenic amino acids for production of energy, even when inadequate protein is consumed in the diet.[1] The hepatic enzymes that catabolize amino acids for energy are always active, and cannot be down regulated in times of decreased intake. Because of this, a fixed level of protein in the diet is always required for catabolism to provide energy.[5] Although these changes impair the cat's ability to conserve protein when dietary sources are limited, on their natural diet it ultimately conserves energy by eliminating the cost of enzyme synthesis and degradation.[1] There are four essential amino acids that are especially important for cats, they are: arginine, taurine, methionine, cysteine.[5]

In 1986, National Research Council recommended a minimum of 240 grams of protein/kg in the diets of growing kitten and 140 grams of protein/kg in the diets of adult cats. This is equivalent to 26% of metabolizable energy in the diet for kittens and 23% of metabolizable energy for adult maintenance. Keep in mind, these are minimum recommendations, and they assume a highly digestible protein source is provided in the diet. You cannot expect optimal results when you are feeding to meet minimal requirements.

Taurine

Taurine, which is an essential amino acid for cats, is not incorporated into proteins or degraded by mammalian tissues, but is essential for conjugation of bile salts, vision, cardiac muscle function, and proper function of the nervous, reproductive and immune systems.[3,6,8] Taurine is found as a free amino acid in the natural diet of cats (i.e. rodents, small birds), but is found in lower concentrations in large animals such a cattle.[5]

Cats can only conjugate bile acids with taurine to make bile salts. Taurine continues to be lost in the gastrointestinal tract through this conjugation with bile, this coupled with a low rate of synthesis contributes to the obligatory requirement for cats.[1,3,6,8] A carnivorous diet supplies abundant taurine; however cereal and grains supply only marginal or inadequate levels of taurine for cats.[3] Therefore, diets based on these types of protein sources may be lacking or limited in taurine.

Taurine is either more available or better retained by cats fed dry food diets. Because of the wide spread use of taurine within the body, changes from deficiency can be seen in virtually all body systems.[3] Three syndromes have been identified related strictly to taurine deficiency; feline central retinal degeneration, reproductive failure and impaired fetal development and feline dilated cardiomyopathy.[1] Clinical signs of taurine deficiency occur only after prolonged periods of depletion (from 5 months to 2 years).[1]

Methionine and Cystine

Methionine is an essential amino acid for cats; this species has a higher requirement than do dogs or other omnivores. Methionine and cystine are sulfur-containing amino acids, and are considered together because cystine can replace up to half of the requirement for methionine.[5] Cystine is also required for production of hair and felinine, an amino acid found in cat urine. Felinine is found in largest amounts in intact male cats and is thought to be used for territorial marking.[1,6] Methionine tends to be the first limiting amino acid in many food ingredients.[1] Meaning that when breaking down proteins for use into their various amino acid components, methionine would "run-out" first, limiting the amount of proteins made in the body that need methionine for formation.

Nutritional deficiencies are possible, especially in cats fed homemade, vegetable based diets or human enteral diets. Clinical signs of methionine deficiency include poor growth and a crusting dermatitis at the mucocutaneous junctions of the mouth and nose.[1,6]

Arginine

Arginine deficiency in cats can be one of the most dramatic responses seen. Cats cannot synthesize sufficient ornithine or citrulline for conversion to arginine. Arginine is required for the urea cycle to work properly.[5] After consuming a meal, their highly active hepatic protein catabolism enzymes produce ammonia. Without sufficient arginine in the diet, the urea cycle cannot convert the ammonia to urea, resulting in ammonia toxicity. This hyperammonia can result within 1 hour of consuming a deficient meal.[5]

Signs consistent with ammonia toxicity include vocalization, emesis, ptyalism, hyperactivity, hyperesthesia, ataxia, muscle rigidity and spasms, apnea and cyanosis. Death may ensue within 2–5 hours of ingestion of a deficient meal.[5] Luckily, meat-based diets are high in arginine, and deficiencies have only been reported in cats fed experimental foods specifically designed to be arginine deficient or in cats fed casein-based human enteral diets.[5]

Fats

Cats are able to digest high levels of fat as would be found in meat-based diets. Like other obligate carnivores, cats have a dietary requirement for arachidonic acid, an essential fatty acid. They have limited ability to convert linoleic acid to arachidonic acid as do dogs and other omnivores.[5] A preformed, exogenous source of arachidonic acid is especially important during the more stressful stages of a cat's life such as gestation and lactation. Arachidonic acid is abundant in animal tissues, especially organ and neural sources, but is absent in plant-based proteins.[5]

Vitamin Metabolism

The cat is unable to convert beta-carotene to retinol (vitamin A) because of a lack of intestinal enzymes necessary for the conversion, and therefore cats require a dietary source of pre-formed vitamin A. Vitamin A is necessary for the maintenance of vision, bone and muscle growth, reproduction and healthy epithelial tissues.[1] Because vitamin A is a fat soluble vitamin and is stored in the liver, deficiencies are slow to develop, and are only seen in cats with severe liver failure or gastrointestinal disease resulting in fat malabsorption.[6]

Cats also lack sufficient enzymes to meet the metabolic requirements for vitamin D photosynthesis in the skin; therefore they require a dietary source of vitamin D.[1] For indoor cats, this conversion of D2 to the active form D3 requires direct exposures to the sun, this cannot happen through a window. The primary function of vitamin D is calcium and phosphorus homeostasis, with particular emphasis on intestinal absorption, retention and bone deposition of calcium.[6] As with vitamin A, deficiency is rare and slow to develop.[1,6]

Vitamin A, vitamin D and arachidonic acid are found in plentiful amounts in animal fats and liver. Dietary fat is important not only for provision of fuel for energy, but also for increasing palatability and acceptance of food and provision of fat-soluble vitamins.[6]

Cats require increased amounts of many dietary water-soluble B vitamins, including thiamin, niacin, pyridoxine (vitamin B6), and in certain circumstances cobalamin (vitamin B12). The requirement for niacin and pyridoxine is four times higher than that for dogs.[1,6] Cats are unable to convert sufficient amounts of tryptophan to niacin. Although cats have the metabolic pathway necessary to convert tryptophan to niacin, their requirement exceeds the rate of synthesis.[5] Because most water-soluble B vitamins are not stored (except cobalamin, which is stored in the liver), a continually available dietary source is required to prevent deficiencies.[6] Deficiencies are rare in cats eating appropriate diets because each of the B vitamins is found in high concentrations in animal tissue.[6]

Conclusion

The cat may be seen as one of our most visible "specialists." As an obligate carnivore, they have evolved to such a point that many of the redundant metabolic systems that we have are no longer required. Instead of seeing cats as "inferior," I think we need to acknowledge that they have surpassed both humans and dogs, and have streamlined their lives. We need to appreciate this unique and wonderful creature that continues to enrich our lives and protect our houses and yards.

References

1 Kirk CA, Debraekeleer J, Armstrong PJ (2000) Normal cats. In MS Hand, CD Thatcher, RL Remillard *et al.* (eds), *Small Animal Clinical Nutrition* (4th edn), pp. 291–337, Marceline, MO: Walsworth Publishing.

2 Case LC, Carey DP, Hirakawa DA, Daistotle L (2000) Nutritional idiosyncrasies for cats. In *Canine and Feline Nutrition* (2nd edn), pp. 71–3, St Louis, MO: Mosby Publishing.

3 Voith V (1994) Feeding behaviors. In J Wills, KW Simpson (eds), *The Waltham Book of Clinical Nutrition of the Dog and Cat*, pp. 119–27, Tarrytown, NY: Elsevier.

4 Horwitz D, Soulard Y, Junien-Castagna A (2008) The feeding behavior of the cat. In P Pibot, V Biourge, D Elliott (eds), *Encyclopedia of Feline Clinical Nutrition*, pp. 440–67, Aimarges, France: Aniwa SAS.

5 Armstrong J, Gross K, Becarova I, Debraekeleer J (2010) Introduction to feeding normal cats. In MS Hand, CD Thatcher, RL Remillard *et al.* (eds), *Small Animal Clinical Nutrition* (5th edn), pp. 321–52, Marceline, MO: Walsworth Publishing.

6 Zoran, DL (2002) *JAVMA* **221**(11): 1559–66.

7 Welborn MB, Moldawer LL (1997) *Glucose metabolism*. In JL Rombeau, RH Rollandelli (eds), *Clinical Nutrition Enteral and Tube Feeding*, pp. 61–80, Philadelphia, PA: WB Saunders.

8 Wills JM (1996) Adult maintenance. In N Kelly, J Wills (eds), *Manual of Companion Animal Nutrition and Feeding*, pp. 44–6, Ames, IA: Iowa State Press.

30   Nutrition Myths

Introduction

With the ready availability of the internet, clients have an even greater access to information. Where previously they had relied on information from their friends, breeders and news sources, now they can add the "net" to their source network. Unfortunately, they don't tend to "filter" out the information, taking everything in their source network as gospel, and do not look at the source or references. Many clients feel uncomfortable talking to their veterinary team about nutrition questions, or feel that they know as much as the veterinarian and technicians do. This has led many a well-intentioned client to follow poor recommendations. Some of the more common "myths" are presented below, followed by the truth.

Myth: Meat By-products Are Inferior in Quality Compared to Whole Meat in a Diet ...

When listed on an ingredient label, meat is defined by the American Association of Feed Control Officials (AAFCO) as "any combination of skeletal striated muscle or that muscle found in the tongue, diaphragm, heart, esophagus with or without the accompanying and overlying fat, and the portions of the skin, sinew, nerve and blood vessels which normally accompany the muscle derived from part of whole carcasses."[1] It also must be suitable for use in animal foods. This definition *excludes* feathers, heads, feet and entrails.[2] Meat by-products are defined as "non-rendered, clean parts of the carcass which may contain lungs, spleen, kidneys, brain, liver, blood, bone, heads, feet (of poultry), partially defatted fatty tissue, stomach and intestines emptied of their contents." It does not include hair, horns, teeth or hooves.[2] Depending on the supplier

and the type of refining process that the manufacturer uses, by-products can vary greatly in the amount of nondigestible material they contain.

The ash content can give you an idea of the quality of the by-products. High ash content is an indicator of a poorer quality protein with lower digestibility. The presence of by-products does not indicate a poor quality diet, a higher ash to protein ratio would. Feeding trials evaluating nutrient content and digestibility will help greatly in evaluating the quality of the ingredients. Feeding trials can establish digestibility levels. The higher the digestibility, the better the quality of the ingredients found in the diet. This information is available in most product reference guides, on-line references and by contacting the manufacturer.

Foods that have not undergone feeding trials will not have digestibility information available. Knowing the reputation of the manufacturer is your best indicator of a good quality diet.

Myth: Feeding Trials Are Not Necessary ...

Feeding trial protocol as established by the AAFCO for adult maintenance, lasts 6 months, requires only 8 animals per group and monitors a limited number of parameters. These parameters are set at the minimum nutrient requirements as defined by the National Research Council (NRC).[1,2] These levels tend to be lower than the recommended daily intake (RDI). Requirements are the minimum level of a nutrient, which over time, is sufficient to maintain the desired physiological functions of the animals in the population. RDI is the level of intake of a nutrient that appears to be adequate to meet known nutritional needs of practically all healthy individuals. The NRC recommendations are to serve as a guide to diet formulations, but they do not account for digestibility or nutrient availability.

Nutrition and Disease Management for Veterinary Technicians and Nurses, Second Edition. Ann Wortinger, Kara M. Burns
© 2015 John Wiley & Sons, Inc. Published 2015 by John Wiley & Sons, Inc.
Companion Website: www.wiley.com/go/wortinger/nutrition

AAFCO feeding trials provide reasonable assurance of nutrient availability and sufficient palatability to ensure acceptability. They also provide some assurance that the product will support certain functions such as gestation, lactation and growth.[2]

A feeding trial is also the only way to accurately access the quality of the protein in a diet, as this is the only valid way to determine digestibility of a protein, and therefore its quality. Passing a feeding trial does not ensure that the food will be effective in preventing long-term nutrition/health problems or detect problems with a low prevalence in the general population. A feeding trial is also not designed to ensure optimal growth or maximize physical activity.

If a diet has not gone through a feeding trial by the manufacturer, you will be conducting the feeding trial for them using your patients and pets. While feeding trials especially on therapeutic diets can not be expected to detect all deficiencies or excesses (which may also be due to disease processes, malabsorption or maldigestion) they give you an added advantage of having someone else evaluate the diets before you offer them to your clients.

Feeding trials are conducted on healthy dogs and cats, with controls that are the same breed and gender. During the trials, the animals must receive the test food as their only source of nutrition. The same formula must be fed throughout the entire trial. The trials are conducted by measuring the daily food consumption, weekly body weight measurement, stated lab parameters measured at the end of the trial, and a complete physical exam by a veterinarian at the beginning and end of the trial. A number of animals, not to exceed 25%, can be removed for nonnutritional reasons or poor food intake, with a necropsy conducted on any animal which dies during the trial with findings recorded. Reproducing animals need the additional following information recorded: body weight within 24 hours of delivery, offspring's body weight within 24 hours of birth, litter size at birth, 1 day later and at end of study, as well as a recording of any stillborn or congenital abnormalities.[1,2]

At the end of the feeding trial, the results obtained are compared to the results from a control group, a historical colony average or to reference values published by the AAFCO.[1,2]

All premium manufacturers conduct feeding trials on their foods, and continue to conduct them as the foods are changed and updated both for palatability

and as new evidence is discovered regarding nutritional requirements. To verify if feeding trails have been conducted on a food, check the product label to find the source of AAFCO certification: if feeding trials have been done, it will be stated on the label as such. Feeding trials are designed to ensure the food meets the minimal requirements, not to ensure they are able to provide optimal results. Therefore quality of a diet should not be based solely on the presence of feeding trials.

Myth: Pet Food Preservatives Are Bad …

Preservatives are defined as any substance that is capable of inhibiting or retarding the growth of microorganisms or of masking the evidence of such deterioration.[2,3] The primary nutrient requiring protection from preservatives during storage is dietary fat. These fats can be in the form of vegetable oils, animal fats or the fat-soluble vitamins A, D, E and K. These nutrients have the potential to undergo oxidative destruction, called lipid peroxidation, during storage. Antioxidants are included in foods to prevent this lipid peroxidation.[2,3] Oxidation of fats in pet foods also results in loss of calorie content and the formation of toxic forms of peroxides that can be harmful to the health of the pets.

The FDA defines an antioxidant as any substance that aids in the preservation of foods by retarding deterioration, rancidity or discoloration as the result of oxidation processes.[2,3] Various types of antioxidants have been accepted for use in human and animal foods since 1947. Antioxidants do not reverse the oxidative effects on foods once they have started, but rather retards the oxidative process and prevents destruction of the fats in the food. Because of this, for antioxidants to be fully effective they must be included in the food when it is initially mixed and processed. This inclusion helps prevent rancidity, maintains the food's flavor, odor, and texture and prevents accumulation of the toxic end products of lipid degradation.[2,3]

Antioxidants can be divided into two basic types-natural derived products and synthetic products. Natural-derived products are commonly found in certain grains, vegetable oils and some herbs and spices. While these products do exist in nature, all of these compounds are processed in some way to make them available for use in commercial foods. The most common natural derived antioxidants include mixed tocopherols (vitamin E compounds), ascorbic acid (vitamin C), rosemary extract and citric acid.[2,3]

Alpha tocopherol has the strongest biologic function on tissues, but is a poor antioxidant in foods. Delta and gamma tocopherols both have low biologic activity but are more effective than alpha tocopherol as antioxidants. Tocopherols used in foods are obtained primarily from distillation of soybean oil residue. Tocopherols are rapidly decomposed as they protect the fat from oxidation, for this reason food preserved with mixed tocopherols has a shorter shelf life than food preserved with a mixture of antioxidants.[3]

Ascorbic acid (vitamin C) is a water soluble antioxidant and is not easily soluble with the fatty portion of foods. It does work synergistically with other antioxidants, such as vitamin E and butylated hydroxytoluene (BHT). Ascorbyl palminate is similar in structure to ascorbic acid, though it is not normally found in nature. When hydrolyzed it yields ascorbic acid and the free fatty acid (FFA) palmitic acid, both of which are natural compounds.[3]

Rosemary extract is obtained from the dried leaves of the evergreen shrub, *Rosemarinus officinalis*. It is effective as a natural-derived preservative in high-fat diets and has been shown to enhance antioxidant efficiency when combined with mixed tocopherols, ascorbic acid and citric acid. Much processing of the plant oil is needed before addition to foods due to the taste associated with the oil affecting the taste of the food.[3]

Citric acid is found in citrus fruits such as oranges and lemons, and is often included in combination with other natural derived antioxidants.[3]

Due to the high cost of using these compounds they are usually used in conjunction with synthetic antioxidants as preservatives in pet foods. It is difficult to attain the necessary level of natural derived antioxidants without the food becoming cost prohibitive to the client.[3]

Synthetic antioxidants are more effective than natural derived antioxidants and better withstand the heat, pressure and moisture during food processing, this is called "carry through." By being more effective they better preserve the fat-soluble vitamins A, D and E for activity in the body rather than being used in the food as antioxidants.[2,3]

Synthetic antioxidants include butylated hydroxyanisole (BHA), butylated hydroxytoluene (BHT), tertiary butylhydroquine (TBHQ) and ethoxyquin. BHA and BHT are approved for use in both human and animal foods and have a synergistic antioxidant effect when used together. BHA and BHT also have good carry-through and a high efficiency in protection of animal fats, but are slightly less effective when used with vegetable oils. TBHQ is an effective antioxidant for most fats and is approved for use in human and animal foods in the United States but is not approved for use in Canada, Japan or the European Union. Because of this, it is not usually used in pet foods sold in the international market.

Ethoxyquin has been approved for use in animal feeds for more than 30 years, and has been used in pet food manufacturing for more than 15 years. It is approved for both human and animal foods, has good carry-through and has especially high efficacy in the protection of fats in foods. Ethoxyquin is more efficient as an antioxidant than BHA or BHT, which allows lower levels to be used. It is especially effective in protection of oils that contain high levels of polyunsaturated fatty acids (PUFA).[2,3]

If the use of synthetic antioxidants has clients concerned, they should be made aware that most canned foods do not contain antioxidants, and that many commercially prepared dry foods use natural derived antioxidants. There are no studies that support the contention that synthetic antioxidants in general or ethoxyquin in particular are responsible for the variety of health problems reported by owners to the FDA.

The proper use of antioxidants prevents the occurrence of rancidity and the production of toxic peroxide compounds in foods. In most cases, synthetic antioxidants are the best choice because of their efficacy, good carry-through and cost. In contrast, poor carry-through, instability and the high levels needed for effective protection make natural-derived antioxidants difficult to use as the sole source in pet foods.[2,3]

Myth: All Foods Are Created Equally

Food quality cannot be determined by the label, the commercial or the celebrity endorsement. When trying to compare two different foods whether they are canned, dry or somewhere in between, comparing products using metabolizable energy (ME) gives a better idea of caloric distribution, and allows you to accurately compare dissimilar diets. ME does not take into account digestibility of the diet in the animal, this

Table 30.1 Determination of metabolizable energy content in foods

To determine ME:
Total calories in 100 grams of food
    Protein grams x 3.5 kcal/gram = protein kilocalories in food
    Fat grams x 8.5 kcal/gram = fats kilocalories in food
    Carbohydrate grams x 3.5 kcal/gram = carbohydrate kilocalories in food
Total calories/100 gram = protein calorie + fat calorie + carbohydrate calorie

Percentage of ME contributed by each nutrient (caloric distribution)
Protein = (protein calories/100 gram ÷ by total calories/100 gram) x 100 = % ME
Fat = (fat calories/100 gram ÷by total calories/100 gram) x 100 = % ME
Carbohydrate = (carbohydrate calories/100 gram ÷ by total calories) x 100 = % ME

Table 30.2 Calculating energy density from the guaranteed analysis

Energy density from guaranteed analysis
% in diet of nutrient x modified Atwater factor = kcal/100 gm of food
Divide % nutrient by total calories to get nutrient distribution

Modified Atwater factors are the amounts of energy/gram of nutrient
Protein and carbohydrates are 3.5, fats are 8.5
    If the kilocalories/100 grams is not given, a rough estimate of the ME can be determined from the guaranteed analysis. This is also called a "proximate analysis" and is the same as "percent as fed."
% in diet of protein x 3.5 = protein/100 grams of food
% in diet of fat x 8.5 = fat/100 grams of food
To find carbohydrates: (100 %−(% protein− % fat− % crude fiber− % moisture− % ash)) x 3.5 = carbohydrate/100 grams of food.
Add these three numbers together to get an estimate of total calories/100 grams. Calculate percent ME as above.

can only be determined through the use of feeding trials (Table 30.1).

If the grams of nutrients/100 gram of food are not given, than using the guaranteed analysis and kilocalories/100 grams the following formula can be used. Remember that the guaranteed analysis only provides minimums and maximums of a small number of nutrients and is used as a reference only. Because you are not accounting for metabolic or fecal/urine losses, these values are not as accurate as the metabolizable energy values (Table 30.2).

As with human grade foods and products, the same factory can produce multiple foods of varying quality. Factories may also produce food for multiple pet food manufacturers. The food manufacturer does not necessarily determine the quality of the food any more than a parts manufacturer for a car determines the quality of the final product. It is also important when comparing foods to see if feeding trials have been done on the product and look at digestibility, if given. If you chose to feed a food that has not had feeding trials done by the producer, then you are doing the feeding trials for them.

Myth: Corn Is Just Filler

Botanically speaking, corn is a grain and as such is able to provide carbohydrates, proteins and fats to whatever animal is consuming it. The corn used in most pet foods is a type called dent corn. On average dent corn contains 70% carbohydrates 9% protein and 4.5% oil. According to Penn State's Agronomy Guide, approximately 56% of the corn grown in the United States is used as livestock feed, 18% is exported and 13% is used for the production of ethanol for energy. The remaining 13% is used for food, seed or for industrial purposes.[4]

As a protein source it is a good source of protein, with a biologic value of ~59. This means that corn contains 59% of the essential amino acids required for dogs and cats. When compared with egg (BV 100) corn is a less complete protein. Plant-based proteins typically have lower biologic values than do meat-based proteins and corn is no exception. For comparison, skeletal meat, regardless of animal source has a BV of ~74, soybean meal BV of ~73, wheat BV of ~65, and white rice BV of ~64.

Biologic value is determined by the first limiting amino acid found in a food, this is the first essential amino acid that the food "runs out of" when digested. The first limiting amino acid found in corn is lysine, the second is histidine and the last is valine.[1] A limiting amino acid just indicates that plant-based proteins need to be combined with a complementary protein to provide all the essential amino acids. This concept is not a new one, and one that is used daily by many healthy vegetarians. Many foods use multiple protein sources to improve overall quality and amino acid profile of the final food product. Corn and soy bean meal are often combined to take advantage of protein complementation.[5]

When digesting food, the animal is concerned with amino acids profile and nutrients, not with protein source or type. If all the amino acids are provided for, it makes no difference to the animal where that protein source came from.

Meat-based proteins tend to be more digestible since they lack the outside cellulose layer found in most plants, but they are more expensive to produce since the animal whose meat is being eaten must consume the plant-based protein and reassemble it into an animal protein.[5]

The time to harvest for most types of corn is 65–90 days. For most meat-based protein sources, who eat the corn to obtain their amino acids to make their protein the time to harvest can be as low as 16–20 weeks for chickens to as long as 2 years for cattle. Obviously, the longer it takes to obtain the final product, the more expensive the protein source will become.

As a "green conscious" and economical protein, carbohydrate and fat source, you would have a hard time beating corn. Corn also contains high levels of poly-unsaturated fatty acids, B vitamins, minerals and natural antioxidants that can benefit the animal consuming it; this is hardly the description of a "filler."[5]

Conclusion

Once clients are given the facts regarding pet foods, all our jobs should become easier! After all, a well-informed client is our best friend. With proper information, they will be able to pick a pet food that contains quality ingredients, has undergone feeding trials and is properly preserved so that all the ingredients are available to their pet. They may also learn that their veterinary team is the best source for nutrition information!

References

1 Case LP, Carey DP, Hirakawa DA, Daristotle L (2000) Digestion and absorption, nutrient content of pet foods. In *Canine and Feline Nutrition* (2nd edn), pp. 60–3, 175–85, St Louis, MO: Mosby.

2 Gross KI, Wedekind KJ, Cowell CS *et al.* (2000) Nutrients. making commercial pet foods. Making pet foods at home. In MS Hand, CD Thatcher, RL Remillard, P Roudebush (eds), *Small Animal Clinical Nutrition* (4th edn), pp. 58–60, 140–6, 167–9, Marceline, MO: Walsworth Publishing.

3 Case LP, Carey DP, Hirakawa DA, Daristotle L (2000) Nutrient content of pet foods. In *Canine and Feline Nutrition* (2nd edn), pp. 175–85, St Louis, MO: Mosby.

4 Penn State Agronomy Guide 2009–2010. Part 1, Section 4: Corn. http://agguide.agronomy.psu.edu/cm/sec4/sec41.cfm (accessed 9/3/2010).

5 Gross KL, Jewell DE, Yamka RM *et al.* (2010) Macronutrients. In MS Hand, CD Thatcher, RL Remillard *et al.* (eds), *Small Animal Clinical Nutrition* (5th edn), pp. 89–96, Marceline, MO: Walsworth Publishing.

31 Nutritional Support

Introduction

Many hospitalized and critically ill dogs and cats are at risk of becoming severely malnourished because they lack an appetite or the ability to eat. Decreased food intake can be caused by any number of factors ranging from primary medical problems such as Diabetes mellitus, Inflammatory Bowel Disease or Chronic Renal Failure, but also by fear, anxiety and untreated pain.[1]

We have many studies that have shown positive outcomes from instituting nutritional support in animals. Despite the presence of all these studies, one very important study shows that negative energy balances were very common in a population of hospitalized dogs.[2] Reasons for this negative energy balance included inadequate feeding orders, orders to repeatedly withhold food for testing, and the patient's refusal to eat.[2] While we can't force an animal to want to eat, we can affect the quality of the feeding orders and hospital protocols that result in prolonged periods of starvation. We can also use methods to introduce nutrition that remove the animal's willingness to cooperate with us through the use of feeding tubes and parenteral nutrition.

Who Is at Risk?

Dogs and cats of any age or life stage may become malnourished from inadequate nutrient intake.[3] Malnutrition is any disorder with inadequate or unbalanced nutrition that is associated with either nutritional deficiencies or excessive nutrient intakes.[3] Protein and energy malnutrition can also result from diets that are inappropriate for the physiological status of the patient (i.e. low-protein diet when increased protein is required, such as during gestation or lactation) (Figure 31.1).[3]

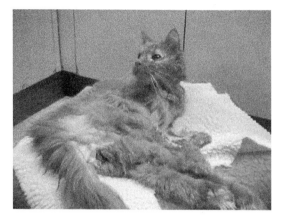

Figure 31.1 Extreme starvation in a cat. This was taken 1 week after hospitalization, shaved areas were sites of decubital ulcers present at admittance.

Insufficient nutrient intake can cause impaired immunity, decreased resistance to infection, inability to withstand shock, surgery and the effects of drugs, decreased wound strength, muscular weakness, organ failure and death.[1]

Nutrition Goals

The goals of nutritional support are to meet the patients nutritional needs, and if possible to prevent further deterioration. This can be done by providing protein, carbohydrate, fat, and other nutrients in a formula that can be utilized by the body with maximum efficiency, minimal adverse effects and minimum discomfort.[4] When the body uses exogenous (those provided outside of the body) rather than endogenous (those provided by the animal's own body stores) nutrients, the breakdown of lean body mass is slowed down and the patient's

Nutrition and Disease Management for Veterinary Technicians and Nurses, Second Edition. Ann Wortinger, Kara M. Burns
© 2015 John Wiley & Sons, Inc. Published 2015 by John Wiley & Sons, Inc.
Companion Website: www.wiley.com/go/wortinger/nutrition

response to therapy is optimized.[5] Increased protein breakdown in response to illness or injury depletes the body of protein stores, thereby affecting wound healing, immune and cellular functions, and cardiac and respiratory functions.[6]

When subjected to starvation, body tissue (except the brain and bone) loses cell mass in varying degrees.[4] Tumors and wounds may act as additional burdens, and can further increase the patient's caloric and nutritional requirements.[4] Malnutrition from inappropriate diets can impair immune function and wound healing, decrease organ function, and affect the prognosis for recovery.

The magnitude of metabolic aberration is determined by the severity of the illness or injury and associated tissue damage.[6] Even with initiation of adequate nutritional support, muscle wasting and negative nitrogen balance can occur.[6]

Guidelines for Support

General guidelines for initiating nutritional support include the loss or anticipated loss of more than 10% of the body weight; anorexia for longer than 3 days; conditions that may preclude eating for the next 2–3 days, such as oral surgery or facial trauma; any other trauma; surgery (including elective surgeries); severe systemic infiltrative disease such as cancers, inflammatory bowel disease or liver failure; increased nutrient loss through diarrhea, vomiting, draining wounds, or burns associated with decreased serum albumin.[2,6]

Other issues that must be considered include gastrointestinal tract function, whether the patient can tolerate tube or catheter feeding (i.e. presence of any organ failure, ability to protect their airway) and the physical or chemical restraint required for placing the tube or catheter, venous accessibility, whether the patient is at risk for pulmonary aspiration (i.e. megaesophagus), availability of nursing care and equipment, and client cost.

Nutritional Assessment

The cornerstone of nutritional assessment are conducting a complete physical examination, obtaining a

Table 31.1 Nutritional questions[5]

- When was the last time your pet ate or drank? How much was offered? How much was consumed?
- What type of food is usually fed (canned, dry, table food, scraps)? How much and how often?
- What brand of food is usually fed? For how long?
- Have there been any recent changes in your pets eating or drinking habits? If so, what changes over what period of time?
- Have there been any recent changes in body condition (e.g. muscle loss, swollen abdomen, hair loss or poor grooming)?
- Has your pet recently taken, or is currently taking any medication? Were there any changes in your pet's condition while taking these medications? Is so, what? (4)

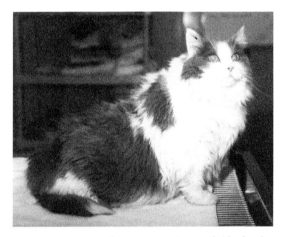

Figure 31.2 Obese cat. This cat is at an increased risk of malnutrition when compared to a normal weight animal.

detailed patient history, recording body weight, assessing the patient's body condition, and evaluating blood chemistry profiles.[5] The blood profiles required depend on the patient's condition (Table 31.1).

The body condition scores used for healthy animals often do not apply to sick animals. When an animal is physiologically stressed, lean body mass is its preferred energy source; in contrast, healthy animals use stored body fat for energy. The result is increased catabolism of body protein (Figure 31.2).[1]

A patient may present with increased amounts of body fat but still be at serious risk of malnutrition-associated complications caused by protein catabolism. Careful examination, including palpation of skeletal muscles over bony prominences (e.g. the scapula, vertebrae, hips and cranial crest), can help identify any muscle wasting consistent with increase protein catabolism.[3] Other indicators of poor nutritional status include edema and ascites, which may reflect low plasma protein levels secondary to malnutrition. Poor hair coat and skin condition can also result from inadequate food intake or micronutrient deficiencies.[3]

Calculating Energy Requirements

Caloric requirements are determined by body weight and function and can be calculated by using the resting energy requirements (RER) for healthy adults at rest in environmentally comfortable cages.[4] The application of illness factors to the RER are now thought to be a source of more complications rather than improving clinical outcome and are therefore discouraged.[7] Water requirements equal those for energy (1 ml = 1 kcal).[8] Patients that eat more than the calculated RER amounts should not be discouraged from doing so while recovering from surgery or trauma.

Routes of Administration

The gut is generally the safest and most natural route for administering nutrients. Maintaining the intestinal mucosa may also help prevent bacterial translocation from the gut to the rest of the body. This is best accomplished with enteral feeding.[9] Voluntary oral intake is the preferred route for enteral nutrition; however, patients must be able to consume at least 85% of their calculated RER for this method of feeding to be effective.[4,8] Technicians often need to devise ways to encourage patients to accept oral feedings (Table 31.2).

Pharmacologic appetite stimulants such as cyproheptidine, prednisolone, benzodiazepines, mirtazapine propofol, megesterol acetate and dronabinol can be utilized as a short-term means of increasing caloric intake. They are not appropriate for long-term use as they usually do not result in consumption of adequate calories to sustain the animal.[2] Syringe feeding, forced feeding or assisted feeding are commonly used to get food into an animal. Again this is not ideal due to the stress involved to both the patient and if done at home, the client. In addition to the stress involved in feeding,

Table 31.2 Hints for increasing oral intake of food[8]

- Hand-feed or pet the patient during feeding.
- Warm the food to slightly below body temperature, if microwaving be sure food is stirred well before feeding.
- Add warm water to dry food or make a slurry from canned foods by adding warm water.
- Use baby food meats as a top dressing, dogs may also like cat food used as a top dressing.
- Try various shapes and types of bowls. Shallow dishes for cats and brachycephalic dog breeds, plastic may have a strange smell to the animals.
- Use foods that have a strong smell or odor.
- Add appetite stimulants to "jump start" the feeding process(usually ineffective over the long term). (7)

the chance of aspiration of food, development of food aversions and choking present real dangers.[2] There is also significant risk to the feeder of being scratched or bitten during the feeding process. Trying to get an accurate calculation of the volume of food actually consumed by the animal during an assisted feeding episode is also quite a challenge, as most of the food will be on the floor, towels, hair coat, cupboard doors and even the ceiling.

If a patient is unwilling or unable to eat voluntarily, tube feeding should be considered. Tube feeding, however, is limited by diet selections. In most instances, only liquid or gruel diets can be fed through the tube due to the small internal diameter. In addition, tubes can become clogged and must be flushed with water frequently to help prevent this.[3] While it is tempting to administer medications, the chances of clogging a small diameter feeding tube are significant. Liquid medications are preferred; if administering ground up pills ensure that they are fully dissolved in a water suspension and that grinding them up will not change their pharmacokinetic properties (Figures 31.3, 31.4 and 31.5).

Parenteral Nutrition

When enteral nutrition is not an option as with gut failure, when enteral nutrition could exacerbate a disease (e.g necrotic hemorrhagic pancreatitis), intractable vomiting and/or diarrhea, poor anesthetic candidate for enteral feeding tube placement, inability to meet

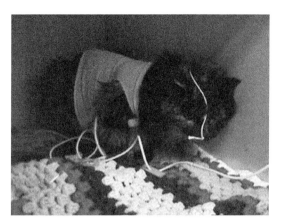

Figure 31.3 A cat receiving nasoesophageal feedings in hospital.

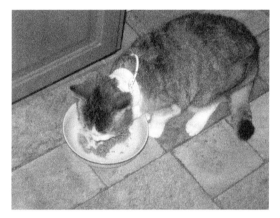

Figure 31.4 A cat at home, eating with an esophagostomy tube in place.

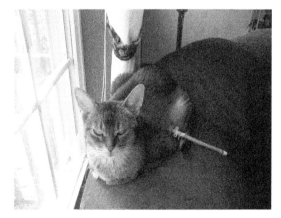

Figure 31.5 A cat at home with a percutaneous endoscopic gastrostomy (PEG) tube in place.

the full energy requirements enterally, or the animals airway can not be protected and aspiration pneumonia is a concern, parenteral nutrition is an option.[3,10] For patients with chylothorax, TPN allows administration of lipids in the diet as this method of feeding bypasses the lymphatic system and thoracic duct.[10] The most commonly reported disease states in which PN is used include pancreatitis, gastrointestinal disease, and hepatic diseases including hepatic lipidosis.[10]

Parenteral nutrition uses a modified solution with nutrients that can be absorbed by the cells without passing through the gut first. Parenteral solutions can be used alone (i.e. total parenteral nutrition-TPN) or as a supplement to enteral feedings (i.e. partial parenteral nutrition-PPN) when insufficient caloric intake is seen. Using parenteral nutrition as the only means of calories is recommended only for patients that cannot be fed enterally. Due to the expense associated with set up and use and the difficulty in obtaining the solutions, short term use is usually not justified, and most animals started on PN should need support for a least 5 days including a transition period back to enteral feeding.[3]

There are commercially prepared PPN solutions that can be given through a peripheral catheter, which allows use as needed for any animal with a catheter in place. These solutions typically lack the lipid portion of the solution making their osmolality lower, and allowing administration though a peripheral rather than a central catheter. Since the solutions do not need to be compounded, and can sit on a shelf in the same way as crystalloid fluids, they are more convenient than other PN fluids (Figure 31.6).[10]

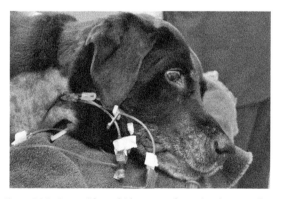

Figure 31.6 Dog with multi-lumen catheter in place to allow TPN administration.

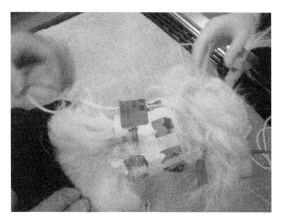

Figure 31.7 To avoid serious complications, the port being used for TPN should be labeled and treated aseptically.

Parenteral nutrition has several disadvantages. A dedicated central venous catheter is required for TPN, and the special nutrient solution must be properly and aseptically prepared. Some clinics have onsite pharmacies that can prepare the solutions, but this is not the norm. Intensive monitoring is necessary; thrombophlebitis and sepsis are serious complications if strict aseptic technique is not followed during the entire time the PN is being provided.[11] Lack of nutrients in the intestinal lumen may lead to breakdown of the bacterial barrier in the gut, further increasing the incidence of sepsis.[4] Lastly, a transitional period is necessary to wean the patient from parenteral back to enteral feedings (Figure 31.7).[4]

Because parenteral solutions have a very high osmolality (often greater than 800–1200 mOsm), a central venous catheter should be used to help prevent phlebitis. If a peripheral catheter is use, the solutions must be substantially diluted to decrease the osmolality, this will also dilute the caloric content. Administration must also be adjusted to prevent fluid overload.[11] Line separation or breakage must be avoided to decrease the incidence of introducing bacteria into the solution or the patient.[11]

Diets

Patients with stress starvation can be glucose intolerant and if so, use glucose less efficiently as an energy source. Therefore, protein and fat are important sources of energy.[11] Before evaluating the need for fat, protein and carbohydrate, however, a good diet strategy

Table 31.3 Practices that adversely affect nutritional status[3]

- Failing to record weight daily
- Failing to observe, measure and record amounts of food consumed
- Allowing diffusion of responsibility for patient care during staff rotation
- Prolonging administration of dextrose and electrolyte containing solution without providing additional nutritional support
- Delaying nutritional support until a patient reaches an advanced state
- Withholding food to conduct multiple diagnostic tests or procedures
- Failing to recognize and treat increased nutritional needs
- Failing to appreciate the role of nutrition in prevention and recovery from infection and placing unwarranted reliance on drugs
- Allowing surgery to be performed without verifying whether the patient is optimally nourished
- Providing inadequate nutritional support after surgery
- Failing to use laboratory tests to assess nutritional status (2)

should address the animal's requirement for water and correct any preexisting fluid, electrolyte and acid–base deficits.[11] After these needs have been satisfied, sufficient fat, carbohydrate and protein should be provided to meet the animal's energy requirements and minimize the gluconeogenesis of amino acids (Table 31.3).[11]

Commercial pet foods are specifically designed to meet the dietary requirements of cats and dogs and contain ingredients (e.g. glutamine, taurine, carnitine) not usually found in liquid or parenteral diets.[11] The route of entry for the food is equally important. What can be fed orally may not be able to be fed through a feeding tube. The type of food being fed through a feeding tube will vary based on the location of the tube, as well as the internal diameter (ID) of the tube and the caloric requirements of the animal.

Liquid diets have gained favor in human medicine, and many different types are available both OTC and prescription. The principal differences between human and animal liquid diets are the extent that the ingredients are subject to hydrolysis and the protein contents.[11] For example, most human enteral diets contain 14–17% ME protein, which is insufficient for both dogs and cats. In addition, arginine and methionine levels in human enteral diets tend to be too low, especially for cats.[11]

Table 31.4 Recommended levels of protein, fat, and carbohydrate in critical care diets[11]

Species	Protein % ME	Fat % ME	Carbohydrate% ME
Dogs	20–30	30–55	15–50
Cats	25–35	40–55	15–25

It is better for the animal and easier on the technician or client to use a veterinary formulated enteral liquid diet rather than try to rebalance a human enteral diet to match the nutrient profile required for a cat or dog. Few, if any of us, have the proper equipment to ensure we've done this correctly, let alone be able to figure out what the final caloric content of the solution really is (Table 31.4).

Pediatric or growth pet diets are often recommended as recovery diets because they are highly digestible, have high fat and protein contents, and are very palatable.[9] Meat-based baby foods contain 30–70% protein and 20–60% fat. However, because they are deficient in calcium, vitamin A, and thiamine, baby foods should not be used as the sole dietary source.[6] The presence of onion flavoring in many of the meat-based baby foods would also prohibit their extended use, as this will result in hemolytic anemia in our patients (Table 31.5).

Rate of Diet Initiation

Because nutritional support is not an emergency procedure, the general guidelines are to start slowly.[9] Food intake should be gradually increased over a 2–3 day period until the estimated caloric intake is met.[11] If the patient shows discomfort, vomits, is nauseous, or becomes distressed, the diet and the route and rate of delivery need to be assessed.

Generally, 50% of the RER, divided into multiple small meals, is offered the first day. If this amount is well tolerated, then 100% of the RER can be fed the second day. If the feedings are not well tolerated, the increases should be more gradual over the next 2–3 days. Smaller meals tend to be better tolerated because they do not cause over distension of the stomach and subsequent delayed gastric emptying or aggravate nausea as can occur with larger meals.[3]

With patients receiving assisted feedings via nasoesophageal, esophageal or gastrostomy tube, delivering the food using a syringe pump for a continuous rate infusion will allow more food to be fed than if bolus feedings were used, and significantly decrease the incidence of nausea because only small amounts of food are in the stomach at any given time. This also is much easier on the nursing staff than if frequent small bolus feedings are being fed every 2–4 hours. The feeding line does still need to be flushed every 4–6 hours to ensure the tube remains patent.[2] If using a CRI feeding, ensure that the patient is not vomiting, and could not redirect the terminal end of the tube from the esophagus into the trachea. If a syringe pump is being used, the animals will require constant monitoring, and should not be housed in the kennel where only periodic monitoring is available.

Refeeding Syndrome

Refeeding syndrome is an electrolyte disturbance that can occur in patients with depleted intracellular cations (e.g. potassium, phosphorus, magnesium and calcium), and can be seen with malnutrition, starvation as with feline hepatic lipidosis, or prolonged diuresis as seen with uncontrolled diabetes or renal failure. Patients at greatest risk are severely malnourished with significant loss of lean body mass.

Reintroduction of nutrition results in a rapid shift of these cations from the plasma (where levels may be normal prior to feeding) to the intracellular space. Profound hypophosphatemia, hypokalemia and/or hypomagnesemia may result and can lead to muscle weakness, intravascular hemolysis and possible cardiac and respiratory failure.

This syndrome can be avoided by monitoring the patient closely, introducing feeding cautiously (continuous rate infusion of a commercial recovery diet), monitoring electrolytes frequently (every 12–24 hours), and supplementing the diet as needed when deficiencies in the electrolytes are seen.[4] Monitoring should begin before food is introduced, and that includes PN as well as EN. Typically the phosphorus, potassium, glucose and PCV are checked every 12 hours for the first 24–36 hours. If any decreases are seen, supplementation should be made immediately of the affected electrolyte.[2] If deficiencies are seen in more than one

Table 31.5 Comparison of various recovery diets

Food	Protein % ME	Fat % ME	Carb % ME	Nutrient density	Kcal/ml
Hill's Prescription Diet® a/d® (1)	33	55	12	180/5.5 oz can	1.1
Hill's Prescription Diet® m/d® feline canned (1)	46	41	3	156/5.5 oz can	0.9
Royal Canin® Recovery RS™ canned canine/feline (2)	37.8	55.7	6.5	183/5.8 oz can	1.0
Iams Veterinary Formula™ Maximum Calorie Plus™ (3)	29	68	3	333/ 6 oz can	2.1
Purina Veterinary Diets® DM® canned feline (4)	38.8	58	3.3	191/5.5 oz can	1.1
Abbott Clinicare® liquid canine/feline (5)	28.7	43.3	28	237/8 oz can	1.0
Virbac Rebound® liquid canine/feline (5)	4	16	40	200/8 oz can	0.8
Evsco Nutrical® canine/feline (5)	2	94	4	30/tsp	6

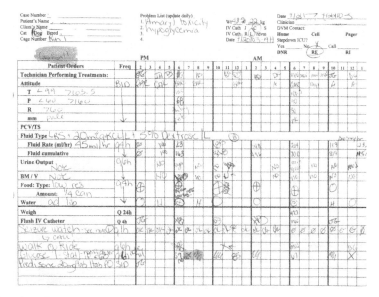

Figure 31.8 Sample flow chart showing accurate food intake notes.

electrolyte, calculations are done to replace the most deficient one as when using KPhos for supplementation.

Implementing Feeding Orders

Technicians responsible for patient treatments should be given instructions listing the type of food to be offered along with how much to give and how often. A flowchart can be used to record the amount eaten, the technique used to feed the patient, and the food that was offered (e.g. ½ can of slightly warmed dog food offered by hand at 3:00 pm, ate well). The technician can then draw a circle on the flow chart and fill in the amount of food the patient consumed (e.g. filling in a quarter of the circle if the patient ate ¼ of the amount offered); if the patient refused to eat, the technician should record an R in the circle. The technician should also note whether any food, amount or technique recorded differs from the instructions. Such record-keeping provides veterinarians with an accurate measurement of food intake and technicians with feeding methods that succeed on a per-patient basis, especially helpful during shift changes (Figure 31.8).

Diet Transitions

Although diet transitions may occur while the patient is hospitalized; typically this is done 2–6 weeks after discharge from the hospital. Transitions depend on the diet being fed, condition of the patient, its response to therapy, and the comfort level of the owner. As with diet initiation, it is best to proceed slowly. For example, when shifting from a support diet to a maintenance diet, each dietary change should represent an decrease of one quarter of the current diet every 3–4 days. For days 1–4, feed 3/4 of the therapeutic diet and 1/4 of the maintenance diet; days 5–8, feed 1/2 of the therapeutic diet and 1/2 of the maintenance diet; days 9–12, feed 1/4 of the therapeutic diet and 3/4 of the maintenance diet; day 13, feed 100% maintenance diet (i.e. transition phase of 12–16 days). If a problem develops at any stage, the owners should be instructed to return to the last diet combination that worked, and to contact the veterinary team for further instructions.

Technicians should supply owners with well-written, concise discharge instructions and reasonable expectation of what the diet being fed can do. Unfortunately, therapeutic diets can not "cure" inflammatory bowel disease, chronic renal failure or diabetes, though they are often used to help control the signs of these diseases. It is very important that owners are aware of this.

Conclusion

Being aware of the nutritional aspects of patient care can improve the long-term outcome of the patient's health as well as the client–patient–veterinary team relationship. Technicians can assume a primary role in providing excellent nutritional support to our patients. Even if we are not able to save our patients every time, the clients understand that we do care and want what is best for their pet.

References

1 Buffington CA, Hollaway C, Abood SK (2004) Clinical dietetics. In *Manual of Veterinary Dietetics*, pp. 54–60, St Louis, MO: Elsevier.

2 Larsen JA (2012) Enteral nutrition and tube feeding. In S Delaney, A Fascetti (eds), *Applied Veterinary Clinical Nutrition*, pp. 329–47, Ames, IA: Wiley-Blackwell.

3 Remillard R, Armstrong PJ, Davenport D (2000) Assisted feeding in hospitalized patients: Enteral and parenteral nutrition. In M Hand, C Hatcher, R Remillard, P Roudebush (eds), *Small Animal Clinical Nutrition* (4th edn), pp. 352–70, Marceline, MO: Walsworth Publishing.

4 Donaghue S (1989) Nutritional support of hospitalized patients. *Veterinary Clinics of North America Small Animal Practice* **19**(3): 475–93.

5 Abood SK (1997) Nutritional assessment of the critical care patient. In *Purina Nutrition Forum*, St Louis, MO: Ralston Purina Co.

6 Wingfield WE (1997) The essentials of life in critically ill animals. In *Purina Nutrition Forum*, St Louis, MO: Ralston Purina Co.

7 Chan DL (2005) In-hospital starvation: Inadequate nutritional support. In *11th International Veterinary Emergency & Critical Care Symposium Proceedings*, pp. 515–18.

8 Torrance AG (1996) Intensive care nutritional support. In *Manual of Companion Animal Nutrition and Feeding*, pp. 171–80, Ames, IA: Iowa State University Press.

9 Hill RC (1994) Critical care nutrition. In JM Wills, KW Simpson (eds), *The Waltham Book of Clinical Nutrition of the Dog and Cat*, pp. 39–57, Tarrytown, NY: Pergamon Press.

10 Perea SC (2012) Parenteral nutrition. In S Delaney, A Fascetti (eds), *Applied Veterinary Clinical Nutrition*, pp. 353–69, Ames IA: Wiley-Blackwell.

11 Tennant B (1996) Feeding the sick animal. In *Manual of Companion Animal Nutrition and Feeding*, pp. 171–80, Ames, IA: Iowa State University Press.

32 Assisted Feeding in Dogs and Cats

Introduction

Addressing the nutritional needs of our hospitalized and critical care patients can dramatically improve their outcomes, but also allows them to return home sooner. Oral enteral nutrition is the ideal route, but if the patient is unable or unwilling to consume at least 85% of their calculated resting energy requirements (RER) then another route needs to be utilized.

When oral nutrition is not an option, what other options are available? There are a number of different types of feeding tube available, and most of them do not require special equipment or skills to place. The choice of tube will be dependent on the condition of the patient, the disease being addressed, and expense of administration, availability of intensive care facilities, the preferred food and anticipated length of feeding assistance.

The first step would be to calculate the RER for the individual patient. The most widely used formula is: (weight in kilograms × 30) + 70 = RER

This formula can be utilized in both cats can dogs over 2 kilograms to 45 kilograms.[1-3] For animals outside this range, one of the logarithmic formulas can be used to calculate RER.

Feeding Tube Materials

The best feeding tubes for prolonged use are made of polyurethane or silicone. For short-term feeding, usually less than 10 days, polyvinylchloride (PVC) tubes can be used. These are not appropriate for long-term feeding because they tend to become stiff with prolonged use causing additional discomfort for the patient. Silicone is softer and more flexible than other tube materials and has a greater tendency to stretch and collapse. Polyurethane is stronger than silicone, allowing for thinner tube walls and a greater internal diameter, despite the same French size. Both the silicone and polyurethane tubes do not disintegrate or become brittle in situ, providing a longer tube life. Latex (rubber) feeding tubes are soft and comfortable for the patient, but due to their composition, tend to have larger tube wall thicknesses, decreasing the internal diameter of the tube. They also tend to become brittle in situ, and will undergo significant material disintegration ~12–16 weeks after placement. If the anticipated length of use is less than this period of time, this would not pose a significant problem. Latex is inexpensive, non-irritating to the animal and comfortable to long-term use.[4]

The French unit measures the outer lumen diameter of a tube and is equal to 0.33 mm. Because the outer diameter is being measured, a thinner tube wall can produce a larger internal lumen making feeding easier on the nursing staff or owner.[2] The type of material the feeding tube is composed of can also affect the easy of passage for the food. Silicon and polyurethane are "slick" and offer less resistance to food passage, latex offers slightly more resistant, and PVC tubes can offer more resistance than latex.[4]

While force feeding can be used to provide the necessary nutrition, this is usually too stressful to the patient, not to mention the stress to the owner. Seldom is this method able to deliver the volume of nutrients necessary to meet the patients' needs.

Enteral feeding tubes include tubes that enter through a natural opening (the nares) to those where surgical openings are made, such as esophagostomy, gastrostomy and jejunostomy tubes. They may terminate anywhere

Nutrition and Disease Management for Veterinary Technicians and Nurses, Second Edition. Ann Wortinger, Kara M. Burns
© 2015 John Wiley & Sons, Inc. Published 2015 by John Wiley & Sons, Inc.
Companion Website: www.wiley.com/go/wortinger/nutrition

Table 32.1 Tube feeding comparisons

Type of tube	Condition	Disease	ICU costs	Food type used	Length of time
Nasoesophageal/ Nasogastric	Not recommended for patients that are vomiting or those with respiratory disease	Short-term anorexia, supplement oral intake	$	Liquid +/− thinning required; CRI or bolus	Short-term, in-hospital use only (3–7 days)
Pharyngostomy/ esophagostomy	Not recommended for patients that are vomiting or those with respiratory disease	Hepatic lipidosis, anorexia, oral surgery or trauma, cancer	$$	Liquid, recovery diet or gruel commercial diet based on tube size; CRI or bolus	Long-term, in-hospital and at-home use (1–20 weeks, depending on tube type used)
Gastrostomy	Can be used on patients that are vomiting or that have respiratory disease	Pancreatitis, hepatic lipidosis, anorexia, esophageal strictures, oral surgery or trauma, cancer	$$$	Liquid, recovery diet or gruel commercial diet based on tube size; CRI or bolus	Long-term use, can be permanent, depending on tube type used
Jejunostomy	Can be used on patients that are vomiting or that have respiratory disease	Pancreatitis, intestinal anastomosis, coma	$$$$	Liquid diet; CRI or bolus	Short-term, in-hospital use only (3–10 days)

from the mid-esophagus to the jejunum, dependent on what type of tube is being placed and the desired placement site (Table 32.1).

Nasoesophageal/Nasogastric Tube

Nasoesophageal tubes are useful for providing short term nutritional support, usually less than 10 days. They can be used in patients with a functional esophagus, stomach and intestines. Nasoesophageal tubes are contraindicated in patients that are vomiting, comatose or lack a gag reflex.[2,5] Because of the requirement of passage through the nose, they are typically a smaller diameter tube (5–8 fr). These tubes offer the advantage of placement without general anesthesia (topical is recommended in the nose), and no specialized equipment is required. Nasoesophageal tubes can also be of benefit for those animals with confirmed or suspected coagulopathies, as no incisions are needed for placement.[4]

On the con side of use, they can be quite irritating to the patient due to the facial sutures, the sight line of the tube on the animal's face, and the potential need of an Elizabethan collar to ensure the tube is not "accidentally" removed.[4] Due to the requirement for a liquid diet being fed frequently, they are also impractical

for use by owners at home, and are only practical for short-term use.[4]

Complications include epistaxis, lack of tolerance of the procedure, inadvertent removal by the patient. These tubes should not be used in vomiting patients or those with respiratory disease as the potential exists that the tube can be vomited up from the esophagus, and displaced into the trachea causing aspiration pneumonia during feeding.[1–3,5]

Due to the small internal diameter of these tubes, only liquid enteral diets can be used. They can either be fed through a syringe pump as a continuous rate infusion or bolus fed. If feeding through a syringe pump, completely change the delivery equipment every 24 hours to help prevent bacterial growth within the system. Tube clogging is a common problem; a syringe pump may help to decrease the incidence as will flushing well before and after bolus feeding. If the tube becomes clogged, replacement may be necessary. Diluting the liquid with water may also help, though this further decreases the caloric concentration of the diet, increasing the volume necessary to meet the caloric needs.

Nasogastric tubes are placed in the same manner as a nasoesophageal tube, but the terminal end is located in the stomach rather than the distal esophagus. By passing through the cardiac sphincter into the stomach, the risk of gastroesophageal reflux increases, therefore increasing the incidence of esophageal strictures.[4]

Esophagostomy Tube Placement

Esophagostomy tube placement does require anesthesia to perform, but it does not need to be surgical depth of anesthesia. They need to be deep enough to place a mouth gag in without causing pain or complications.[4] These tubes are generally well tolerated by the patient, and don't require any special equipment to place. The biggest advantages of these tubes include the large size that can be placed (12–14 fr for cats and 14 fr or higher for dogs), and the ability to discharge the animal for continued care with the owner at home. Polyethylene tubes appear to be quite irritating for this use, and should be avoided, as should PVC tubes if long-term use is anticipated.[4] If there is tube clogging or other failure, a new tube can be placed through the existing stoma site if nutritional support is still needed.[4]

Complications include tube displacement due to vomiting or removal by the patient, skin infection around the exit site and biting off of the tube end by the patient after vomiting. There may be some signs of discomfort seen with the neck bandage, and many softer, long-term bandages are commercially available for use.[4]

The large bore of these catheters allow for feeding of a gruel recovery diet, sometimes without dilution with water. These catheters are also easy for clients to use and maintain at home as long as vomiting is not a problem. Since the incision is located in the neck, feeding can begin immediately after recovery from anesthesia with no additional time needed for a temporary stoma to form.[4]

When removing, the tube may be simply pulled out after the sutures are removed. The exit hole is allowed to heal by second intension. A light bandage may be applied for the first 12 hours (Figure 32.1).

Gastrostomy Tube

Gastrostomy tubes can be placed either endoscopically, blindly or surgically. All three techniques require general anesthesia, but again this does not need to be surgical depth of anesthesia. Endoscopic placement allows for visualization of the esophagus and stomach as

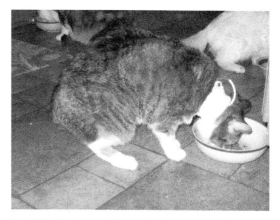

Figure 32.1 Neck wrap being used at home on an esphagostomy tube.

well as biopsy collection from the stomach and proximal duodenum and foreign body removal. Blind biopsy allows placement of a gastrostomy tube without the investment in an endoscopic unit. Surgical placement is useful during surgical exploratory or when the scope can not be passed through the esophagus due to trauma or esophageal strictures.

A minimum of 12 hours is needed for a temporary stoma to form before feeding can begin. The feeding tube should be left in place for a minimum of 7–10 days to allow a permanent stoma to form before removal. The tubes can be left in long term (1–6 months) without replacement. When replaced with another PEG tube, low profile silicone tube or foley type feeding tube, the stoma can be used for the rest of the patient's life.

Complications associated with PEG tubes include those seen from tube placement such as splenic laceration, gastric hemorrhage and pneumoperitoneum. Delayed complications can also be seen such as vomiting, aspiration pneumonia, tube removal, tube migration, and peritonitis and stoma infection.[2]

Blind percutaneous gastrostomy tube placement involves basically the same technique as endoscopic placement, but a large plastic or steel tube is used instead of the endoscope and a firm wire is used instead of the suture. The catheter is the same as in the endoscopic insertion technique. Reported complications are the same as for PEG tubes, though the risk of splenic, stomach or omental laceration is greater. Contraindications to using the blind technique include severe obesity that would make palpation of the end of the tube difficult and esophageal disease.

Surgical placement has been largely superseded by endoscopic placement because of the ease and speed of placement, lower cost and decreased morbidity. A surgical approach may be indicated in obese animals, those with esophageal disease or when laporatomy is already scheduled. To place a surgical gastrostomy a larger incision is needed into the stomach and the exit location is sometimes hard to locate because of the position on the surgical table. Surgical placement involves placing purse string sutures around the catheter to secure it as well as attaching the stomach to the body wall.

Gastrostomy tube placement is the technique of choice of long-term enteral support. These tubes are well tolerated by the patient, produce minimal discomfort, allow feeding of either gruel recovery diets or blenderized commercial foods, and can be easily managed by owners at home.[5] Patients are able to eat normally with gastrostomy tubes in placed and can easily be used as a nutritional supplement until the patient is totally self feeding. For patients that are difficult to medicate and require long-term medications, many medicines can also be given thought the feeding tube. The major disadvantage of gastrostomy tubes is the need for general anesthesia and the risk of peritonitis.[5]

For animals requiring long-term management, the initial Pezzer catheter can be replaced with either low-profile silicone tubes or with foley type gastrostomy tubes. Both of these types can be placed through the external stoma site without the endoscope. Sedation or anesthesia may be necessary based on the individual patient.

For removal, if the tube has been in place 16 weeks or less the tube may be simply removed. This is best accomplished by placing the patient in right lateral recumbency. The tube is grasped with the right hand close to the body wall, with the left hand holding the animal. Pull firmly and consistently to the right in an upward motion. Some force may be required for this. It is also helpful to ensure that the patient has been fasted, and placing a towel over the tube site to catch any "stuff." If the tube has been in longer than 16 weeks, the incidence of tube breakage is much higher. Depending on where the breakage occurs, the remaining tube pieces may need to be endoscopically retrieved. Larger patients can easily pass retained parts; smaller patients may need to have them retrieved.

The exit hole is allowed to heal by second intension. A light bandage may be applied for the first 12 hours.

Jejunostomy Tube

Jejunostomy feeding is indicated when the upper gastrointestinal tract must be rested or when pancreatic stimulation must be decreased. Jejunal tubes can be placed either surgically or threaded through a gastrostomy tube for transpyloric placement. Standard gastojejunal tubes designed for humans are unreliable in dogs due to frequent reflux of the jejunal portion of the tube back into the stomach. Investigation is ongoing involving endoscopic placement of transpyloric jejunal tubes through PEG tubes.

Due to the small diameter of these tubes (typically 5–8 fr) and the location, liquid enteral diets are recommended. Because the jejunum has minimal storage capacity compared to the stomach, continuous rate infusion using a syringe pump is the preferred method of delivery.

Common complications include osmotic diarrhea, vomiting, premature removal of the tube, retrograde tube movement out of the jejunum, focal cellulitis, leakage of gastrointestinal contents and tube obstruction.

It is recommended that the jejunal tube be left in place for 7–10 days to allow adhesions to form around the tube site and prevent leakage back into the abdomen.[1,5] Completely changing the delivery equipment every 24 hours will help prevent bacterial growth within the system. Clogging is a common problem; a syringe pump may help to decrease the incidence as will flushing well every 4 hours.

When removing, the tube may be simply pulled out after the sutures are removed. The exit hole is allowed to heal by second intension. A light bandage may be applied for the first 12 hours.

Beginning Enteral Feeding

Tube placement is only the beginning of the feeding for these animals. Next we have to start feeding, and be able to maintain it for the length of time the animal requires to recover or begin eating on their own again. Initially we will start feeding a liquid or gruel recovery diet at a consistency that will easily pass through the feeding tube. With nasoesophageal or nasogastric tubes, feeding can begin immediately after tube placement. For esophagostomy tubes, feeding can begin after anesthetic recovery. For gastrostomy and jejunostomy tubes, feeding must be delayed for 12 hours post placement to allow a temporary stoma to form around the tube placement site.[4]

Depending on the physical condition of the patient and the disease processes being addressed feeding frequency and volumes may need to be adjusted. For animal's who are at a normal BCS and do not have concurrent disease processes (i.e. HBC, post-surgical) feeding can be started at 50% RER, divided into 3–4 equal feedings. For those that are physically debilitated or have significant disease processes (i.e. hepatic lipidosis, diabetes mellitus, and renal failure), feedings can be started at 25–30% RER with frequency of q 4 hr or as a CRI.[4]

As the recovery progresses, the feeding volume can be increased while the feeding frequency decreases (Table 32.2).

This is a typical feeding schedule for a moderately severe hepatic lipidosis cat from the time of the initial feeding until it is ready for discharge from the hospital.

Diet Choices

There is no best diet for enteral tube feeding, but there are many options.[4] When looking for a diet you need to evaluate the disease process you are treating, the size of the tube you wish to use and the cost and availability of the food if using by the owners at home.

Table 32.2 Feeding schedule for a 12# cat with a DER calculated at 280–303 kcal/day. The food has 2.1 kcal/ml

---

Total feeding volume will be 280–303/2.1 = 133–144 ml/day
- Day 1 – 1.8 ml/hr CRI (30%)
- Day 2 – 3 ml/hr CRI (50%)
- Day 3 – 3.6 ml/hr CRI (60%)
- Day 4 – 14 ml q 4 hr (60%)
- Day 5 – 18 ml q 4 hr (75%)
- Day 6 – 27 ml q 6 hr (75%)
- Day 7 – 36 ml q 6 hr (100%)
- Day 8 – 48 ml q 8 hr (100%)

Feedings are only increased in volume or time between feedings if the patient tolerates the schedule without vomiting.
Typically, either the volume is increased or the time between feedings is increased but not both.

Gruel, liquid, canned and dry foods can all be used for enteral feeding, but not every food can be used with every tube. Liquid diets can usually go through tubes larger than 5 fr, gruel diets need a 10–12 fr tube, and may still have some clogging problems with this size. For blenderized diets, whether they are canned or dry food a 14 fr or larger is usually advised.[4] The finer the diet can be processed, the less chance of tube clogging. Ideally recovery diets do not need additional processing, but if using a canned or dry diet additional processing will be needed.

For canned diets, they are usually processed in a food blender with a ratio of 1 can of food to 1 can of water, mix well. You need to get the particles fine enough to pass easily through the feeding tube and a consistency that can be drawn up and administered with a feeding syringe.[4]

For a dry diet add the dry food to the blender dry, pulverize the food well then add an equal amount of water. Mix well again. Due to the dry carbohydrates found in this type of diet, allow the food to site for 20–30 minutes to allow the carbohydrates to soak up the water. Additional water may need to be added to thin out the consistency to allow passage through the syringe.

When blenderizing foods, the calories will not be calculated on a per mL amount, as we may not know what the final volume will be as the amount of water to add may vary. We will know what the calorie content will be on a per can or per cup basis, and will need to figure out our volumes from there.

Example:

Our patient needs 1 can of Dog Gruel/day through their feeding tube divided into 3 equal meals. Each can is 13.5 oz. When we blenderize 1 can of food with 1 3/4 cup of water we get a final mixture of ~ 3.5 cups. If we divide 3.5 cups/3 meals we get 1.16 cups/meal. There are 240 ml in a cup. 1.16 cup × 240 ml = 278 ml/meal. 278 ml/meal × 3 meals = 835 ml/day.

The higher the caloric density of the food, the lower the volume that must be fed to reach their DER. When using OTC foods (canned or dry), the caloric density will be inherently lower than that found in therapeutic recovery diets, necessitating feeding of higher volumes of food. In the long run, feeding a commercial diet to a feeding tube animal may not be less expensive or easier on the owner.

Mechanical Complications

Mechanical complications include both tube obstruction and premature removal of the tube or dislodgement from the site of placement.[6] The most common problem, tube obstruction can be prevented in most cases by proper tube maintenance. Food should never be allowed to sit in the tube, and the tube should be flushed with warm water after *every* feeding, or whenever gastrointestinal contents as aspirated through the tube as when checking residuals. When using the feeding tube to administer medications, only one medication at a time should be given through the tube, and it should be given separately from the food.[6] This will help to prevent drug-to-drug interactions as well as drug-to-food interactions as not all medications and enteral foods are compatible with one another.

If the feeding tube becomes clogged either from insufficient flushing after feeding, or from hair accumulation through the holes in the end of the tube, first try to flush the clog out using warm water and the feeding syringe.[2] Hold the tube firmly and push the water with force. If the clog is not bad, this may work. If it is still clogged, try switching to a carbonated cola beverage in the feeding tube, and allow this to sit for a period of time. Some practitioners have suggested the use of pancreatic enzymes mixed with water and various other mixtures instilled into the tube to break up the clog.[6]

Premature tube removal or dislodgement is best prevented by choosing the most appropriate tube for the animal and using Elizabethan collars and wraps when appropriate.[2] Whenever the location of the tube is in doubt, it should be checked radiographically. While most tubes are radiopaque, a sterile contract media (i.e. Omnipaque) can be infused through the tube to check for leaks into the peritoneal or thoracic cavity.[6]

Gastrointestinal Complications

Some of the gastrointestinal complications seen with tube feeding are related to the feeding itself. Food that is administered too quickly, in too large an amount or at the wrong temperature can all cause nausea, vomiting or abdominal discomfort.[6] These signs can also be related to the patient's underlying disease process or a complication of medications the patient is receiving.

Liquid enteral diets are typically very low residue, and are likely to cause a soft stool if not actual diarrhea in a normal animal let alone one who is already ill. Likewise, most recovery diets, both liquid and gruel forms, are high in fat, a patient with impaired fat digestion and absorption may develop steatorrhea when fed these diets.[4]

One cause of diarrhea not typically thought of is the medications that we are giving to the animals, whether they are orally or through the feeding tubes. Many liquid oral forms of medications are hypertonic or contain sorbital, a nonabsorbable sugar, and may cause, at least in part diarrhea.[6] We also need to remember that a number of commonly used antibiotics, analgesic agents and other drugs can cause nausea, vomiting and gastrointestinal ileus and may contribute to the discomfort our patients are feeling. Canned pumpkin, 5–15 ml per feeding, will usually resolve the diarrhea. Since canned pumpkin is typically sold in large cans, you can suggest to the client that they measure out the volume of pumpkin needed for each meal, place this in an ice cube trays and freeze it. When frozen they can be removed from the ice cube trays, placed in a plastic freezer bag and stored until needed. The amount used at each feeding will need to be adjusted for that individual animal.

Constipation is not an unusual complication seen in patients with feeding tubes. As they can be fairly weak from muscle loss and metabolic derangement, the development of constipation is not unexpected.[6] Adding Lactulose to the diet will often solve this problem, 1–2 ml per meal, adjusted as needed to maintain stool consistency.

Metabolic Complications

There are two types of metabolic complications that our patients can develop. The first is the result of the patient's inability to assimilate certain nutrients.[2] This can best be anticipated by doing a proper nutritional assessment of the patient before developing the nutritional plan. The other type is seen with "Refeeding Syndrome."

Keeping in mind the changes the body has undergone while in starvation, when reintroducing food several areas need to be monitored closely to prevent the "Refeeding Syndrome." During recovery, excessively rapid refeeding (or hyperalimentation) can overwhelm the patient's already limited functional reserves.[4,6]

Refeeding or reintroduction of nutrition causes a shift in the body from a catabolic state where protein is the primary energy source to an anabolic state where carbohydrates are the preferred energy source. Administration of enteral or parenteral nutrition stimulates the release of insulin; this causes dramatic shifts in serum electrolytes from the extracellular space to the intracellular space, primarily phosphorus, potassium and to a lesser degree magnesium.[2,6] Insulin promotes intracellular uptake of glucose and phosphorus for glycolysis. These electrolyte shifts can have a profound impact on metabolic functions within the body, phosphorus is used by the red blood cells as their primary source of energy in the form of 2,3 DPG, without this they die and you have hemolysis. Phosphorus is integral in the formation of ATP-the power source for most cells within the body, without this they cannot function properly. Potassium is involved in the sodium/potassium pump, without adequate amounts, no muscle contraction/ relaxation can occur.

Serum cobalamine (B12) is often low in cats that have small intestinal disease, pancreatic disease and hepatic lipidosis. Supplementation may be necessary even before enteral nutrition is started to allow adequate assimilation of nutrients within the intestine. The CRI method of feeding will help prevent many of the problems associated with Refeeding Syndrome.[6]

Serum electrolytes, phosphorus and packed cell volume should be monitored closely. A base line value should be established before treatment is started then once daily thereafter, unless dramatic changes are seen. If changes are seen in any of these values, supplementation needs to be started immediately. This can either be intravenous or through the feeding tube. Refeeding Syndrome is one of the most dramatic "side-effects" and can lead very quickly to death.[6]

Metabolic complications of any type are less likely to occur if estimated caloric needs are conservative. Current recommendations are to initiate feeding at caloric amounts equal to the patient's calculated resting energy requirements (RER) without the addition of any "illness requirements." As recovery progresses, we can increase the amount to DER.

Infectious Complications

The types of infectious complications that can occur in tube fed patients include contamination of the enterally fed formulas, peristomal cellulitis, septic peritonitis and aspiration pneumonia.[6]

Microbial contamination of the food is easily avoided by following basic hygiene in preparation and storage of the food. Blenderized foods should be prepared daily, and opened commercial liquid diets should be kept refrigerated and discarded after 48 hours. When food is being delivered via a syringe pump, no more than 6 hours' worth of food should be set-up at a time. One of the biggest sources of contamination is inadequate cleaning of equipment used for preparation and delivery of foods. Syringes, containers, and tubing used for preparing, storing and delivering food should be discarded after use.[6] Things that are reused, such as blenders and storage containers, should be cleaned thoroughly and preferably sterilized each time they are used. The equipment used to deliver the food should also be replaced every 24 hours; this includes the syringes and delivery tubes and if the food is hung, the administration bag.

Peristomal cellulitis can be seen with esophagostomy, gastrostomy and jejunostomy tubes. This can usually be avoided by insuring that the tube is not secured too tightly to the body wall, and by keeping the site clean and protected.[6] Septic peritonitis can develop in patients where the gastrostomy or jejunostomy tube has become dislodge or removed before a permanent stoma had formed.[4] Proper tube selection can help prevent this problem; button or balloon size should be large enough to secure the tube in the stomach lumen. Wraps or Elizabethan collars may be necessary to prevent the patient from accidentally or intentionally prematurely removing the tube. Ensuring that a mature stoma has formed prior to tube removal can help to prevent peritonitis. Patients that are malnourished (hypoalbunemic) or are receiving medications that impair wound healing may take longer to develop a mature stoma than would healthy patients.

Aspiration pneumonia can be seen with patients that have previously developed aspiration pneumonia, those with impaired mental status, patients with neurologic injuries, reduced or absent cough or gag reflexes and those on mechanical ventilation. Feeding patients in any of these categories pre-pylorically puts them at risk of aspiration of food.[5] Viable alternatives would include jejunostomy tubes and parenteral nutrition. Lastly, caution should be used when feeding patients with nasoesophageal or esophagostomy tubes using constant rate infusion. These types of tubes can be vomited up and the tip of the tube could relocate in the pharynx and place the patient at risk for pulmonary aspiration.

Hospital Management

Patients should be allowed out to exercise for 20–30 minutes approximately 1 hour before feeding, 2–3 times daily. This can be started even while the CRI feedings are being done, just disconnect the syringe pump, flush the line with water and cap. Exercise has been found to greatly enhance both gastric motility and patient attitude.[4]

Potential Post-discharge Complications

Very few patients do poorly after discharge, particularly if good communication is established with the owners and regular rechecks are scheduled. Recheck frequency should be based on the type of tube being used, the condition of the patient and how their recovery is going. It may be as frequent as every 2 weeks or as long as every quarter for long-term tube usage (Figure 32.2).

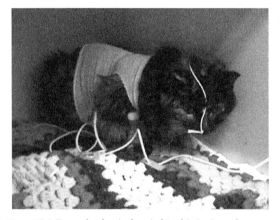

Figure 32.2 Example of an in-hospital "t-shirt" using tube gauze. Be sure to place 1" tape folded over the neck edge to keep the shirt from sliding down the cat's torso.

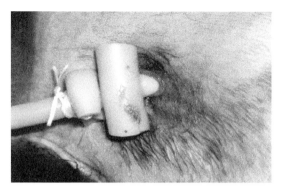

Figure 32.3 Hair regrowth around a tube site.

Granulation tissue normally forms around the tube site on the outside and may be quite pink and can even bleed when handled.[4] It is important to let clients know this is normal and to expect it, this tissue is what allows the hole to close after the tube is removed. It has been found in cats with dark hair coats (including tabbies) that the hair will grow in a dark ring around the tube site and thicker than the surrounding hair regrowth.[4] Many clients will think that this is necrosis and become very concerned, a quick warning to expect this will greatly ease their minds (Figure 32.3).

What do you do about the patient that insists on chewing on its tube? A simple solution is to place a baby's t-shirt on a cat, usually an infant's size 6–9 months works well for most. For large patients, larger shirts can be used. Use a t-shirt that has a fitted neck, not the lap shoulders. Once the t-shirt is on, place a piece of 1" porous tape near the end of the feeding tube, tuck the tube up under the t-shirt and use a safety pin to pin the tape to the t-shirt. This makes removal easier for feeding, and decreases the risk of pinning through the tube and damaging it.

Once the patient goes home, tube feedings are continued – even after the patient begins self-feeding. Owners are given instructions to always have fresh food and water available for the convalescing patient and when the desired weight is reached, tube feedings are decreased by 25–50% depending on the oral intake. The tube can be removed after the patient has reached its desired weight, has recovered from the trauma or has finished chemotherapy treatment and has been totally self-feeding for 2 weeks without showing any signs of weight loss. Many feeding tubes can be maintained long

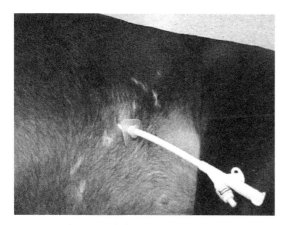

Figure 32.4 This stoma hole is almost 3 years old. The Great Dane developed esophageal strictures when she was 8 years old. She was managed for over 3 years with a gastrostomy tube and eventually died of heart failure.

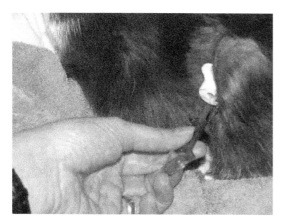

Figure 32.5 An example of a low-profile feeding tube being used in an oral cancer patient. Placement of this type of feeding tube requires a mature stoma hole.

term, and the same stoma hole used for repeated tube placements (Figures 32.4 and 32.5).

Conclusion

The enteral route is the preferred method of nutritional support in patients with functional gastrointestinal tracts. Many tube and food choices are available and can be tailored to fit the individual patient and condition.

Typically owners are very happy with the results they see when using a feeding tube and the animals feel much better. They do require routine daily care such as cleaning around the tube site and flushing of the feeding tube with water, but the tubes need not be used every day to feed the patient. The use of feeding tubes can give many clients the benefit of enjoying their pet for a longer period of time, and having a better quality of life for both of them.

References

1 Willard M (1992) The GI system. In RW Nelson, CG Couto (eds), *Essentials of Small Animal Internal Medicine*, pp: 305–9, St Louis, MO: Mosby.

2 Marks SL (2000) Enteral and parenteral nutritional support. In SJ Ettinger, EC Feldman (eds), *Textbook of Veterinary Internal Medicine Volume 1* (5th edn), pp. 275–82, Philadelphia, PA: WB Saunders.

3 Appendix V: Assisted feeding techniques. In MS Hand, CD Thatcher, RL Remillard, P Roudebush (eds), *Small Animal Clinical Nutrition* (4th edn), pp. 1145–53, Marceline, MO: Walsworth Publishing.

4 Larsen J (2012) Enteral nutrition and tube feeding. In S Delaney, A Fascetti (eds), *Applied Veterinary Clinical Nutrition*, pp. 329–48, Ames, IA: Wiley-Blackwell.

5 Nutritional management of gastrointestinal disease. In WG Guilford, SA Center, DR Strombeck (eds), *Strombeck's Small Animal Gastroenterology* (3rd edn), pp. 904–8, Philadelphia, PA: WB Saunders.

6 Michel K (2006) Monitoring the enterally fed patient to maximize benefits and minimize complication. In IVECCS Proceedings, pp. 495–8.

SECTION 4
Nutritional Management of Disease

33 Nutritional Management of Gastrointestinal Disorders

In veterinary hospitals around the world, gastrointestinal (GI) problems are one of the most common reasons that pet parents bring their pet to the hospital. The main challenge to the veterinary healthcare team presented with a pet that has GI dysfunction is to determine whether an emergency situation exists or is the presentation leading to a potentially serious problem versus a chronic or intermittent problem. The GI tract is known for its resiliency and the veterinary healthcare team has seen numerous pets with clinical signs of acute vomiting and/or diarrhea resolve uneventfully, sometimes without any supportive care. However, this is not true of all acute GI events as some may be life-threatening disorders, which if not identified and treated, could lead to poor patient management and/or death of the pet.

Vomiting is a clinical sign seen frequently in small animals and vomiting is associated with GI disorders; however, vomiting may occur with nongastrointestinal conditions as well. Thus it is difficult to identify the etiology of the vomiting and may require extensive diagnostic workup in some dogs and cats. Vomiting is the forceful discharge of ingested material from the stomach and sometimes proximal small intestines. Vomiting truly consists of three stages: nausea, retching, and subsequently vomiting. Nausea is the first stage. Outward signs of nausea for which the healthcare team should be aware may include depression, shivering, hiding, yawning, and licking of the lips. Increased salivation and swallowing occur, subsequently lubricating the esophagus. Retching often helps distinguish the episode from regurgitation, gagging, or coughing. Retching is the forceful contraction of the abdominal muscles and diaphragm. Negative intrathoracic pressure and positive abdominal pressure changes cause the movement of gastric contents into the esophagus and

out the mouth. This vomiting process is initiated by the central nervous system.

In addition to vomiting, diarrhea is one of the most common reasons owners bring their pets to the veterinary hospital. Diarrhea is the passage of feces containing an excessive amount of water thus resulting in an abnormal increase in stool liquidity and weight. Patients may also experience an increase in the frequency of their defecation. This would lead to the broad description of too rapid evacuation of too loose stools. It is important for the veterinary technician to gain a thorough understanding of the owner's definition of diarrhea as it may not be as accurate as the healthcare team's definition. This would incorporate a very involved discussion with the owner while gathering the history. Diarrhea is the trademark sign of intestinal dysfunction. It is important for healthcare team members to determine acute from chronic problems when assessing animals with diarrhea. Acute diarrhea is typically the result of diet, parasites, or infectious disease (e.g., parvovirus, coronavirus, etc.). Chronic diarrhea is termed as such when it has not responded to conventional therapy within a two to three week time frame.

The next step is to determine the origination of the diarrhea – small intestine or large intestine. A thorough history by the veterinary technician is again the best tool. Increased frequency of defecation resulting in larger than normal amounts of soft-to-watery stool is often seen in small bowel diarrhea. Failure to lose weight or body condition is typically indicative of large bowel disease. Weight loss usually indicates small bowel disease although severe large bowel diseases such as malignancy, histoplasmosis, and pythiosis may result in weight loss. Animals with weight loss from severe large bowel disease usually have signs associated with colonic

Nutrition and Disease Management for Veterinary Technicians and Nurses, Second Edition. Ann Wortinger, Kara M. Burns
© 2015 John Wiley & Sons, Inc. Published 2015 by John Wiley & Sons, Inc.
Companion Website: www.wiley.com/go/wortinger/nutrition

involvement such as fecal mucus, marked tenesmus, and hematochezia. Fresh blood (bright red in color) in the stool or evidence that the pet is straining to defecate is indicative of a large bowel disorder. Hematochezia (bright-red blood) typically originates in the anus, rectum, or descending colon. Melena is described as coal tar black stools that result from digested blood. Melena may originate from the pharynx, lungs (coughed up and swallowed), esophagus, stomach, or upper small intestine. Tarry stools are the result of bacterial breakdown of hemoglobin. Dyschezia is difficult and/or painful defecation. Tenesmus refers to persistent and/or prolonged straining, typically with no effect. Owners may mistake tenesmus with constipation, so it is important to question the owner further to determine which clinical sign truly is manifesting in their pet. Dyschezia and tenesmus are most often associated with large bowel disorders.

Diagnosis

A complete history is the first step (and it is a crucial step) in trying to establish a cause for vomiting and diarrhea. The signalment and history, as well as a description of the vomiting episodes, are important. First, one must determine whether the animal truly is vomiting. The healthcare team should differentiate the owner's report of vomiting from gagging, coughing, dysphagia, or regurgitation. The description of retching is characteristic for vomiting. Signalment may also be helpful. For example, young, unvaccinated pets are more susceptible to infectious disease, such as parvovirus. Vaccination status, travel history, previous medical problems, and the medication history should be determined. Many drugs can result in vomiting, such as nonsteroidal antiinflammatory drugs (NSAIDs), which are known to cause gastrointestinal ulceration and vomiting. The healthcare team member should also explore the possibility of toxin or foreign body ingestion and of other concurrent signs that often arise with systemic or metabolic disease. An example: polydipsia, polyuria, and weight loss are typical of vomiting associated with diabetic ketoacidosis or chronic kidney failure.

The history should then focus on the actual vomiting episodes. The duration, frequency, and relationship of the episodes to eating or drinking should be ascertained. A complete physical description of the vomited material should be documented. A dietary history, including the type of diet or recent dietary changes, is important because vomiting may be associated with an adverse reaction to food. Vomiting of an undigested or a partly digested meal more than 6–8 hours after eating, a time at which the stomach should normally be empty, suggests a gastric outflow obstruction or gastric hypomotility disorder. The description of the vomit should include the volume, color, consistency, odor, and the presence or absence of bile or blood. Undigested food suggests a gastric origin, whereas vomit-containing bile makes a gastric outflow obstruction unlikely. Vomit having a fecal odor is suggestive of a low-intestinal obstruction or bacterial overgrowth in the small intestine. Hematemesis (either as fresh, bright-red blood or as digested blood with the appearance of coffee grounds) is indicative of gastrointestinal erosion or ulceration. Gastric ulceration is caused by metabolic conditions such as hypoadrenocorticism, reaction to certain drugs, clotting abnormalities, gastritis, or neoplasia (Table 33.1 and Figure 33.1).

A complete physical examination should begin with an evaluation of the mouth and oral cavity. The presence of a fever is suggestive of an infectious or inflammatory process. Bradycardia or cardiac arrhythmias in a vomiting animal may be a sign of a metabolic disturbance, such as hypoadrenocorticism. Careful palpation of the abdomen should be part of the physical examination to rule out; distention or tympany (e.g., gastric dilatation–volvulus [GDV] syndrome), effusion (e.g., peritonitis), masses or organomegaly (e.g., neoplasia, intussusception, or foreign body), and pain (e.g., peritonitis, pancreatitis, or intestinal obstruction). Obstruction is suggested when there are gas- and fluid-filled intestines, whereas bunching of the bowel is characteristic of intestinal plication from a linear foreign body obstruction. A rectal examination provides characteristics of colonic mucosa and feces. Melena suggests upper-gastrointestinal bleeding while the presence of foreign material in the feces supports a possible foreign body etiology.

Performing a complete blood count (CBC) is extremely important for GI patients, especially in those animals at risk for neutropenia (e.g., parvoviral enteritis), infection, and anemia (e.g., melena, hemataemesis). Patients should also have a serum chemistry profile performed upon presentation. A serum biochemistry profile, especially in patients

Table 33.1 GI history questionnaire

- When did the GI issues begin?
- Was the onset acute?
- Any other animals at home?
  - If yes – are others showing signs of diarrhea?
- Has the patient been to areas where there are large numbers of other animals? Obedience, dog parks, pet stores, pet shows, etc.?
- Has there been access to drinking from a pond or streams?
- Describe the environment where the pet spends their time?
- What is the breed?
- Typical temperament of the pet?
- Did the pet get into/ingest any of the following: trash, toxins, other pet foods, foods that have spoiled, etc.
- Have any drugs been prescribed or administered recently that could result in diarrhea? For example, antibiotics.
- Have there been any changes in the pet's environment that may be stressful to the pet? New pet, change in family dynamics, alteration in home environment, boarding, day care, etc.
- Has there been any change in diet?
  - Dry to can?
  - New bag or case of food?
  - Raw food?
  - Treats?
  - People foods? Added? Part of diet?
- Describe the diarrhea
- What is the size, volume of the feces?
- Consistency of stool? Watery? Soft, formed
- Are there any normal stools passed during the day?
- Frequency of stools?
- Blood or mucus seen?
- Timing? Increased defecation? Unable to make it outside? Increased during nighttime? Urgency?
- If feline – does cat use litterbox? Does it defecate near the or away from the litterbox?
- Other symptoms present? Lethargy, fever, vomiting?
- Vomiting
- How often does the pet vomit? Describe the vomitus?
- Can the pet keep any food or water down?
- When is the last time the pet has taken anything in by mouth?
- Other family in the home – human, animal?

presenting with severe vomiting, diarrhea, ascites, unexplained weight loss, and/or anorexia should include alanine transaminase, alkaline phosphatase, blood urea nitrogen, creatinine, total protein, albumin,

total CO_2, cholesterol, calcium, phosphorous, magnesium, bilirubin, and glucose concentrations, along with electrolytes; sodium, chloride, and potassium.

Vomiting may result in significant fluid, electrolyte, and acid-base alterations. The most common electrolyte disturbance in vomiting cats and dogs is hypokalemia. Acid-base changes generally are minimal or, if abnormal, tend toward an acidosis. If metabolic alkalosis is identified and is associated with hyponatremia, hypochloremia, and hypokalemia, the most likely cause will be gastric outflow or high-duodenal obstruction. Rarely animals with gastrinomas or with frequent and unrelenting vomiting have a metabolic alkalosis. When routine diagnostic testing fails to identify an obvious etiology, additional tests may be necessary. Additional tests may include viral or heartworm serology, thyroid hormone testing, adrenocortical testing for hypoadrenocorticism, bile acid determination for liver disease, toxologic testing (e.g., lead poisoning), and a neurologic examination.

When testing fails to identify a nongastrointestinal cause for the vomiting, the focus should move to investigation of gastrointestinal disease as a possible etiology. The diagnostic approach includes contrast radiography, ultrasonography, endoscopy, or laparotomy. Frequently, inflammatory gastrointestinal lesions are a cause of chronic vomiting; these conditions include chronic gastritis, *Helicobacter* gastritis, inflammatory bowel disease (IBD), and chronic colitis. Cats with inflammatory bowel disease often have vomiting as the main clinical sign and diarrhea as a minor clinical component. Conditions such as gastric antral pyloric mucosal hypertrophy, antral polyps, foreign bodies, or neoplasia can cause gastric outflow obstruction. These conditions cause gastric retention and vomiting. Such gastric lesions can be easily identified endoscopically or using contrast radiography.

Nutritional Factors

Following a diagnosis by the veterinarian, the vomiting and/or diarrhea will need to be managed. The healthcare team should be cognizant of key nutritional factors and their impact when managing a patient nutritionally. Nutritional management of patients suffering with vomiting and/or diarrhea should consider the following nutritional factors:

FECAL SCORING CHART

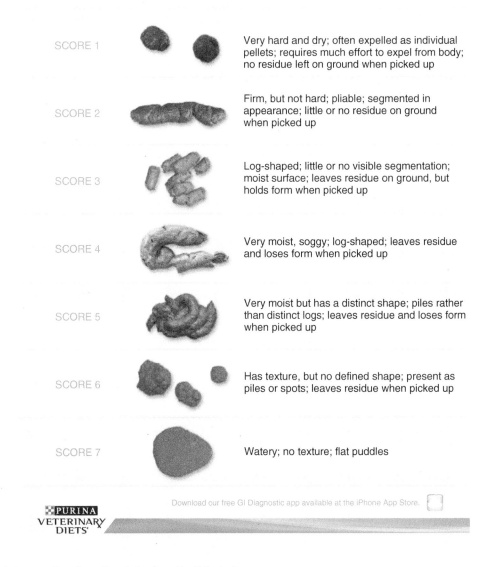

SCORE 1 — Very hard and dry; often expelled as individual pellets; requires much effort to expel from body; no residue left on ground when picked up

SCORE 2 — Firm, but not hard; pliable; segmented in appearance; little or no residue on ground when picked up

SCORE 3 — Log-shaped; little or no visible segmentation; moist surface; leaves residue on ground, but holds form when picked up

SCORE 4 — Very moist, soggy; log-shaped; leaves residue and loses form when picked up

SCORE 5 — Very moist but has a distinct shape; piles rather than distinct logs; leaves residue and loses form when picked up

SCORE 6 — Has texture, but no defined shape; present as piles or spots; leaves residue when picked up

SCORE 7 — Watery; no texture; flat puddles

Download our free GI Diagnostic app available at the iPhone App Store.

PURINA
VETERINARY
DIETS

Figure 33.1 Feces grading chart. (Permission from Nestlé Purina).

Water

Water is extremely important when working with patients with acute vomiting due to the potential for life-threatening dehydration from excess fluid loss and inability of the patient to replace the lost fluid. Patients with persistent nausea and vomiting should be supported with subcutaneous or intravenous rather than oral fluids. Where applicable, moderate to severe dehydration should be corrected with appropriate parenteral fluid therapy.

Electrolytes

Gastric and intestinal secretions differ from extracellular fluids in electrolyte composition, so their loss can result in systemic electrolyte abnormalities. Dogs and cats presenting with vomiting and diarrhea may have abnormal serum potassium, chloride and sodium concentrations. Serum electrolyte concentrations are useful in tailoring appropriate fluid therapy and nutritional management of these patients. Mild hypokalemia, hypochloremia and either hypernatremia or hyponatremia are the electrolyte abnormalities most commonly associated with acute vomiting (and diarrhea). Initially, electrolyte disorders should be addressed and corrected with appropriate parenteral fluid and electrolyte therapy. Patients experiencing vomiting and/or diarrhea should begin nutritional therapy ideally containing levels of potassium, chloride and sodium above the minimum allowances for normal dogs and cats. Recommended levels of these nutrients are 0.8 to 1.1% potassium (dry matter [DM]), 0.5 to 1.3% DM chloride and 0.3% to 0.5% DM sodium).

Protein

Nutritional therapy for patients exhibiting vomiting and/or diarrhea should probably not provide excess protein (no more than 30% for dogs and 40% for cats). Products of protein digestion (peptides, amino acids and amines) increase gastrin and gastric acid secretion. "Hypoallergenic" or elimination foods for patients with vomiting/diarrhea have been recommended as dietary antigens are suspected to play a role in the etiopathogenesis.

Ideal elimination foods should: (1) avoid protein excess (16 to 26% for dogs; 30 to 40% for cats), (2) have high protein digestibility (≥87%) and (3) contain a limited number of novel protein sources to which the patient has never been exposed. On the other hand a food containing a protein hydrolysate may be utilized in nutritional management of the patient.

Fat

Solids and liquids higher in fat empty more slowly from the stomach than comparable foods with less fat. Fat in the duodenum stimulates the release of cholecystokinin, which delays gastric emptying. Foods with less than 15% DM fat for dogs and less than 25% DM fat for cats are appropriate for dietary management.

Fiber

Foods containing gel-forming soluble fibers should be avoided in vomiting and/or diarrhea patients as these fibers increase the viscosity of ingesta and slow gastric emptying. These fibers include pectins and gums (e.g., gum arabic, guar gum, carrageenan, psyllium gum, xanthan gum, carob gum, gum ghatti and gum tragacanth). Overall, the crude fiber content should not exceed more than 5% DM.

Food Form and Temperature

Moist foods are considered to be the best form since they reduce gastric retention time. For the same reason, the veterinary healthcare team should educate clients to warm foods to between room and body temperature (70–100°F (21– 38°C)).

Vitamins and Trace Minerals

Iron, copper, and B vitamins may benefit patients with gastroduodenal ulceration and GI blood loss. Hematinics should be used in patients with nonregenerative, microcytic/hypochromic anemias attributable to iron deficiency. However, they probably are not necessary in most animals that have received a blood transfusion.

Acid Load

Alkalemia should be expected if vomiting patients lose hydrogen and chloride ions in excess of sodium and bicarbonate. Hypochloremia perpetuates the alkalosis by increasing renal bicarbonate reabsorption. A common finding is mild alkalemia in vomiting patients; however profound alkalemia is more likely to occur with pyloric or upper duodenal obstruction. Acidemia may occur in vomiting patients if the vomited gastric fluid is relatively low in hydrogen and chloride ion content (e.g., during fasting) or if concurrent loss of intestinal sodium and bicarbonate occurs. It is best to correct severe acid-base disorders with parenteral fluid and electrolyte therapy. Foods for patients with acute vomiting and diarrhea should avoid excess dietary acid load. Foods that normally produce alkaline urine are less likely to be associated with acidosis.

Gastrointestinal disorders are a common reason for pet parents to bring their pets to the hospital. It is essential for the veterinary healthcare team to identify these clinical signs and perform a complete history and evaluation regarding these frequent signs when pets present. Nutritional management is a crucial part of therapy in the management of vomiting and/or diarrhea. Certain key nutritional factors play a role in managing vomiting and diarrhea in cats and dogs – through enteral and parenteral nutrition – and veterinary technicians should recognize the circumstances and reasoning for the KNF's to insure a positive outcome for the vomiting and diarrheic patient.

Further Reading

Allenspach, K, Gaschein, FP (2008) Small intestinal disease. In JM Steiner (ed.), *Small Animal Gastroenterology*, pp. 187–202, Germany: Schlutersche.

Burns KM (2012) Gastrointestinal disorders. In L Merrill (ed.), *Internal Medicine for Veterinary Technicians*. Ames, IA: Wiley-Blackwell.

Davenport DJ, Remilliard RL. (2010a) Introduction to small intestinal disease. In MS Hand, CD Thatcher, RL Remilliard, *et al.* (eds), *Small Animal Clinical Nutrition* (5th edn), pp. 1047–9, Marceline MO: Walsworth Publishing, Mark Morris Institute.

Davenport DJ, Remillard RL. (2010b) Acute gastroenteritis and enteritis. In MS Hand, CD Thatcher, RL Remilliard, *et al.* (eds), *Small Animal Clinical Nutrition* (5th edn), pp. 1053–61, Marceline MO: Walsworth Publishing, Mark Morris Institute.

Hall EJ, German, AJ (2010) Diseases of the small intestine. In SJ Ettinger, EC Feldman (eds), *Textbook of Veterinary Internal Medicine* (7th edn), pp. 1526–72, St Loius, MO: Elsevier.

Tams TR (2003) Chronic diseases of the small intestine. In TR Tams (ed.), *Handbook of Small Animal Gastroenterology* (2nd edn), pp. 211–50, St Louis, MO: Saunders.

Willard MD (2009) Disorders of the intestinal tract. In Small Animal *Internal Medicine* (4th edn), pp. 441–76, St Louis, MO: Mosby.

34   Hepatic Disease

The liver is the central metabolic organ of the body. The liver is the second largest organ in the body and is responsible for approximately 1500 essential biochemical functions. The liver's main responsibility is maintaining homeostasis and removing waste products that have accumulated within the body. The liver also plays a key role in digestion and metabolism of food and nutrients. The liver has a large storage capacity as well as functional reserve and regenerative capability. Hepatic disease is typically severe before clinical signs and/or laboratory tests reveal/confirm the disease. Consequently, the patient is often suffering significant metabolic alterations by the time an appropriate feeding plan is implemented by the healthcare team. Nutritional management of liver disease usually is directed at the clinical manifestations of the disease as opposed to the specific cause of the disease. There are five goals of nutritional management of hepatic disease: (1) maintaining normal metabolic processes, (2) correction of electrolyte disturbances, (3) providing substrates to support hepatocellular repair and regeneration, (4) avoiding toxic by-product accumulation, and (5) avoiding and managing hepatic encephalopathy (HE).

Regardless of the primary liver disease, the hepatic reaction pattern is similar; thus, most of these disorders, if severe and/or longstanding, often lead to a few syndromes with potentially serious metabolic consequences (e.g., cholestasis, icterus, portal hypertension, ascites and hepatic encephalopathy).

As with all patients and disease conditions, assessment of the patient with hepatic disease includes a history and physical examination (including body weight and body condition scoring), laboratory evaluation, and imaging of the liver. There are a wide range of hepatobiliary diseases which also differ in severity therefore making it difficult to recommend one nutrient profile for all liver patients.

Key Nutritional Factors in Hepatobiliary Diseases

General recommendations of key nutritional factors can be made to benefit the majority of patients with hepatic disease. The foundation of adequate nutritional management in hepatic patients is the provision of adequate calories. It is prudent to think first of the total caloric need of the patient and then consider protein requirement.

Malnutrition is a very common feature of chronic hepatic disease, and correct nutrition should be evaluated in each individual patient. Protein malnutrition is seen in patients with hepatic disease, manifesting clinically as weight loss, muscle atrophy, and hypoalbumineria. The amount of protein fed to hepatic patients must be finely balanced. The biological value or digestibility of the proteins should be increased. Higher biological value proteins help to fulfill the patient's needs while producing minimally nitrogenous waste. Small frequent meals help the patient optimize blood flow through the liver, manage fasting glucose, and minimize hepatic encephalopathy.

Additionally, there are a number of other key nutritional factors to consider when managing patients with hepatic disease. The liver plays an important role in the regulation of carbohydrate homeostasis and serum glucose levels through its ability to remove glucose from and release glucose into the circulation. Therefore, it is important to have highly digestible carbohydrate sources. This will reduce protein breakdown and the resulting gluconeogenesis. Vitamin K and zinc are recommended in dietary management of liver disease to help avoid deficiencies commonly found in patients suffering with hepatic disease. Soluble fiber is essential to help promote colonic evacuation and to encourage nitrogen fixation by enteric bacteria thus reducing the amount of ammonia production and absorption.

Nutrition and Disease Management for Veterinary Technicians and Nurses, Second Edition. Ann Wortinger, Kara M. Burns
© 2015 John Wiley & Sons, Inc. Published 2015 by John Wiley & Sons, Inc.
Companion Website: www.wiley.com/go/wortinger/nutrition

Hepatic Lipidosis

In felines, hepatic lipidosis (HL) is a well-recognized syndrome. HL is characterized by the accumulation of excess triglycerides in hepatocytes resulting in choleostasis and hepatic dysfunction. Lipidosis may occur secondary to diabetes mellitus, diseases resulting in anorexia and weight loss (e.g., pancreatitis or inflammatory bowel disease) or as an idiopathic disorder of unknown etiology. Cats with idiopathic hepatic lipidosis often present with a history of prolonged anorexia after a stressful event. The biochemical mechanisms responsible for causing hepatic lipidosis during fasting are not completely understood. Potential causes include protein deficiency, excessive peripheral lipolysis, excessive lipogenesis, inhibition of lipid oxidation and inhibition of the synthesis and secretion of very low-density lipoproteins. The prognosis for this life-threatening disorder has improved dramatically during the past several years as a result of long-term enteral feeding (i.e., three to eight weeks or longer). Hepatic lipidosis is considered a reversible process but resolution of hepatic lipidosis secondary to pancreatitis, infection, or other causes depends on the success of treating the underlying disorder and providing appropriate nutritional support. It is important for the veterinary healthcare team to remember that success may take weeks to months and consistency and patience are assets to managing HL.

Chronic Hepatitis and Cirrhosis

Chronic hepatitis in dogs is a poorly defined group of clinicopathologic entities characterized by parenchymal necrosis with associated lymphoplasmacytic inflammation. Chronic hepatitis may result from a myriad of causes including copper accumulation, infectious diseases, drugs, breed-associated hepatitis and possibly autoimmune disease. Unfortunately, the majority of the time a cause is never determined. Lymphoplasmacytic inflammation suggests an immune mediated mechanism. Autoantibodies have been recognized in dogs with chronic hepatitis but it is unknown if such an immune reaction is the cause or result of the disease. The subtle onset contributes to the poor understanding of the pathogenesis because most patients have an advanced stage of the disease when it is recognized. Hepatic fibrosis is an accumulation of extracellular collagen and connective tissue within the liver and is a sequela to hepatic inflammation. Fibrosis not only results in distortion of normal hepatic structural design, but also becomes a barrier to movement of substances back and forth between blood and hepatocytes. Cirrhosis is defined as fibrosis with loss of normal acinar liver design and with regenerative nodules. The architectural changes in cirrhosis impair blood and bile flow and nutrient exchange, thus perpetuating hepatocellular injury.

Canine Copper Associated Hepatotoxicosis

Hepatic copper storage disease is an inherited autosomal recessive trait that impairs biliary excretion of copper. Veterinary medicine sees this disease most prevalently in the Bedlington terrier breed. Affected dogs progressively accumulate copper. Evidence of hepatic necrosis is observed when copper concentrations exceed approximately 2000 ppm (µg/g) DW liver (normal copper concentrations are <400 µg/g DW). As copper concentrations increase, damage progresses to chronic hepatitis and ultimately cirrhosis. Rarely, massive widespread hepatic necrosis can result in some dogs presenting with acute liver failure. Without appropriate treatment with dietary management and copper chelation, affected dogs usually do not live longer than 7–10 years of age. The gene responsible for this defect has been identified and it has become possible to distinguish affected, homozygous normal and carrier Bedlington terrier dogs using DNA markers. It was once estimated that about 25% of Bedlington terriers were affected with copper toxicosis and another 50% were carriers. Now, through genetic testing and responsible breeding programs, the incidence of this disease is significantly lower.

Hepatic mitochondria are important intracellular targets of copper toxicosis. Functional abnormalities of mitochondria associated with oxidative injury (i.e., lipid peroxidation) have been documented to occur in people, rats and Bedlington terriers with copper-induced hepatic injury. Oxidative injury and abnormal hepatic mitochondrial respiration may be involved in the pathogenesis of copper toxicosis. This theory forms the basis for using vitamin E and other antioxidants as potential therapeutic agents in addition to chelation therapy.

The role of copper in hepatic diseases observed in other dog breeds is less clear. Abnormal concentrations of copper in the liver can result secondary to cholestatic liver disease or as a primary defect in hepatic copper excretion resulting in hepatic injury. Breeds that are currently thought to have primary copper-associated hepatopathies include Skye terriers, West Highland white terriers, Doberman pinschers, Dalmatian dogs, and Labrador retrievers. The liver diseases in these dogs differ from copper toxicosis in Bedlington terriers in that hepatic copper concentrations are generally lower and do not always increase with age. Other factors may be responsible for hepatic damage in some breeds. The exceptions might be Doberman pinschers and Dalmatian dogs because they tend to accumulate hepatic copper in concentrations similar to Bedlington terriers, suggesting defects in hepatic copper excretion.

Cholangitis

Cholangitis (i.e., inflammation of the biliary ducts, especially the intrahepatic ducts and the surrounding liver tissue) is the most common feline inflammatory liver disease. The World Small Animal Veterinary Association Liver Pathology Standardization Working Group categorized the two most common forms of cholangitis into neutrophilic and lymphocytic forms. Bacterial infection from enteric bacteria (especially *Escherichiacoli*) ascending through the bile ducts is thought to be the cause of most neutrophilic forms, whereas immunologic mechanisms may be involved in the lymphocytic type. Chronic cholangitis may progress to biliary cirrhosis. Many cats with cholangitis develop significant cholestasis and may have sludged or inspissated bile, causing partial or complete biliary obstruction. Concurrent cholecystitis, pancreatitis and inflammatory bowel disease are common in feline cholangitis patients.

Portosystemic Shunts

PSS are vascular communications between the portal and systemic venous circulation. PSS can be either congenital or acquired and are seen in both dogs and cats. Congenital shunts can be further subdivided into intrahepatic shunts, occurring mostly in large-breed dogs or extrahepatic shunts, occurring mostly in smaller dog breeds and cats. Intrahepatic shunts are the remnant of a ductus venosus that did not completely close after birth. Extrahepatic shunts are seen as anomalous embryonic vessels between the portal vein and the systemic circulation. A hereditary basis for congenital shunts has been established in Irish wolfhounds and a number of other breeds have a significant risk for development of congenital shunts, again supporting a hereditary cause. Acquired PSS may develop as multiple shunts in response to portal hypertension caused by cirrhosis or other causes (e.g., tumors or portal vein thrombosis). Both congenital and acquired PSS are seen more often in dogs than in cats.

Primary portal vein hypoplasia (also referred to as microvascular dysplasia) is a second congenital vascular anomaly occurring in dogs, but rarely in cats. This anomaly is a consequence of portal vein hypoperfusion that results in hepatic arterialization in the portal triad and the development of microscopic intrahepatic shunts. Commonly affected breeds include cairn terriers, Yorkshire terriers and Maltese. Affected dogs have abnormal bile acid concentrations and variable liver enzymes but rarely have clinical signs. A less common variant of portal vein hypoplasia associated with fibrosis in the portal triads results in portal hypertension, ascites and PSS.

Polydipsia and polyuria are commonly seen in patients with PSS. Ammonium urate and other purine uroliths occur in some animals because of high urinary excretion of ammonia and uric acid. Stunted growth or failure to gain weight may occur in young animals with congenital shunts. Surgical closure is the treatment of choice for congenital PSS but not for acquired PSS. Dietary management is the cornerstone of successful case management and prevention of HE in the pre- and immediate postoperative phase and in partially closed shunts.

Neoplasia

The most commonly encountered hepatic malignancies in dogs and cats are metastases, lymphoma, hemangiosarcoma, hepatocellular carcinoma and cholangiocarcinoma. The appearance may be localized or diffuse. Due to the liver's tremendous reserve capacity, tumors (especially localized malignancies) may go undetected for long periods. In advanced stages, tumors may be visible or palpable during physical examination. Severe liver dysfunction with icterus, coagulopathies, and portal hypertension may occur especially in diffusely distributed malignancies (e.g., malignant lymphoma and hemangiosarcoma).

The veterinary team plays a crucial role in monitoring, reassessing, and overall management of the hepatic patient. Therefore, It is important to remember that hepatic disease is typically severe before clinical signs and/or laboratory tests reveal/confirm the disease. Consequently, the patient is often suffering significant metabolic alterations by the time an appropriate feeding plan is implemented by the healthcare team. It is imperative that nutritional management of liver disease be directed at the clinical manifestations of the disease as opposed to the specific cause of the disease. Proper nursing care and nutritional management of hepatic patients will help to reduce patient suffering and provide for a better quality of life for these patients.

Further reading

Michel KE (1995) Nutritional management of liver disease. *Vet Clin North Am Small Anim Pract* **25**(**2**): 485–502.

Meyer HP, Twedt DC, Roudebush P and Dill-Macky E (2010) Hepatobiliary disease. In In MS Hand, CD Thatcher, RL Remillard *et al.* (eds), *Small Animal Clinical Nutrition* (5th edn), pp. 1155–92, Topeka, KS: Mark Morris Institute.

Ruauz CG. (2010) Nutritional management of hepatic conditions. In *Textbook of Veterinary Internal Medicine* (7th edn), pp. 682–7, St Louis: Elsevier.

Rothuizen J, Bunch SE, Charles JA, *et al.* (2006) *WSAVA Standards for Clinical and Histological Diagnosis of Canine and Feline Liver Disease*. Oxford, UK: Saunders.

Watson PJ, Bunch SE (2009) Hepatobiliary and exocrine pancreatic disorders. In In MS Hand, CD Thatcher, RL Remillard *et al.* (eds), *Small Animal Internal Medicine* (4th edn), pp. 485–606, St Louis: Elsevier.

35 Weight Management

Pet obesity has reached epidemic proportions in North America as well as other industrialized countries. This mirrors the epidemic in the human population. It is estimated that 35–40% of adult pets and 50% of pets over age 7 are overweight or obese.[1-4] Over the last five years, one US study documents that the number of overweight or obese cats has increased by an astonishing 90%.[5] Obesity can be defined as an increase in fat tissue mass sufficient to contribute to disease. Dogs and cats weighing 10–19% more than the optimal weight for their breed are considered overweight; those weighing 20% or more above the optimum weight are considered obese.[6-8] Obesity has been associated with a number of disease conditions, as well as with a reduced lifespan. A combination of excessive caloric intake, decreased physical activity and genetic susceptibility are associated with most cases of obesity and the primary treatment for obesity is reduced caloric intake and increased physical activity. Obesity is one of the leading preventable causes of illness/death and with the dramatic rise in pet obesity over the past several decades, weight management and obesity prevention should be among the top health issues healthcare team members discuss with every client.

Causes of Obesity

Obesity is a complex polygenic disease involving interactions between multiple genes and the environment. Obesity is caused by an imbalance of energy intake and energy expenditure – it is very simple: too many calories in, not enough calories expended! There are several risk factors that affect energy balance. In today's society, indoor pets (in North America) are typically neutered. While there are many positive health benefits associated with neutering, it is important that metabolic impacts are addressed as well. Studies have demonstrated that neutering may result in decreased metabolic rate and increased food intake, and if energy intake is not adjusted, body weight, body condition score and amount of body fat will increase resulting in an overweight or obese pet. Other recognized risk factors for obesity include breed, age, decreased physical activity, and type of food and feeding method.[6-9]

Specific breeds of dogs and cats are more likely to become overweight. In dogs these include Shetland Sheepdogs, golden retrievers, dachshunds, cocker spaniels, Labrador retrievers, Dalmatians, Rottweilers and mixed breeds. In cats, mixed breeds and Manx cats have been found more likely to be obese compared to most purebred cats. Veterinary technicians should begin discussions on maintaining appropriate/optimal weight in pets, particularly in at-risk breeds, during the initial puppy/kitten health and wellness examination.

Health Risks Associated with Obesity

Healthcare team are well aware of the many health conditions associated with obesity in pets including arthritis, diabetes mellitus (DM), cancer, respiratory conditions, cardiovascular disease, skin diseases, lower urinary tract problems, and hepatic lipidosis. Obese pets are also more difficult to manage in terms of sample collection (blood, urine) and catheter placement. Also obese pets may be more prone to treatment complications including difficulty intubating, respiratory distress, slower recovery time, and delayed wound healing. It is widely believed that obesity affects quality of life and leads to reduced life expectancy. The dramatic impact of excess body weight in dogs and cats has been demonstrated. In cats, it is estimated that 31% of DM and 34% of lameness cases could be eliminated if cats

Nutrition and Disease Management for Veterinary Technicians and Nurses, Second Edition. Ann Wortinger, Kara M. Burns
© 2015 John Wiley & Sons, Inc. Published 2015 by John Wiley & Sons, Inc.
Companion Website: www.wiley.com/go/wortinger/nutrition

were at optimum body weight. Lifespan was increased by nearly 2 years in dogs that were maintained at an optimal body condition.[10] It's important to recognize and to communicate to our clients that fat tissue is not inert and that obesity is not an aesthetic condition that only affects our pet's ability to interact with us on a physical activity level. Fat tissue is metabolically active and in fact is the largest endocrine organ in the body and has an unlimited growth potential. Fat tissue is an active producer of hormones and inflammatory cytokines and the chronic low-grade inflammation secondary to obesity contributes to obesity related diseases.[3,10]

The Largest Endocrine Organ

Adipose tissue is more than a storage site for energy; it is now recognized as a multifunctional organ. Adipose tissue plays an active role in a variety of homeostatic and pathologic processes. As an organ, adipose tissue responds to nutrient, neural and hormonal signals, and secretes adipocytokines.[11] Adipocytokines (i.e., leptin and adiponectic) function as hormones to influence energy homeostasis in humans. They also regulate neuroendocrine functions. Adipose tissue secretes a variety of cytokines such as TNF-α, IL-6, resistin, and visfatin that affect immune functions and inflammatory processes throughout the body. Adipocytokines have numerous functions including satiety regulation, carbohydrate and lipid metabolism, and insulin sensitivity as well as many aspects of inflammation and immunity.[12]

Evaluating Weight and Nutrition

Obesity is a difficult disease to talk with owners about because most pet owners do not recognize (or want to admit) that their pet is overweight. All members of the healthcare team need to commit to understanding and communicating the role of weight management in pet health and disease prevention. In particular, the veterinary technician is the primary source for client education; the interface between the client, the doctor, and the rest of the hospital team; and is the key advocate for the patient.

The healthcare team should assess every patient that comes into the hospital, every time they come in to the hospital to establish nutritional needs and feeding goals. These goals will vary depending on the pet's physiology, obesity risk factors, and current health status. Designing and implementing a weight management protocol supports the team, the client, and most importantly the patient.[6,8,9]

The first steps in patient evaluation are as follows: a complete history including a detailed nutritional history and a complete physical examination including a complete blood count, serum chemistry and urinalysis. Signalment data should include species, breed, age, gender, neuter status, weight, activity level, and environment. The nutritional history should determine the type of food (all food) fed, the feeding method (how much, how often), who is responsible for feeding the pet and any other sources of energy intake (no matter how small or seemingly insignificant).[6,8,9]

The following questions should be part of every nutritional assessment:

- Tell me everything that your pet eats in a day.
- What brand of food do you feed your pet (try to get specific name)?
- Do you feed moist or dry or both?
- How do you feed your pet – feeding method (how much, how often)?
- Does your pet receive any snacks or treats of any kind? If so, what and how often?
- Do you give your pet any supplements?
- Is your pet on any medications, including chewable medications? If so, obtain name and dosage.
- What type of chew toys does your pet play with?
- What foods or treats not specifically designated for pets (such as human foods) does your pet receive? What and how often?
- Does your pet have ANY access to other sources of food (neighbor, trash, family member, etc.)?

Obtaining a complete nutritional history supports consistency and accuracy of patient information, provides key insights to barriers in client compliance, guides client discussion, and supports the optimal weight management program for the pet.

Be sure to weigh the pet and obtain a body condition score at *every visit* and record the information in the patient's medical record. It's helpful to use the same scale and chart the findings for the client. Body condition scoring (BCS) is important to assess a patient's fat stores and muscle mass. A healthy and successful weight management program results in loss of fat tissue while maintaining lean body mass and consistent and accurate assessment of weight and BCS are important tools to track progress. The use of body condition charts and breed charts are helpful tools in discussing the importance of weight management with clients and helps them visualize what an optimal weight would look like on their pet.

Body Condition Scoring (BCS)

The BCS is a subjective assessment of an animal's body fat that takes into account the animal's frame size independent of its weight. A variety of scoring systems with defined criteria have been published. All are useful tools for assessing body condition. In general, dogs and cats in optimal body condition have: (1) normal body contours and silhouettes, (2) bony prominences that can be readily palpated but not seen or felt above skin surfaces and (3) intra-abdominal fat insufficient to obscure or interfere with abdominal palpation. In addition to body weight, the BCS should always be recorded in the hospital record whenever an animal is examined. Body weight alone does not indicate how appropriate the weight is for an individual animal. A Labrador retriever weighing 30 kg, or a domestic short-hair cat weighing 4 kg, may be underweight, optimal weight or overweight. The BCS puts body weight in perspective for each individual patient (Table 35.1).

Owners should be taught to perform BCS at home. This is helpful both during a weight loss program and for long-term maintenance. However, it is important to recognize that owners are often reluctant to objectively evaluate their pets. Several studies have demonstrated that both dog and cat owners consistently underestimate their pet's body condition score.[13,14]

However, by reinforcing the health risks associated with obesity and educating owners on performing a BCS on their own pet, we can help pets maintain their ideal body weight. It is important to remind owners to report their pet's BCS monthly and then insure that this is documented in the medical record.

Body Fat Index Risk Chart Validation

Recent studies by veterinary nutritionists and scientists at the University of Tennessee College of Veterinary Medicine compared a variety of diagnostic methods used to assess body composition with DEXA-scans in dogs and cats presented for weight management programs.[15,16] The primary goal of these studies was to develop practical methods to better diagnose body composition in obese pets. The hypothesis was that a more accurate diagnostic test would promote more effective weight loss in client owned pets. In addition to current BCS methods, pets were assessed using bioelectric impedance, morphometric measurements and a newly developed Body Fat Index (BFI) Risk Chart.

Eighty-three client-owned dogs, representing 27 breeds weighing from 11 to 162 lb (5–73.6 kg), and 39 client-owned cats, representing 9 breeds ranging from 6 to 25 lb (2.7–11.4 kg), were enrolled in these studies. Bioelectric impedance was found to be an unreliable tool for predicting body composition. Body condition scoring was inaccurate in 60% of pets.[16] The findings from these studies indicated that when traditional BCS was used to estimate ideal body weight and consequently food dose, over half of the pets received a recommendation to ingest excess calories. By incorporating expanded definitions, using the BFI Risk Chart improved the accuracy of prediction of ideal for both dogs and cats, particularly those pets with greater than 45% body fat.

Weight Management Program

As with many aspects of healthcare, designing a successful weight management program is not a "one program fits all" for our patients. A successful weight management program includes consistent and accurate weight measurement/patient monitoring, effective and educational client communication, identification of compliance gaps, and utilization of tools to reinforce compliance, client and patient support and program restructure as needed.

Setting a goal for weight loss and calculating the appropriate energy intake start with determination of the pet's ideal body weight. Ideal body weight is a starting goal that is adjusted for appropriate body condition as the pet loses weight. The healthcare team must determine the number of daily calories that will result in weight loss while subsequently providing adequate protein, vitamins and minerals to meet the pet's daily energy requirement (DER). The DER reflects

Table 35.1 Body condition scoring system

Canine	Body Condition Score	Feline
	1: Very Thin *Ribs:* easily visible and felt with no cover *Waist:* severe waist *Tail Base:* lumbar vertebrae and pelvic bones are raised with no fat between the skin and bone *Side View:* severe abdominal tuck *Overhead View:* accentuated hourglass shape	
	2: Underweight *Ribs:* easily felt with minimal fat cover *Waist:* easily noted *Tail Base:* bones are raised with minimal fat between the skin and bone *Side View:* prominent abdominal tuck *Overhead View:* marked hourglass shape	
	3: Ideal *Ribs:* easily felt with slight fat cover *Waist:* observed behind ribs *Tail Base:* smooth contour but bones can be felt under a thin layer of fat *Side View:* abdominal tuck *Overhead View:* well-proportioned waist	
	4: Overweight *Ribs:* difficult to feel with moderate fat cover *Waist:* poorly discernible *Tail Base:* some thickening but bones can be felt under a moderate layer of fat *Side View:* no abdominal tuck *Overhead View:* back is slightly broadened	
	5: Obese *Ribs:* difficult to feel under thick fat cover *Waist:* absent *Tail Base:* thickened and difficult to feel bones beneath prominent layer of fat *Side View:* fat hangs from the abdomen *Overhead View:* markedly broadened and prominent paralumbar fat deposits	

Source: Candyce J, Patricia W (2014) *Veterinary Technician's Daily Reference Guide: Canine and Feline* (3rd edn), John Wiley & Sons, Inc.

the pet's activity level and is a calculation based on the pet's resting energy requirement (RER).[7,8]

There are a couple of basic formulas that all technicians should memorize or have on laminated note cards in every exam room (along with a calculator)! The most accurate formula to determine the RER for a cat or a dog is:

$$\textbf{RER kcal/day} = \textbf{70(Ideal Body Weight in Kg)}^{0.75}$$

or

$$\textbf{RER kcal/day} = (\textbf{kg} \times \textbf{kg} \times \textbf{kg}, \sqrt{}, \sqrt{}) \times \textbf{70}$$

After RER is determined, DER may be calculated by multiplying RER by "standard" factors related to energy needs. The calculations used to determine energy needs for obese prone pets or for pets needing to lose weight are:[7−9]

Obese prone dogs DER = 1.4 × RER

Weight loss/dogs DER = 1.0 × RER

Obese prone cats DER = 1.0 × RER

Weight loss/cats DER = 0.8 × RER

Gathering the above information is crucial to success and only takes a few minutes. This information is the foundation for developing a weight loss program that includes:

1 target weight or weight loss goal
2 maximum daily caloric intake
3 specific food, amount of food, and method of feeding.

The weight management program should also include detailed protocols for monitoring the pet's weight (schedule these before the client leaves and send reminder cards), adjusting the pet's energy intake accordingly, and exercise guidelines/suggestions.

Determining Ideal Weight Matters

We have discussed the fact that appropriate calorie reduction is required for successful weight loss. It must be noted that slight inaccuracies can make big differences, especially in smaller pets. For example, a 10 lb (4.5 kg) cat consuming just 10 kcal/day more than RER will gain nearly 1 lb (0.5 kg) or 12% of body weight per year. In other words eating the equivalent of 10 extra kibbles of a typical dry cat food will cause weight gain in a cat which is equal to a 150 lb (68 kg) person gaining almost 20 lb (9 kg) in a year.[17] Overestimating ideal weight will lead to feeding recommendations that may actually promote weight gain rather than weight loss.

Client/Behavioral Factors

For weight loss programs to be successful, everyone involved in feeding the pet must make a commitment to accomplish that goal. Weight loss will not occur unless the pet owner recognizes the problem and is willing to take corrective steps. Several strategies exist to help owners make this commitment. Careful consideration must be given to the powerful relationship between feeding and the human animal bond.

Calorie Restriction

Incorporating a detailed food diary is a crucial diagnostic step in developing a weight-loss program. The diary can help in determining how severe caloric restriction will need to be to produce weight loss. Simply calculating estimated energy requirements for cats or dogs will often lead to inaccurate results because of wide variation between individual animals. In practice, individual animals are encountered that need precisely the same, markedly fewer, and occasionally, markedly more calories than calculations suggest. Caloric restriction may be insufficient to produce weight loss or may even produce weight gain in some animals if calculations for caloric restriction are applied without taking into account the calories being eaten to maintain the animal's current weight. There is also a wide range of therapeutic and wellness foods designed for weight control. Calorie density of these products is quite variable. A therapeutic weight loss food should be selected based on the individual needs of each patient.

Exercise

Exercise is the only real-world way to increase energy expenditures. Exercise may also benefit obese patients by lessening the loss of lean body mass and maintaining or improving RER. Additionally, increased physical activity may improve metabolic abnormalities even without significant alterations in body weight. In humans, increased physical activity has been shown to improve insulin sensitivity, partially reverse leptin resistance and suppress the enhanced proinflammatory response induced by obesity.[18] In some cases, pets fail to lose weight unless exercise is included as part of the weight reduction plan, regardless of the severity of caloric restriction. One recent study evaluated the effects of environmental enrichment designed to increase physical activity in obese cats. Cats that received enrichments had increased activity and a trend toward increased % weight loss. Most importantly, owners of cats that received enrichments had greater satisfaction with the weight loss program.[19]

There are many ways for an owner to get their pet active and it is healthcare team member must discuss these with the client and determine which could work for that specific patient and client. Exercise should start simply – having the owner walk their dog to the end of the driveway for example. Also, starting to play with interactive toys with their cat for a few minutes a day would be a great way to begin to get cats more engaged in exercise. Gradually you want to educate the owner to build up the distance and time spent exercising.[6] If the owner is excited and takes the dog on a 3 mile walk on the first day, the dog may tire easily and the owner may find this frustrating and not want to walk with their dog again. Remember to advise owners that exercise needs to begin in moderation. By following this, a more successful outcome will result.[14]

Weight Management Guidelines

We have discussed the sensitivity around communicating and implementing a weight management program for dogs and cats. Healthcare teams know how an effective customized weight loss program provides a consistent and healthy rate of weight loss to reduce risk of disease, prevent malnutrition, and improve quality of life. The American Animal Hospital Association produced the AAHA Weight management Guidelines in early 2014 to aid veterinary healthcare teams by offering guidelines and tools for the management of weight loss and long-term maintenance of healthy weight. These guidelines are aimed at raising awareness of the health consequences from pets being overweight or obese. The guidelines also promote the prevention of excess weight, and offer suggestions and tools for the management of weight loss and long-term maintenance of healthy weight. The guidelines are downloadable for free to veterinary hospitals.[20]

There are several specific recommendations that support a successful weight loss program including:

1 Emphasizing feeding consistency including feeding the pet from its designated dish only.
2 Be sure the client is using an 8 ounce measuring cup.
3 Recommend the appropriate weight loss food and calculate the initial feeding amount.
4 Discuss the importance of total energy intake (do not feed anything other than the recommended food at the designated amount).

5 If the client wants to "treat" their pet, make appropriate recommendations and adjust the caloric intake of the base food accordingly.
6 Encourage client's to feed their pet's separately if possible.
7 Recommend appropriate exercise for the pet.
8 Offer your client's suggestions on ways other than food to reward or bond with their pet.
9 Evaluate, adjust, communicate, and encourage on a consistent basis.
10 Celebrate success!

Summary

Successful weight management begins with recognition of the disease of overweight and obesity as well as the importance of weight control in our pets. It is essential that the ideal weight of the pet be determined to avoid feeding the fat instead of the pet within. The healthcare team, must communicate the serious effects that even a few excess pounds can have on the health and longevity of their pet's lives. Weight management should be a cornerstone wellness program in every hospital and the veterinary technician the champion of the program and advocate for the patient.

References

1 Rosenthal M (2007) Obesity in America: Why Brune and Bessie are so heavy and what you can do about it, *Vet Forum* **24**: 26–34.
2 Lund E, Armstrong P, Kirk C *et al.* (2005) Prevalence and risk factors for obesity in adult cats from private US veterinary practices, *International Journal of Applied Research in Veterinary Medicine* **3**: 88–96.
3 Lund E, Armstrong PJ, Kirk CA, et al. (2006) Prevalence and risk factors for obesity in adult dogs from private US veterinary practices, *International Journal of Applied Research in Veterinary Medicine* **4**: 177–86.
4 Armstrong PJ, Lusby AL (2011) Clinical importance of canine and feline obesity. In TL Towell (ed.), *Practical Weight Management in Dogs and Cats*, pp. 3–21, Ames, IA: Wiley Blackwell.
5 Klausner JS, Lund E (2012) *Banfield Pet Hospital State of Pet Health* 4.
6 Burns KM, Towell TL (2011) Owner education and adherence. In TL Towell (ed.), *Practical Weight Management in Dogs and Cats*, pp. 3–21, Ames, IA: Wiley Blackwell.

7 Burns KM (2006) Managing overweight or obese pets, *Veterinary Technician*. June: **385–9**.

8 Burns KM (2013) Why is Rocky so stocky? Obesity is a disease!, *NAVTA Journal*. Convention Issue, **16–19**.

9 Toll PW, Yamka RN, Schoenherr WD, Hand MS (2010) Obesity. In MS Hand, CD Thatcher, RL Remillard *et al.* (eds), *Small Animal Clinical Nutrition* (5th edn), pp. 501–42, Marceline, MO: Walsworth Publishing, Mark Morris Institute.

10 Laflamme DP (2006) Understanding and managing obesity in dogs and cats, *Vet Clin Small An Pract* **36**: 1283–95.

11 Ahima RS (2006) Adipose tissue as an endocrine organ, *Obesity* **14** (Suppl 5): 242S–249S.

12 Tilg H, Moschen AR (2006) Adipocytokines: mediators linking adipose tissue, inflammation and immunity, *Nature* **6**: 772–83.

13 Sing R, Laflamme DP, Sidebottom-Nielsen M (2002) Owner perceptions of canine body condition score, *J Vet Intern Med* **16**(3): 362.

14 Kienzle E, Bergler R (2006) Human–animal relationship of owners of normal and overweight cats, *J Nutr* **136**: 1947S–1950S.

15 Toll PW, Paetau-Robinson I, Lusby AL *et al.* (2010) Effectiveness of morphometric measurements for predicting body composition in overweight and obese dogs, *Journal of Veterinary Internal Medicine* **24**: 717.

16 Lusby AL, Kirk CA, Toll PW *et al.* (2010) Effectiveness of BCS for estimation of ideal body weight and energy requirements in overweight and obese dogs compared to DXA (abstract), *Journal of Veterinary Internal Medicine* **24**: 717.

17 Michel K, Scherk M (2012) From problem to success: Feline weight loss programs that work, *J Feline Med Surg* **14**: 327–36.

18 Berggren JR, Hulver MW, Houmard JA (2005) Fat as an endocrine organ: influence of exercise, *J Appl Physiol* **99**: 757–64.

19 Trippany JR, Funk J, Buffinton CA (2003) Effects of environmental enrichments on weight loss in cats, *J Vet Intern Med* **17**: 430.

20 American Animal Hospital Association (2014) Weight Management Guidelines for Dogs and Cats. https://www.aahanet.org/Library/WeightManagement.aspx (last accessed 12/02/2014).

Feline Lower Urinary Tract Disease

Feline lower urinary tract disease (FLUTD) is a term used to describe any condition affecting the urinary bladder or urethra of cats and is a common reason for hospital visits and veterinary evaluation of our feline patients. Regardless of underlying cause, FLUTD is characterized by the following signs: dysuria, pollakiuria, stranguria, hematuria, and/or periuria (urination in inappropriate places). It is important that veterinary technicians are aware of signs and symptoms of FLUTD when talking with clients.

Over the course of the last decade, knowledge of specific causes of FLUTD has increased in the veterinary profession, allowing diagnostic and therapeutic efforts to be directed toward identification and elimination of specific underlying disorders. The most common cause of FLUTD in cats less than 10 years of age is feline idiopathic cystitis (FIC). This is followed by uroliths, and urethral plugs. The common causes of FLUTD are divided into two overall categories, with these categories established on (1) the presence or (2) the absence of an identifiable cause.[1,2] A diagnosis of FIC is made by excluding all other causes of FLUTD. In older cats (those over 10 years), urinary tract infection and/or uroliths are the most common cause of FLUTD.

In 1981, 78% of feline uroliths were composed of struvite and only 2% were calcium oxalate. In the mid- to late-1980s, the occurrence of calcium oxalate uroliths began to increase. Between 1994 and 2002, approximately 55% of uroliths were calcium oxalate and only 33% were struvite. Since 2001, however, the number of struvite uroliths has continued to increase while occurrence of calcium oxalate uroliths has decreased. Based on 10 093 feline uroliths analyzed at the Minnesota Urolith Center in 2006, the most common mineral types were struvite (50%) and calcium oxalate (39%), followed by purine (5%). These trends have continued into 2011. In 2006, 88% of urethral plugs evaluated at the Minnesota Urolith Center were composed of struvite, 9% were matrix, < 1% were calcium oxalate, and 2% were of other mineral compositions.

Diagnostic Evaluation

Urinalysis and diagnostic imaging should be standard protocol in the evaluation of cats with recurrent or persistent lower urinary tract signs . If there is a history of urinary tract manipulation (e.g., urethral catheterization), evidence of urinary tract infection (e.g., pyuria, bacteriuria, malodorous urine), or the cat is older (usually over 10 years), a urine culture is warranted. More advanced procedures (e.g., contrast radiography) are appropriate in some cases.

As stated, urinalysis is an important part of evaluating patients with signs of lower urinary tract disease. It is ideal to perform the urinalysis in-house since fresh urine samples analyzed within 30 minutes of collection are preferred. Urine specimens evaluated after 30 minutes may form crystals that are not in fact present in the patient. Samples may be refrigerated for up to 8 hours and then evaluated (after the sample has returned to room temperature). However, this method is not best for evaluating crystalluria and should be avoided.

Although it may be tempting to only perform dipstick analysis, measure urine specific gravity, and omit urine sediment examination, it is very important to perform complete urinalysis. Sediment examination is the only way to accurately detect pyuria, hematuria, bacteriuria, and crystalluria. Healthcare team members cannot rely solely on urine dipstick analysis since results for detection of pyuria are often false positive in cats and the occult blood reagent pad on the dipstick is not

Nutrition and Disease Management for Veterinary Technicians and Nurses, Second Edition. Ann Wortinger, Kara M. Burns
© 2015 John Wiley & Sons, Inc. Published 2015 by John Wiley & Sons, Inc.
Companion Website: www.wiley.com/go/wortinger/nutrition

specific for hematuria (in addition to red blood cells, it also becomes positive with hemoglobin and myoglobin). Pyuria (>5 WBCs/hpf) indicates inflammation which can be the result of several disorders (urolithiasis, bacterial infection). Pyuria is less commonly observed in cats with FIC.

A number of crystals may be identified on urine sediment examination, but the most commonly identified are struvite (triple phosphate) and calcium oxalate. The presence of crystals indicates that the urine is supersaturated with that substance and the patient is at risk for forming uroliths. It is worth noting that cats also may have crystals and never develop uroliths. Without other findings such as uroliths or urethral plugs, the presence of crystals alone is not diagnostic of urolithiasis or struvite disease. Struvite crystals may be present in normal cats and cats with struvite uroliths (sterile or infection-induced), nonstruvite urolithis (including some cats with calcium oxalate uroliths), urethral plugs, as well as other urinary disorders such as FIC.

Survey radiographs are helpful for identifying radiopaque uroliths and crystalline-matrix urethral plugs. Positioning should also include the caudal abdomen (urethra) in the radiograph; or there may be risk of missing potentially important information. Normal survey radiographs do not exclude FIC, radiolucent uroliths (urate/purine), small uroliths (<2 mm), neoplasia, blood clots, or anatomic defects. In these cases, abdominal ultrasonography and/or contrast urethrocystography is useful. After thorough diagnostic evaluation if no cause is found, a diagnosis of FIC is very likely.

When managing cats with FLUTD, it is recommended that a multimodal approach be used to attain the best results. This approach includes identifying and treating underlying medical conditions, modifying the home environment, addressing behavioral issues, and managing nutritional factors.

It has been determined that the most common cause of FLUTD in cats less than 10 years of age is feline idiopathic cystitis (FIC). Diagnosing FIC is through exclusion of other FLUTD causes. In older cats (over 10 years), urinary tract infection and/or uroliths are the most common cause of FLUTD.

Factors that have been found to be significantly associated with FIC development appear to fall into the following categories:[3,4]

- psychogenic (e.g., anxiety, fearfulness, nervousness, etc.);
- physiologic (e.g., sedentary, decreased water intake, increased BCS);
- environmental (e.g., indoor vs. outdoor, less hunting activities, using a litterbox, etc.).

Pathogenesis of FIC

Although FIC is suspected when all other causes are ruled out, the following steps have been theorized to play a major role in the pathogenesis of FIC [5,6]

1 The stress response system (SRS) is activated when a cat perceives stress in its environment.
2 The SRS heightens activity in the sympathetic nervous system and increases outflow down the spinal cord to the urinary bladder. In otherwise healthy cats, this response is regulated/dampened by activity of the hypothalamic/pituitary/adrenal input.
3 Increased sympathetic input to the bladder is believed to cause neurogenic "inflammation," which leads to:
   ○ increased permeability of the urinary bladder mucosa;
   ○ greater access of substances in the urine to sensory neurons in the bladder wall;
   ○ increased pain receptors/fibers in the bladder;
   ○ release of inflammatory cytokines from cells in the bladder wall and increased sensitivity of afferent nerves.
4 Sensory input via afferent input from the bladder is transmitted back to the brain and perceived as pain, which causes additional stress

The result is a vicious cycle affecting the brain and the urinary bladder. Therefore, to increase success of managing cats with FIC, treatment approaches should be aimed at both the brain and the bladder.

Nutritionally Managing Cats with FIC

The goals of managing cats with FIC are as follows:
1 reduce stress;
2 provide pain relief;
3 decrease severity of clinical signs;
4 increase the interval between episodes.

Feeding moist food (>60% moisture) has been associated with a decreased recurrence of clinical signs in cats with FIC. During a 1-year study, clinical signs recurred less often in cats with FIC when fed a moist food compared with cats fed the dry formulation of the same food.[7] Beneficial effects have been observed in cats with FIC when urine specific gravity values decrease from 1.050 to values between 1.032 and 1.041. Additional methods for increasing water intake (e.g., adding broth to foods, placing ice cubes in the cat's water, and providing water fountains) also may be helpful for some cats.

A recent study shows that consistently feeding a therapeutic urinary food was associated with a reduction in recurrent episodes of FIC signs. This is the first study to definitively show that foods of different nutritional profiles impact the expression of acute episodes of FIC signs in cats. Additionally, the addition of L-tryptophan, a precursor of serotonin that inhibits neurotransmitters in the brain to balance mood, as well as hydrolyzed casein, a bioactive peptide that helps relieve anxiety in cats has been presented as nutrients that will aid in managing the stress component of FIC.

Increasing salt content of food is an effective method of causing urine dilution in cats, but the potential for adverse effects should be considered. At this time, there are differing opinions regarding role of sodium in cats with kidney disease. In a recent study, the effects of high-salt (1.2% sodium, dry matter basis (DMB)) intake for 3 months were evaluated in 6 cats with mild azotemia due to naturally occurring chronic kidney disease. These cats had progressive increases in BUN, serum creatinine, and serum phosphorus compared with consumption of food with 0.4% sodium (DMB). Based on all findings to date, further study is needed to better determine the role of sodium in healthy cats fed long-term as well as cats with hypertension, chronic kidney disease, and calcium oxalate uroliths. Pending further studies, it is sensible to avoid high-salt foods in cats with chronic kidney disease and monitor kidney function when high-salt foods are fed to cats at risk for kidney disease.

Inflammation plays a role in many causes of FLUTD, especially FIC and urolithiasis. Therefore, a key nutritional factor for managing cats with FLUTD includes omega-3 fatty acids, specifically EPA & DHA, which are known to have potent anti-inflammatory effects. Additionally, vitamin E and beta carotene are helpful for counteracting oxidative stress and reducing free radical damage, conditions that often accompany inflammation.

Managing stress and anxiety nutritionally involves foods that contain specific nutrients with proven anti-anxiety benefits and offers an innovative approach for management of FIC. Nutritional management with L-tryptophan and alpha-casozepine is supported by clinical studies in dogs and cats.[8] Additionally, a nutritional approach is beneficial for cats as the owner may no longer need to administer daily treatments causing stress in the owner and the cat. Through nutrition cats can receive the necessary nutrients to decrease anxiety and stress. This will strengthen the human-animal bond and subsequently increase compliance.

Serotonin, a major neurotransmitter in the brain, is responsible for regulating mood and emotion in animals and human beings. Tryptophan is an amino acid that serves as a precursor for the synthesis of serotonin. Serotonin is not able to cross the blood–brain barrier (BBB) to enter the central nervous system. However, tryptophan and 5-hydroxytryptophan are able to cross the BBB by way of a carrier protein. Pro-inflammatory cytokines are linked to many behavioral or psychiatric diseases in animals and human beings.[9] Feline stressors (i.e., those associated with unusual events) can increase the level of pro-inflammatory cytokines.[10] As a result, chronic stress can lead to anxious pathological states and this could be linked with a shift in tryptophan metabolism.

Historically, milk from cows' has been considered to have tranquilizing effects in humans.[9,11] This calming effect was hypothesized to be from a natural component in the cow's milk created via digestion (tryptic hydrolysis) in human babies. Researchers first identified a decapeptide, obtained via tryptic hydrolysis, responsible for the anxiolytic activity.[9] This milk protein is known as alpha-S1 casein. It is converted to a bioactive peptide via hydrolysis (with trypsin) to form hydrolyzed casein. Hydrolized casein has a natural affinity for the benzodiazepine site of the GABA receptor and has been shown to regulate anxious and stressful behavior in multiple species. In felines, a study associated alpha-casozepine with a significant decrease in fearfulness and an increase in contact with people.[12]

Nutritional management aimed at addressing FLUTD, specifically FIC, will lead to improved compliance, overall better health care for cats, and fewer painful FIC recurrences. Nutritional management will help reduce pain associated with FLUTD, and strengthen the human–animal bond between pets and their owners.

The healthcare team must educate owners about the impact of stress in cats and how nutritional management allows the owner to participate in the long term management of urinary health for their feline family member.

Treatment of Cats with Feline Idiopathic Cystitis

The goals of managing cats with FIC are to decrease severity of clinical signs and increase the interval between episodes of lower urinary tract disease. Over the past 40 years, many different treatments have been recommended to control signs in cats with FIC, yet only a few have been evaluated in clinical trials of cats with FIC.

Environmental Enrichment

In addition to nutritional management, the currently recommended treatment for cats with FIC also includes environmental enrichment and stress reduction. Environmental enrichment is also an important adjunct to therapy in all types of FLUTD.[13,14] The veterinary health care team plays a crucial role in educating cat owners about the importance of environmental enrichment, stress reduction, and litter box management. Cats with FIC should avoid stressful situations (e.g., conflict with other cats in the home). Owners should be educated to provide opportunities for play/resting (horizontal and vertical surfaces for scratching, hiding places, and climbing platforms). Any changes (e.g., switching to a new food) should be made *gradually* so the cat has adequate time to adapt and avoid becoming stressed.

A recent prospective study evaluating effects of multimodal environmental modification was reported in 46 client-owned cats with FIC. The findings showed significant reductions in lower urinary tract signs, fearfulness, and nervousness after treatment for 10 months. With cats that are suffering with FIC, stressful situations (e.g., conflict with other cats in the home) should be avoided or minimized. Owners should provide opportunities for play/resting (horizontal and vertical surfaces for scratching, hiding places, and climbing platforms). Any changes (e.g., switching to a new food) should be made gradually so the cat has adequate time to adapt and avoid becoming stressed.

Another critical component of managing cats with FLUTD, especially FIC, involves appropriate use and maintenance of litter boxes in the home. The majority of cats prefer clumping, unscented litter; however, it may be necessary to give cats several choices and let them select their preference. It may be possible to have cats within the home that prefer different types of litter or litter boxes. In general, uncovered litter boxes are recommended because they are less likely to trap odors inside. For older cats with mobility issues, the owner should select a litter box with low sides to facilitate the cat getting in and out of the box. Litter boxes should be scooped daily and washed every few weeks with warm, soapy water. Because plastic can absorb odors over time (months to years), owners should consider replacing litter boxes with new ones periodically. Finally, there should be an adequate number of litter boxes (the 1 + 1 rule = 1 more than the number of cats) in the home and they should be located on multiple floors where cats can enter and exit readily. More detailed information about environmental enrichment and litter box management is available in the suggested reading. It may be helpful to encourage owners to read this additional information as well because their involvement is critical for a successful outcome. Finally, health care team members, especially technicians, play a crucial role in educating cat owners about the importance of environmental enrichment and litter box management.

Managing Cats with Struvite Uroliths or Urethral Plugs

Treatment options for cats with struvite uroliths include physical removal of uroliths or dissolution via nutritional management. Only two foods have been evaluated in cats with struvite uroliths (Prescription Diet® s/d® Feline, Hill's Pet Nutrition, Topeka, KS and Medi-Cal® Dissolution Formula, Veterinary Medical Diets, Guelph, Ontario, CANADA); mean time required for dissolution of sterile struvite uroliths using these foods is approximately 1 month. For cats with suspected struvite uroliths, it is appropriate to transition to feeding a canned calculolytic food over a 7-day period. Cats should be re-evaluated every 2–4 weeks (urinalysis and abdominal radiographs). Urine pH should remain <6.1 and specific gravity should be <1.040 if canned food is being fed exclusively. Nutritional management (dissolution) should be continued 1 month beyond radiographic resolution of the urolith.

After dissolution or removal of struvite uroliths or urethral plugs, nutritional management should continue to prevent recurrence. There are several commercially available foods for struvite prevention; however, only one (Prescription Diet® s/d® Feline, Hill's Pet Nutrition) has been evaluated in cats with struvite disease. Several other foods formulated for struvite prevention have been evaluated in healthy cats by measuring urine saturation values of struvite. A dissolution (calculolytic) food is appropriate for initial management (1–3 months) after relieving urethral obstruction; this should be followed by feeding a struvite preventive food indefinitely, with the cat being evaluated routinely by the veterinary healthcare team.

Managing Cats with Calcium Oxalate Uroliths

The treatment of choice for calcium oxalate urolithiasis is urolith removal, followed by methods to prevent recurrence. At present, the standard of care for preventing calcium oxalate urolith recurrence is to feed moist therapeutic food and encourage water intake. There are several commercially available therapeutic foods for prevention of calcium oxalate uroliths in cats.

All cats should be monitored for recurrence including urinalysis every 3 months to detect calcium oxalate crystalluria and diagnostic imaging every 6 months to detect uroliths. If uroliths recur, less-invasive procedures such as voiding urohydropropulsion are more likely to be effective when uroliths are smaller.

Summary

Increased understanding of specific causes of FLUTD has allowed diagnostic and therapeutic efforts to be directed toward identification and elimination of specific underlying disorders. The most common cause of FLUTD in cats <10 years of age is feline idiopathic cystitis (FIC), followed by uroliths, and urethral plugs. A diagnosis of FIC is made by excluding all other causes of FLUTD. In older cats (>10 years), urinary tract infection and/or uroliths are the most common cause of FLUTD. It is imperative that veterinary technicians have a thorough

understanding of FLUTD and the how the various treatments affect the different types of FLUTD. Veterinary technicians play a very important role in the treatment of FLUTD. The history obtained from discussions with the pet owner aids in the diagnosis of FLUTD. The technicians' discussion of the treatment plan with the client is key to the client's understanding and compliance with the veterinarian's recommendation and ultimately the health of the pet.

References

1 Grauer, G (2013) Current thoughts on pathophysiology and treatment of feline idiopathic cystitis, *Today's Veterinary Journal*, Nov/Dec: 38–41.

2 Osborne C, Lulich J *et al.* (2013) Feline urolith epidemiology update: 1981 to 2011. Tracking the trends of mineral composition in cats with urolithiasis, *DVM360*. June.

3 Forrester, SD (2007) FLUTD: How important is it? In *Proc 2007 Hill's FLUTD Symposium* 2007: 5–11 (http://www.hillsvet.com/conferenceproceedings).

4 Lulich JP (2007) FLUTD: Are you missing the correct diagnosis? In *Proc 2007 Hill's FLUTD Symposium 2007*: 12_19 (http://www.hillsvet.com/conferenceproceedings).

5 Defauw PA, Van de Maele I, Duchateau L *et al.* (2011) Risk factors and clinical presentation of cats with feline idiopathic cystitis, *Jl Feline Med Surg* **13**: 967–75.

6 Westropp JL, Kass PH, Buffington CA (2006) Evaluation of the effects of stress in cats with idiopathic cystitis, *Am J Vet Res* **67**: 731–6.

7 Westropp JL, Welk KA, Buffington CA (2003) Small adrenal glands in cats with feline interstitial cystitis, *Jl Urol* **170**: 2494–7.

8 Markwell PJ, Buffington CA, Chew DJ *et al.* (1999) Clinical evaluation of commercially available urinary acidification diets in the management of idiopathic cystitis in cats, *J Am Vet Med Assoc* **214**: 361.

9 Pereira GG, Fragoso S, Pires E. (2010) *Effect of dietary intake of L-tryptophan supplementation on multi-housed cats presenting stress related behaviors, BSAVA*, April.

10 Beata C, Beaumont G, Coll V *et al.* (2007) Effect of alpha-casozepine (Zylkene) on anxiety in cats, *Journal of Veterinary Behavior* **2**: 40–6.

11 Beata C (2014) L-tryptophan and alpha-casozepine: What is the evidence?, *Hill's Global Symposium on Feline Lower Urinary Tract Health Proceedings*, April, Prague.

12 Stella JL, Lord LK, Buffington CA (2011) Sickness behaviors in response to unusual external events in healthy cats and cats with feline interstitial cystitis, *J Am Vet Med Assoc* **238**: 67–73.

13 Burns, KM (2014) FLUTD – using nutrition to go with the flow, *NAVTA Journal*, Convention Edition, 7–12.

14 Brezinova V, Oswald I (1972) Sleep after a bedtime beverage, *Br Med J* **2**: 431–3.

Further reading

Cameron ME, Casey RA, Bradshaw JW, Waran NK,Gunn-Moore DA (2004) A study of environmental and behavioural factors that may be associated with feline idiopathic cystitis, *J Small Anim Pract* **45**: 144–7.

Buffington CA, Westropp JL, Chew DJ, *et al.* Clinical evaluation of multimodal environmental modification (MEMO) in the management of cats with idiopathic cystitis. *J Feline Med Surg* **8**: 261–8.

Lulich J, Kruger J *et al.* (2013) Efficacy of two commercially available, low-magnesium, urine-acidifying dry foods for the dissolution of struvite uroliths in cats. *JAVMA* **243**(8), Oct. **15**: 1147–53.

37 Dermatology

The management and treatment of skin disorders relies heavily on nutritional management. The use of dietary fatty acids, antioxidants, and novel and hydrolyzed proteins can be beneficial in managing inflammatory skin problems.[1] The veterinary healthcare team plays a large role in improving patient care through understanding of inflammatory skin diseases in dogs and cats, the application of nutritional therapy in managing these disorders, client communication, and enhanced compliance.

The skin, which is the largest organ of the body, protects the animal against water loss as well as physical, chemical, and microbiologic injury. The skin is also a sensory organ and can perceive temperature, pain, touch, pruritus, and pressure. Skin disorders are among the most common conditions treated in veterinary hospitals.[2] Surveys indicate that approximately 15% to 25% of small animal practice involves the diagnosis and treatment of skin and haircoat disorders.[2,3]

Patient History

Obtaining an adequate patient history is the first step in evaluating patients with skin disorders. A complete history should include signalment (i.e., species, breed, age, gender, reproductive status, hair color), presenting complaint, weight and body condition score, nutrition regimen, medical history, and home environment.

A complete nutritional history should determine the quality and adequacy of the food being fed to the pet, the feeding protocol (e.g., meal fed, free choice, amount, family member responsible for the feeding), and a thorough history of the types of foods fed, including access to treats, supplements, and/or other foods. All members of the health care team should be familiar with taking a nutritional history.[4] A nutritional history should include all of the following:

- Tell me everything that your pet eats in a day.
- What brand of food do you feed your pet (try to get specific name)?
- Do you feed moist or dry or both?
- How do you feed your pet – feeding method?
  - how much?
  - how often?
- Does your pet receive any snacks or treats of any kind?
  - what treats?
  - how often?
- Do you give your pet any supplements?
- Is your pet on any medications, including chewable medications?
  - obtain name;
  - dosage.
- What type of chew toys does your pet play with?
- Do you feed your pet any foods or treats not specifically designated for pets?
  - human foods?
  - others?
  - how often?
- Does your pet have *any* access to other sources of food?
  - neighbor?
  - trash?
  - compost?
  - family member (e.g., baby in house, grandparents in house)?

Remember it is imperative that the healthcare team learn everything that enters the pets' mouth. For instance, a dog may be eating a dry commercial food as its main source of nutrition but may also receive pig ears, dog biscuits, flavored monthly oral heartworm prophylactic medication, and table scraps. If the family also includes cats, the dog may have access to commercial food fed to the family cats. Each of these items could

Nutrition and Disease Management for Veterinary Technicians and Nurses, Second Edition. Ann Wortinger, Kara M. Burns.
© 2015 John Wiley & Sons, Inc. Published 2015 by John Wiley & Sons, Inc.
Companion Website: www.wiley.com/go/wortinger/nutrition

be sources of adverse food reactions. Consequently, the pet owner should document everything that enters their pets' oral cavity on a daily basis. This should be done for several weeks prior to the pets' appointment. During the appointment the pet's nutritional history should be reviewed carefully for allergens or ingredients believed to be commonly associated with adverse food reactions.

Physical Examination

The comprehensive physical examination should include a nose to tail evaluation of the pet's skin and hair condition. Any evidence of parasites as well as signs of excessive scratching or licking should be noted in the patient's medical record. The overall health of the patient should be assessed and documented.

Inflammatory skin diseases are typically an allergic (atopy or hypersensitivity) response or an adverse reaction to foods, and the resulting clinical signs often are similar. Clinical signs associated with inflammatory skin diseases include redness, edema, excoriation, hair loss, ulceration, lichenification, pruritus, and dry, flaky skin. The response by the pet is often self-trauma from chronic licking, rubbing, chewing, and scratching of the affected area. Because signs of internal disease may be manifested in skin and haircoat changes, these differentials should not be overlooked because of external lesions. A series of diagnostic tests should be conducted to pinpoint the cause of the skin disorder so that the most effective treatment can be recommended.

Common Skin Disorders in Dogs and Cats

Inflammatory skin diseases define a broad range of skin disorders. The most commonly diagnosed inflammatory skin disorders in dogs include allergy, bacterial infections, parasite infestations, and adverse reactions to food. The list is similar in cats, except cats also develop miliary dermatitis and eosinophilic granuloma complex.

Adverse reactions to food often imitate allergic diseases. An adverse reaction to food is an abnormal response to an ingested food or food additive. Adverse food reactions in dogs typically occur as nonseasonal pruritic dermatitis, occasionally accompanied by gastrointestinal signs.[5,6] The pruritus varies in severity. Lesion distribution is often indistinguishable from that

Table 37.1 Skin lesions in dogs caused by adverse food reactions

- Epidermal collarettes
- Erythroderma
- Excoriations
- Hyperpigmentation
- Otitis externa
- Papules
- Pododermatitis
- Seborrhea sicca

seen with atopic dermatitis; feet, face, axillae, perineal region, inguinal region, rump, and ears are often affected. One-fourth of dogs with adverse food reactions have lesions only in the region of the ears.[7] Therefore, adverse food reactions should always be suspected in dogs with pruritic, unilateral or bilateral otitis externa, even if accompanied by secondary bacterial or *Malassezia* infections.

Adverse food reactions often mimic other common canine skin disorders, including pyoderma, pruritic seborrheic dermatoses, folliculitis, and ectoparasitism.[5] Concurrent allergic disease, such as flea-allergic dermatitis and atopic dermatitis, may be present in 20–30% or more of dogs with suspected adverse food reactions (Table 37.1).[7]

Allergic skin diseases include atopy and flea-bite hypersensitivity. Pruritus is the most common sign in dogs and cats with allergic skin diseases. Atopy initially results in lesions on the face and paws; however, lesions may extend to the ears, axillae, groin, and abdomen. Chronic licking, rubbing, chewing, and scratching commonly result in hair loss, lichenification, excessive pigmentation, scaling, and self-trauma.[8] Flea-bite hypersensitivity is typically characterized by pruritic, papular dermatitis with lesions in the dorsal lumbosacral area, caudomedial thighs, ventral abdomen, and flanks. Lesions involving the ears, footpads, or face strongly suggest a concurrent atopy or adverse food reaction. Secondary bacterial infections, hot spots, and seborrhea are common in chronic hypersensitivity cases.[2,3]

Miliary dermatitis in cats results in numerous small, red papules capped with brownish crusts and associated with varying degrees of hair loss and pruritus. The lesions are typically located in the dorsal lumbar and cervical lesions and are a common response to flea allergy. Miliary dermatitis may also be associated with adverse food reactions and atopy.[9]

Feline eosinophilic granuloma complex describes a skin disorder that involves several syndromes, including indolent ulcers, eosinophilic plaques, and linear granulomas. *Indolent ulcer* is the term used to describe raised, ulcerated lesions in cats seen most commonly on the upper lip and in the mouth. An eosinophilic plaque describes reddened, raised, flat, and firm lesions commonly seen on the abdomen or inner thigh regions. A linear granuloma is a series of raised plaques in a linear configuration often seen on the caudal aspect of a cat's thighs. Feline eosinophilic granuloma complex has been associated with underlying allergies such as flea-bite hypersensitivity, food allergy, and atopy.[10]

Nutritional Management

Key Nutritional Factors

The skin is a metabolically active organ affected by the nutritional status of the animal. Inflammatory skin disorders result in inflammation and infection and require additional nutritional support. An adverse food reaction is an abnormal response to an ingested protein or food additive. Therefore, it is important to ensure that essential nutrients to support normal skin and hair as well as reparative functions are available to the pet. Also, in patients with adverse food reactions, the offending ingredients must be eliminated. Key nutritional factors that help maintain healthy skin and aid in the management of skin disorders are protein, energy, essential fatty acids (EFAs), minerals (copper and zinc), and vitamins (A, E, and B-complex). The pet's food should include optimal levels of these nutrients and the nutrients should be highly digestible and available to the pet.[1]

Protein and energy are essential for development of new hair and skin. It is important for the pet's food to provide optimal protein quality with appropriate levels of essential amino acids, adequate protein quantity, and digestibility. Growth, gestation, lactation, and illness require increased protein and energy; abnormal skin and hair may be noted if nutritionally inadequate foods are fed during these life stages. Inadequate intake of protein and energy may result in depigmentation, dry, dull haircoat and hair loss. Changes in lipid content of the epidermis may affect the protective barrier function of the skin, thereby predisposing the pet to secondary bacterial or yeast infection. Inadequate protein and energy are also associated with impaired wound healing. Pets with severe seborrhea have increased epidermal cell turnover and may have increased protein and other nutrient requirements.

Because most food allergens are thought to be glycoproteins, protein in food is the nutrient of most concern in patients with suspected adverse food reaction. The following should be taken into account:
- types and numbers of diverse proteins in the food;
- protein sources;
- amount of protein;
- digestibility of the protein;
- previous exposure to the protein.

Pet food additives, such as antimicrobial preservatives, colorants, antioxidant preservatives, and emulsifying agents, rarely cause either food intolerance or food allergy.

EFAs are polyunsaturated fatty acids found in phospholipids. They are important in structural function of the lipoproteins of cell membranes allowing conformational responses during temperature fluctuations and providing a barrier function to prevent the loss of water and other nutrients.[11] EFAs are also a source of energy for the skin and are precursors to a variety of important molecules involved in the inflammatory response. EFA deficiencies may result in scaly skin, matting of hair, loss of skin elasticity, alopecia, dry and dull haircoat, erythroderma, hyperkeratosis, interdigital exudation, otitis externa, and poor hair regrowth. These changes affect transepidermal water loss, epidermal cell turnover, poor wound healing, and increased susceptibility to infection. Another important role of EFAs is as antipruritic agents. The inflammation and dermatitis associated with allergic skin disease may be partially caused by abnormal EFA metabolism. The presence of EFA in the cellular membranes may decrease inflammation through competition with arachidonic acid for metabolic enzymes or by antiinflammatory properties.[12] Several studies have looked at the effect of EFAs on pruritus, and on average, 50% of dogs and cats with allergic pruritus improve with modification in EFA intake as long as secondary bacterial and yeast infections are also controlled.[12,13]

Mineral and vitamin imbalances are often associated with skin lesions. Copper deficiency can lead to loss of normal hair coloration, lack of hair, and a dull or rough coat. Zinc is an important enzyme cofactor and modulator of many biologic functions. Zinc deficiency can lead to a dull, rough coat, skin ulcerations, hyperkeratosis, and other dermatoses. Vitamin A, E, and B-complex imbalances are associated with different skin disorders; therefore, foods should be evaluated for appropriate quantity and balance of these vitamins. In general, most commercial pet foods contain excessive vitamins; therefore, skin disorders caused by vitamin deficiencies are rare. However, vitamin deficiency should be considered in animals being fed homemade, noncommercial, or species generic pet foods.

Nutritional Protocol

A complete nutritional protocol in the management of inflammatory skin disorders includes an assessment of the current foods being fed, an assessment of the feeding method, identification of an appropriate feeding plan, and reassessment of the feeding plan.

The pet's food should contain optimal levels of protein, energy, EFAs, minerals, and vitamins for the appropriate life stage of the pet. The nutrients should be high quality to ensure digestibility and availability to meet the pet's nutritional requirements. Assessment of nutritional supplements is also important to identify potential interference with key nutrients or unnecessary supplementation.

The feeding method includes the feeding route, quantity fed, how the food is offered, access to other food, and who is responsible for feeding the pet. This information is gathered when the nutritional history was obtained. It is extremely important when verifying an appropriate feeding method with the pet owner. It is important to thoroughly evaluate the feeding method, although it may not always be necessary to change the nutritional protocol when managing a patient with an inflammatory skin disorder.[4]

Selecting appropriate foods is an important consideration in the nutritional management of patients with inflammatory skin disorders. There are a number of influences which must be considered when treating skin conditions. The patient's access to treats, table scraps, and flavored medicines are a few of the factors which healthcare team should be mindful of when managing skin conditions. For generalized nutritional skin disorders, the diet should be transitioned to a highly digestible food with increased levels of protein and EFAs and an appropriate balance of minerals and vitamins. Oftentimes, the following indications signal a need for change in the pets' diet:

- abnormal hair growth;
- abnormal hair regrowth;
- loss of normal haircoat color;
- adverse reaction to food;
- widespread scaling, crusting;
- dull haircoat or hair loss;
- hyperproliferative skin disorders;
- poor/delayed wound healing;
- decubital ulcers;
- severe and/or generalized inflammatory skin disorders.

The same nutritional management that works for dietary-related skin problems may also help with inflammatory skin disorders and dermatologic signs associated with metabolic diseases in dogs and cats. Research has demonstrated that the use of novel-protein foods with enhanced levels of omega-3 fatty acids and antioxidants is warranted to aid in management of pets with chronic, nonseasonal pruritic dermatitis caused by suspected atopic dermatitis and/or adverse food reaction. Improvements in itchy skin, otitis externa, skin redness, and hair loss were noted by pet owners. Veterinarians recognized the overall improvement in skin and coat condition in the majority of dogs. Novel protein foods with enhanced levels of omega-3 fatty acids and antioxidants should be considered in managing dogs with suspected allergic dermatitis.[14]

Skin disorders caused by nutrient deficiencies usually respond quickly when the pet's diet is changed to a high-quality, highly digestible food. Patient improvement is relatively quick – a few days to a couple of weeks. The healthcare team should closely monitor and document any food and supplement changes. The patient should be examined on a weekly to monthly basis, depending on the diagnosis and severity of the lesions.

A diagnosis of adverse food reaction is more complex and involves a series of elimination trials with novel protein foods or protein hydrolysate foods. Dietary elimination trials are the main diagnostic method used in dogs and cats with suspected adverse food reactions. Ingredients in an ideal elimination food should provide a limited number of highly digestible protein sources, preferably a protein hydrolysate or one to two different types of intact protein to which the animal has not been previously exposed. This recommendation often includes a commercial or homemade food with one animal and one vegetable protein source. An alternate strategy is to use a food containing protein hydrolysate(s). Protein hydrolysates have molecular weights below levels that commonly elicit an allergic response.[15] Caution should be used when recommending a homemade food because most homemade foods fail to meet nutritional requirements because they are made from a minimum of ingredients.[16] If a homemade diet is warranted, this should be done in cooperation with a board certified veterinary nutritionist. It is important to assess the patient for concurrent allergic skin diseases, particularly atopy and flea allergy hypersensitivity because these patients may only partially respond to an elimination trial.

As with any therapeutic protocol, client compliance is critical to a successful outcome. Managing inflammatory skin disorders properly is a long-term investment by the veterinary health care team and the client. Management frequently involves a combination of symptomatic treatment until a definitive diagnosis and appropriate treatment protocol are determined. The technician has a great opportunity to provide vital client support by reinforcing the veterinarian's diagnosis and treatment protocol, educating the client about the importance of and proper application of nutritional protocols and adjunctive therapies, and monitoring patient care through follow-up communications, including call backs and rechecks.

Skin disorders are one of the most common conditions treated in veterinary hospitals. Owners of pets with chronic skin problems often seek veterinary help for symptomatic relief for their pet, resolution of chronic inflammation, and an improvement in the quality and appearance of their pet's haircoat.

Allergic inflammatory skin disorders and adverse reaction to foods are often concurrent and have similar presenting clinical signs. Symptomatic treatment may be necessary while differential diagnoses and appropriate treatment protocols are determined. Nutrition can play an important role in helping to manage and treat skin disorders. The role of the veterinary technician is crucial to optimal patient care through reinforcement of the veterinarian's diagnosis and treatment protocol enhancing client communication and compliance. By encouraging compliance, technicians can help ensure successful patient care, client satisfaction, and improved quality of life for the pet.

References

1 Roudebush PR, Guilford WG, Jackson HA (2010) Adverse reactions to food. In MS Hand, CD Thatcher, RL Remillard *et al.* (eds), *Small Animal Clinical Nutrition* (5th edn), pp. 609–33, Marceline, MO: Walsworth Publishing, Mark Morris Institute.

2 Scott DW, Miller WH, Griffin CE (2001) *Small Animal Dermatology (6th edn)*, Philadelphia, PA: WB Saunders.

3 Miller WH, Griffin CE, Campbell K (2012) *Muller and Kirk's Small Animal Dermatology* (7th edn), Philadelphia, PA: WB Saunders.

4 Burns, KM (2005) *Nutritional management of inflammatory skin disorders*, Veterinary Technician, November:794–800.

5 MacDonald JM (1993) Food allergy. In CE Griffin, KW Kwochka, JM MacDonald (eds), *Current Veterinary Dermatology*, pp. 121–32, St Louis, MO: Mosby.

6 Roudebush P, Schick RO (1994) Evaluation of a commercial canned lamb and rice diet for the management of adverse reactions to food in dogs. *Vet Dermatol* **5**: 63–7.

7 Rosser EJ (2001) Evaluation of a novel carbohydrate and hydrolyzed protein containing diet in previously confirmed food allergic dogs [abstract]. *Vet Dermatol* **12**: 230.

8 Griffin CE, Kwochka KW, MacDonald JM (eds) (1993) *Current Veterinary Dermatology*, St Louis, MO: Mosby.

9 Sousa CA (1995) Exudative, crusting and scaling dermatoses. *Vet Clin North Am Small Anim Pract* **25**: 813–32.

10 Campbell KL (2004) *Small Animal Dermatology Secrets*. Philadelphia: Hanley and Belfus Medical Publishers, pp 220–4.

11 Roudebush PR, Schoenherr WD (2010) Skin and hair disorders. In MS Hand, CD Thatcher, RL Remillard *et al.* (eds), *Small Animal Clinical Nutrition* (5th edn), pp. 638–65, Marceline, MO: Walsworth Publishing, Mark Morris Institute.

12 Miller WH, Scott DW, Wellington JR (1992) Investigation on the antipruritic effects of ascorbic acid given alone or in combination with a fatty acid supplement to dogs with allergic skin disease, *Canine Pract* **17**: 11–13.

13 Harvey RG (1991) Management of feline miliary dermatitis by supplementing the diet with essential fatty acids, *Vet Rec* **128**: 326–9.

14 Allen TA, Fritsch D (2005) A multi-center clinical study of therapeutic foods in dogs with chronic, non-seasonal pruritic dermatitis due to atopy and/or adverse reaction to food. Data on File. Hill's Pet Nutrition Center, Topeka, Kansas.

15 Loeffler A, Lloyd DH, Bond R *et al.* (2004) Dietary trials with a commercial chicken hydrolysate diet in sixty-three pruritic dogs, *Vet Rec* **154**(**17**): 519–22.

16 Roudebush P, Cowell CS (1992) Results of a hypoallergenic diet survey of veterinarians in North America with a nutritional evaluation of homemade diet prescriptions, *Vet Dermatol* **3**: 23–8.

38 Endocrinology

Diabetes mellitus (DM) is a disorder of the endocrine system that is seen in both dogs and cats. DM describes an alteration in cellular transport and metabolism of glucose, lipids, and amino acids as a result of insufficient amounts of insulin released from the pancreas, a lack of insulin receptors, or an inability of the receptors to transduce the signal. The outcome is an elevated glucose level and an inability of the tissues to obtain the glucose they need.[1]

The majority of dogs with diabetes are classified as Insulin Dependent Diabetes Mellitus (IDDM). Cats can be diagnosed with either IDDM or Non-Insulin Dependent Diabetes Mellitus (NIDDM) and may have one form and then over time may revert to the other. The theory being that beta cell function in cats can fluctuate, moving them from one category into the next.[2] Nutritional management in animals with DM is essential. Although nutritional management of IDDM does not eliminate the need for insulin replacement, it may be used to improve glycemic control. In NIDDM patients, nutritional therapy can also improve glycemic control and in some cases may eliminate the need for exogenous insulin therapy. Whether the patient is IDDM or NIDDM, the following factors should be considered in every patient:[2]

- overall health and body condition;
- presence of other diseases;
- type of diet;
- nutrient composition of the diet;
- nutritional adequacy of the diet;
- the animal's caloric requirement;
- feeding schedule.

Dogs and cats with DM typically present to the veterinary hospital with the following signs: polydipsia, polyphagia, weight loss, and lethargy. If the patient is suffering from diabetic ketoacidosis (DKA), the healthcare team will see signs of anorexia, vomiting, diarrhea, weakness, and an overall state of decline. DKA may be brought on by many things including: infection, severe stress, hypokalemia, hypomagnesemia, renal failure, drugs that decrease insulin secretion, drugs that cause insulin resistance, or inadequate fluid intake. A thorough history and physical examination by the healthcare team, including a nutritional assessment is crucial for developing an appropriate management protocol for dogs and cats diagnosed with DKA.

Key Nutritional Factors

Water

Water is one of the key nutrients for all animals. Water is of the utmost importance in animals with diabetes. Patients with DM have increased water losses associated with an osmotic diuresis secondary to glucose and ketone bodies if diabetic ketoacidosis is present. Clean, fresh water should be available at all times.

Energy

Many cats and dogs with diabetes exhibit polyphagia. Despite this, many patients with DM suffer from weight loss. The overall nutritional management of cats and dogs with DM depends upon how well controlled the primary DM is. Another consideration is the presence of concurrent diseases. Weight loss in DM patients may be the result of poorly controlled diabetes or an underlying infection. Weight gain in DM patients may be due to the presence of concurrent disease such as a thyroid disorder or Cushing's disease.

Studies have shown a correlation between obesity and NIDDM in cats. In fact, obesity is well documented as a significant risk factor for DM in cats. Approximately 80% of cats are overweight when diagnosed. Additionally overweight cats have been found to have a fivefold risk increase of developing DM versus cats that are at their optimal weight.[3] The development of feline obesity was accompanied by a 52% decrease in tissue sensitivity to insulin and diminished glucose effectiveness.[4]

Nutrition and Disease Management for Veterinary Technicians and Nurses, Second Edition. Ann Wortinger, Kara M. Burns
© 2015 John Wiley & Sons, Inc. Published 2015 by John Wiley & Sons, Inc.
Companion Website: www.wiley.com/go/wortinger/nutrition

Studies have also shown that baseline insulin levels and insulin response to a glucose load, increases in dogs as their weight increases.[2]

A classification system for food based on its effects on blood glucose levels is referred to as "glycemic index." As a general rule, complex carbohydrates (i.e., barley) have a lower glycemic index than simple carbohydrates (i.e., potatoes) because they are digested and absorbed more slowly.

Fiber

In discussing proper nutritional management of diabetic patients, the amount and type of dietary fiber is often brought up. Dietary fiber is generally classified into two categories: insoluble and soluble. Soluble fibers such as pectins, gums, mucilages, fructooligosaccharides (FOS), etc. have great water-holding capacity, delay gastric emptying, slow the rate of nutrient absorption across the intestinal surface, and are highly fermentable by intestinal bacteria. Whereas insoluble fibers such as cellulose, lignin, and most hemicelluloses have less initial water-holding capacity, decrease gastrointestinal transit time, and are less efficiently fermented by gastrointestinal bacteria. Fiber is believed to slow digestion and absorption of dietary carbohydrates as well as decrease insulin peaks after meals. Soluble fibers are thought to form gels in aqueous solutions, resulting in glucose and water binding; thus preventing their transfer to the intestine's absorptive surface.[1,2]

Although the ideal fiber percentage has not been established, evidence suggests that moderate amounts (approximately 7–18% DMB) of insoluble or mixed insoluble and soluble dietary fiber in high-carbohydrate foods benefits nutritional management of type I and type II diabetes mellitus in dogs and cats. Low carbohydrate/high-protein foods intended for diabetic cats usually contain lower levels of fiber – between 2% and 7% DM.[2]

The amount and structure of carbohydrates used in the nutritional management of DM are different for dogs and cats; mainly due to the fact that dogs are omnivores and tolerate digestible (soluble) complex carbohydrates better than diabetic cats. Foods containing 55% or less digestible carbohydrate (DMB) are suitable for dogs with DM, especially when the food also contains an increased amount of dietary fiber. Conversely, we know that cats are carnivores and have higher dietary protein requirements. The low activity of hepatic enzymes in cats suggests that they generally use gluconeogenic amino acids and fat for energy. It also suggests that diabetic cats may be predisposed to developing higher postprandial blood glucose concentrations following consumption of foods containing a high carbohydrate load and vice versa. Therefore, it is recommended that digestible carbohydrates be less than 20% DMB in low-carbohydrate/high-protein foods for diabetic cats, and increased-fiber/high-carbohydrate foods for diabetic cats should contain less than 40% digestible carbohydrates DMB.[1,2,5] Digestible carbohydrate content in increased-fiber/high-carbohydrate foods for dogs should not exceed 55% DMB. When owners want to provide foods and snacks containing simple sugars, the healthcare team should dissuade them as simple sugars rapidly increase blood glucose concentrations and should be avoided in diabetic pets. Also, in cats fructose is contraindicated as cats do not seem to metabolize fructose. This leads to fructose intolerance, polyuria, and possible damage to the kidneys.[1,2,6] Semi-moist foods and high-fructose corn syrup should be avoided.

Fat

Diabetic animals will often present with abnormalities in lipid metabolism (i.e., hypertriglyceridemia, hypercholesterolemia, etc.). Foods that are high in fat may also lead to insulin resistance and the promotion of hepatic glucose production. Pancreatitis occurs often in many diabetic animals. Pets with alterations in their lipid metabolism or with concurrent pancreatitis should have limited fat in their diet. The amount of fat restriction will be dependent upon the diet history of the pet and the current fat consumption at the time of concurrent disease diagnosis. It is recommended that the fat content be relatively low in fat content, i.e., less than 25% DM. Feeding lower fat foods will help minimize the risk of pancreatitis, control some aspects of hyperlipidemia and reduce overall caloric intake to favor weight loss or maintenance. Foods with a greater fat content may be considered in diabetic dogs and cats when the patient presents as thin or emaciated.

Protein

Diabetic animals may have increased amino acid losses through their urine. Poorly controlled diabetic patients may experience muscle wasting as protein is catabolized to meet energy needs.[1,2] It is important to provide protein quantity and quality that will meet the requirements of diabetic animals in the face of increased amino aciduria while avoiding excess protein content that may enhance renal damage or contribute to excessive insulin secretion. Currently there are two basic approaches to managing diabetes in dogs and cats, high-carbohydrate/moderate-protein foods or low carbohydrate/"high-protein" diets (in some cases "high protein" often only translates into the same amount of protein found in typical maintenance diets). We recognize that as true carnivores, cats primarily use gluconeogenic amino acids rather than dietary carbohydrates for energy. The protein content of foods aimed at managing diabetes is recommended to be 15–35% DMB for dogs and 28–55% DMB for cats.

Hyperthyroidism

Hyperthyroidism is known as the most common endocrinopathy diagnosed in older cats and is seen in cats all over the world. Hyperthyroidism is a clinical condition that results from excessive production and secretion of thyroxine (T4) and triiodothyronine (T3) by the thyroid gland. Management of feline hyperthyroidism has traditionally included thyroidectomy, anti-thyroid medications, and radioactive iodine. Surgery and radioactive iodine therapy are intended to provide long-term solutions, whereas oral anti-thyroid drugs are used to control hyperthyroidism and must be given daily to achieve and maintain their effect. The healthcare team should be familiar with these modalities as well as nutritional management – a new way to manage hyperthyroidism in cats. Recently reported studies reveal that feeding a limited-iodine food normalizes thyroid hormone concentrations and alleviates clinical signs in hyperthyroid cats.[7–10] Now veterinary healthcare teams have a new tool in their toolbox to aid in the management of feline hyperthyroidism.

Feline hyperthyroidism is the result of excessive thyroid hormone production. Thyroid hormone production requires the thyroid gland to take up sufficient amounts of iodine provided by dietary intake.[11] The idea that feline hyperthyroidism could be managed nutritionally through limiting the amount of dietary iodine available for production of thyroid hormone was investigated and introduced to the veterinary profession.[12,13]

Nutritional management of feline hyperthyroidism has been evaluated for approximately 10 years.[10] Three

recently published studies have documented the safety and effectiveness of therapeutic nutrition when used as the only management for cats with naturally occurring hyperthyroidism.[7–9] These studies investigated the magnitude of iodine limitation necessary to return newly diagnosed cats to a euthyroid state;[8] the maximum level of dietary iodine that will maintain cats in a euthyroid state;[7] and the effectiveness of a therapeutic food formulated to control naturally occurring hyperthyroidism in cats.[9] The results of these studies support that feeding ≤0.32 ppm iodine on a dry matter basis (DMB) provides a safe and effective therapy for cats with naturally occurring hyperthyroidism. Serum total thyroxine concentrations decreased within 3 weeks and returned to the reference range within 8–12 weeks of initiating nutritional therapy. When fed ≤ 0.32 ppm iodine DMB as the sole source of nutrition, 90% of hyperthyroid cats remained euthyroid. In all studies to date, indicators of renal function (blood urea nitrogen and serum creatinine) remained stable and no other biochemical abnormalities were observed.[12,13]

Water
Cats with hyperthyroidism often exhibit polydipsia and polyuria. Thus it is important to remind owners to provide fresh, clean water at all times.[1,2]

Energy/Fat
Hyperthyroid patients are typically in an increased metabolic, energy-deficit state. Often, this results in decreased fat stores because of the increased metabolic state. Treatment of the primary disease and use of a food that meets AAFCO nutrient allowances for the desired physiologic state should result in rapid normalization of body weight. If severe wasting of body mass has occurred, the fat content of foods may be increased to achieve higher energy density and enhance weight gain.

Protein
Hyperthyroid cats are in a hypercatabolic state and often present with signs of protein/muscle wasting and protein deficiency.[1,2] Increased protein intake may be needed during the recovery period to replenish body protein. Remember, hyperthyroidism is frequently concomitant with renal failure. Thus a complete evaluation of renal function should be completed before feeding a higher protein food. Provide increased dietary protein for underweight animals. The following protein levels

are adequate unless renal function is compromised: 28–45% DMB. The digestibility of the protein should be greater than 85%.[2]

Fiber

Avoid food with fiber levels greater than 8% DMB in patients with poor body condition.

Nutritional management of feline hyperthyroidism is applicable to cats that are newly diagnosed, currently being managed with anti-thyroid medications, or with recurrence of hyperthyroidism post-thyroidectomy. It is important that healthcare teams educate pet owners regarding the benefits of this new management option. Appropriate and on-going monitoring of the cat is necessary, especially with concurrent diseases (e.g., kidney disease). If patients are newly diagnosed or not currently receiving other therapy for hyperthyroidism, nutritional management may be implemented. As with any new food, transitioning to the limited-iodine therapeutic food is crucial and it is important to educate owners about transition options.[12,13] While the majority of cats require less than 7 days to transition from their current food to a new food, veterinary healthcare team members must educate owners that a longer transition (e.g., several weeks) may be necessary for some cats. The end goal is to have the cat eating the recommended food long-term, therefore, a little time spent initially ensuring a gradual transition is worth the effort. It is important to review each cats' situation and individualize treatment for patients based on all factors, including T$_4$ concentration and the period of time needed to transition to the therapeutic food.

It is imperative that all hyperthyroid cats nutritionally managed with a limited-iodine food not have access to any other food sources. When utilizing the therapeutic food as the sole source of nutrition, 90% of hyperthyroid cats have become and remained euthyroid as long as the cat had no access to other sources of dietary iodine. Should the veterinary healthcare team find persistently increased T$_4$ in a feline patient prescribed the therapeutic food, concerns of poor adherence to dietary recommendations should be considered.[12,13] Discovering the source of dietary iodine intake can be a challenge for the veterinary health care team. Sources of dietary iodine that may alter the response to this therapy include treats, flavored or compounded medications, access to "people food," consumption of wild caught prey, and access to other pet foods. The veterinary technician must perform an in-depth nutritional history to determine exposure to other food sources. The iodine content of compounded medications is of particular concern as many use fish flavoring which may be high in iodine. The iodine content of many over-the-counter supplements may not be known. Therefore, any supplement, treat, homeopathic/holistic therapy or food additive that is fish flavored or derived from ingredients from the sea (fish, shellfish, seaweed etc.) should be questioned and discontinued. Iodine content of water may be considered if all other sources of iodine have been eliminated through a thorough history taken by the technician. This is unlikely if cats are supplied water from municipal water sources. However, it is possible if well water or natural sources of water are available. If iodine in water is suspected, the owner should be counseled to switch to distilled water for one month to assess the response.[12,13]

Hyperthyroidism is a common disease in older cats and thus is seen frequently in veterinary hospitals. While the pathogenesis of feline hyperthyroidism remains unclear, a variety of therapeutic options are available. It is important that veterinary technicians be familiar with all modes of therapy so they can answer questions for pet owners, including advantages and disadvantages of all options. Methods of managing feline hyperthyroidism traditionally have included thyroidectomy, anti-thyroid medications, and radioactive iodine. Nutritional management of hyperthyroidism helps cats return to a euthyroid state and control their clinical signs. Veterinary teams now have a new tool to help manage feline hyperthyroidism.

References

1 Fascetti AJ, Delaney SJ (2011) Nutritional management of endocrine diseases. In AJ Fascetti, SJ Delaney (eds), *Applied Veterinary Clinical Nutrition*, Ames, IA: Wiley Blackwell.
2 Zicker SC, Nelson RW, Kirk CA, Wedekind KJ (2010) Endocrine disorders. In M Hand, C Thatcher, R Remillard *et al.* (eds), *Small Animal Clinical Nutrition* (5th edn), Topeka, KS: Mark Morris Institute.
3 Case LP, Daristotle L, Hayek MG, Raasch MF (2011) Diabetes mellitus. In *Canine and Feline Nutrition* (3rd edn), St Louis, MO: Mosby.
4 Appleton DJ, Rand JS, Sunvold GD (2001) Insulin sensitivity decreases with obesity, and lean cats with low insulin sensitivity are at greatest risk of glucose intolerance with weight gain, *Journal of Feline Medicine and Surgery* **3**: 211–28.
5 Bennett N, Greco DS, Peterson ME *et al.* (2006) Comparison of a low carbohydrate–low fiber diet and a moderate

carbohydrate–high fiber diet in the management of cats with diabetes mellitus, *Journal of Feline Medicine and Surgery* **8**(2): 73–84.

6 Kienzle E (1994) Blood sugar levels and renal sugar excretion after the intake of high carbohydrate diets in cats, *Journal of Nutrition* **124**(12 Suppl): 2563S–2567S.

7 Melendez L, Yamka R, Forrester S *et al.* (2011) Titration of dietary iodine for reducing serum thyroxine concentrations in newly diagnosed hyperthyroid cats, *J Vet Intern Med* **25**: 683 (abstract).

8 Melendez L, Yamka R, Burris P (2011) Titration of dietary iodine for maintaining normal serum thyroxine concentrations in hyperthyroid cats. *J Vet Intern Med* **25**: 683 (abstract).

9 Yu S, Wedekind K, Burris P *et al.* (2011) Controlled level of dietary iodine normalizes serum total thyroxine in cats with naturally occurring hyperthyroidism. *J Vet Intern Med* **25**: 683–4 (abstract).

10 Data on file, Hill's Pet Nutrition, 2011.

11 Mooney CT (2010) Hyperthyroidism. In SJ Ettinger, EC Feldman (eds), *Textbook of Veterinary Internal Medicine: Diseases of the Dog and Cat* (7th edn), pp. 1761–79, St Louis, MO: Saunders.

12 Burns KM (2012) Managing feline hyperthyroidism: As safe and easy as feeding your cat. *NAVTA Journal*, Jan./Feb.: 36–40.

13 Burns KM (2011) A team approach to managing feline hyperthyroidism. *Canadian Vet.* Nov./Dec.: 16–18.

39 Cancer

Cancer diagnoses in humans continue to rise. Approximately 38% of women and 45% of men are likely to develop cancer in their lifetime.[1] Consequently, many pet owners have likely had some experience with cancer – either in themselves or a friend or family member who has had cancer. Therefore the veterinary health care team must remember to approach pets with cancer and their owners with a positive, compassionate, and knowledgeable outlook.

Since pet owners typically understand the importance of nutrition or are willing to learn about it, they are often willing to implement nutritional recommendations that may improve the quality and/or duration of their pets' lives. Additionally, following nutritional recommendations can help pet owners feel like they are participating in the overall management of their pets' cancer.

Metabolic Alterations in Patients with Cancer

Veterinary healthcare teams must remember that patients with cancer may lose weight and have a decrease in body condition due to:
- the location of the tumor (e.g., oral mass);
- complications due to cancer treatment (e.g., radiation of an oral mass);
- cancer cachexia.

Cancer cachexia is a paraneoplastic syndrome manifested by weight loss and a decrease in body condition despite adequate nutritional intake.[2] The numbers of dogs and cats with cancer cachexia are not fully known – but it is imperative for veterinary technicians to remember cachexia when obtaining a patient history and body condition score for pets with cancer.

The metabolic alterations described below have been identified in human and canine cancer patients. To date, studies reviewing metabolic alterations in cats with cancer have not been published. These metabolic alterations in people have been associated with cachexia, a decreased response to therapy, a decreased remission rate, and an increased mortality rate.

Alterations in Carbohydrate Metabolism

Studies have shown that dogs with lymphoma and many other malignant diseases have a significant alteration in carbohydrate metabolism.[3,4] Tumors preferentially metabolize glucose (carbohydrates) for energy and form lactate (lactic acid) as an end product. Therefore the host must expend energy to convert lactate back to glucose. This results in a net energy gain by the tumor and a net loss by the animal. As a result, dogs with cancer lose energy to the tumor and have elevated blood lactate and insulin levels (e.g., laboratory evidence of altered carbohydrate metabolism). Therefore it is important that healthcare team members avoid administering fluids that contain glucose or lactate to pets with cancer.

Alterations in Protein Metabolism

Humans with cancer and weight loss experience a decrease in body muscle mass and an alteration in protein synthesis.[5] Concurrently, to support tumor growth, human cancer patients have increased skeletal muscle protein breakdown, liver protein synthesis, and whole body protein synthesis. If protein intake does not keep pace with use, then immune response, gastrointestinal function, and wound healing are affected.

Cytokines such as tumor necrosis factor–α (TNF-α) are also involved in protein catabolism. An increased level of TNF-α does not induce muscle protein

Nutrition and Disease Management for Veterinary Technicians and Nurses, Second Edition. Ann Wortinger, Kara M. Burns
© 2015 John Wiley & Sons, Inc. Published 2015 by John Wiley & Sons, Inc.
Companion Website: www.wiley.com/go/wortinger/nutrition

catabolism directly but adversely affects important pathways that replenish lost muscle tissue.[6,7]

One study found that compared with normal control dogs, dogs with cancer had altered plasma amino acid profiles.[7] Interestingly, these altered profiles did not return to normal after surgically removing the tumors. This outcome suggests that cancer induces long-lasting changes in canine protein metabolism.

Fat Metabolism Alterations

Catabolism of adipose tissue is the second major feature of cachexia in various chronic diseases, including cancer.[5,7,8] A decrease in fat synthesis or an increase in lipolysis can deplete fat stores. Studies in animal models suggest that production of lipid-mobilizing factor by tumors may account for loss of body fat, especially when this is combined with decreased food intake.

Several cytokines are responsible for altering lipid metabolism. TNF-α is the major cytokine involved in the catabolism of adipose tissue during cachexia in rodents. Altered lipid profiles in dogs with lymphoma suggest that similar changes may occur in pets with cancer.[9]

Unlike host tissues, some tumor cells have difficulty using lipids as a fuel source compared with soluble carbohydrates and protein.[10] This finding has led to the hypothesis that foods relatively high in fat, particularly omega-3 fatty acids, may benefit dogs with cancer compared with foods relatively high in carbohydrates. Pets in North America receive most of their nutrient intake from commercial dry pet foods. These foods are usually high in soluble carbohydrate (25–60%) and relatively low in fat (7–25%). These characteristics may make most commercial dry foods unsuitable for nutritional management of dogs with cancer.

Starvation vs. Cachexia

Cancer associated weight loss differs from that seen with simple starvation. In cachexia there is an equal loss of muscle and fat characterized by increased catabolism of skeletal muscle. During starvation, fat is mobilized first sparing muscle proteins, resting energy expenditure is decreased and glucose metabolism is reduced. In contrast patients with cancer cachexia have normal or elevated resting energy expenditures and glucose turnover. Adequate nutrition will halt and reverse the metabolic alterations that accompany simple starvation but will not completely reverse the metabolic disturbances associated with cancer cachexia.

Prevalence and Diagnosis

Cancer cachexia has been reported to affect 30–85% of human cancer patients. Cachexia is reported as the cause of death in approximately 20% of human patients with cancer.[11] Similar data are not available for veterinary patients. However, one study did document clinically relevant muscle wasting in 15% of dogs presented to a veterinary oncology service. In addition, 4% exhibited cachexia as defined by a body condition score of ≤3/9 and 68% had documented weight loss of 5% to >10%.[12] There are no specific criteria for diagnosis of cachexia in humans but the clinical features which characterize the syndrome include progressive involuntary weight loss with depletion of lean body mass, muscle wasting and weakness, edema, and declines in motor and mental function. There are no specific criteria for diagnosis of cancer cachexia in veterinary patients except weight loss. The diagnosis of cachexia in both human and veterinary patients is complicated by the fact that malnutrition occurs long before clinical signs are evident. Veterinary technicians should suspect cancer associated malnutrition in all tumor bearing animals even in the absence of documented weight loss.

Pathophysiology

Cancer associated malnutrition occurs as a consequence of an imbalance between the nutritional needs of the patient, the demands of the tumor and the availability of nutrients in the body. The competition for nutrients between the tumor and the host promotes a variety of metabolic disturbances including alterations in carbohydrate, lipid and protein metabolism. Cytokines play a key role as the main humoral and tumor derived factors involved in cancer cachexia and may be responsible for the majority of metabolic changes associated with cancer cachexia. Table 39.1 summarizes the effects of cytokines on nutrient metabolism in patients with cancer cachexia.

Table 39.1 Effects of cytokines on nutrient metabolism in patients with cancer cachexia

Carbohydrate	Increased resistance to insulin
	Increased glucose synthesis
	Increased Cori cycle activity (lactate recycling; net energy loss to tumor)
Protein	Increased protein breakdown (catabolism)
	Increased liver (acute phase proteins) and tumor protein synthesis
Fat	Increased lipid mobilization
	Elevated levels of triglycerides

The Ideal Nutritional Profile for Patients with Cancer

Nutritional management of dogs and cats with cancer is part of a multimodal approach to therapy that the veterinary team should consider when initiating treatment. Providing appropriate nutrition may improve quality of life, enhance the effectiveness of treatment, and increase survival time. Alterations in carbohydrate, protein, and fat metabolism precede obvious clinical disease and cachexia in dogs with cancer and may persist in animals with clinical remission of, or apparent recovery from, cancer. Until research results show differently, pathophysiologic and therapeutic principles for cats with cancer should follow those of people and dogs with cancer.[1]

Key nutritional factors in animals with cancer include soluble carbohydrates, fiber, protein, arginine, fat, and omega-3 fatty acids (Table 39.1). These factors should be incorporated in the nutritional management of every patient with cancer.

Soluble Carbohydrates and Fiber

Although most dogs and cats do not require soluble carbohydrates in their diet, ingredients containing these carbohydrates, such as starch, are used in commercial pet food because they are efficient energy sources and have properties that aid in manufacturing and cooking processes. However, soluble carbohydrates may be poorly used by animals with cancer and can contribute to increased lactate production .Thus, soluble carbohydrates should make up less than 25% of a food's dry matter content.

Soluble (fermentable) and insoluble (poorly fermentable) fiber sources are important to help maintain intestinal health, especially in animals undergoing chemotherapy, radiation therapy, or surgery. Increased dietary fiber may help prevent and resolve abnormal stool quality (soft stools, diarrhea) encountered when changing from a high-carbohydrate commercial dry food to a high-fat commercial or homemade food. A crude fiber level greater than 2.5% dry matter is recommended.

Protein and Arginine

Because patients with cancer experience altered protein metabolism, resulting in loss of lean muscle mass (cachexia), dietary protein should be highly digestible and exceed the level normally used for maintenance of adult animals. The protein level should be 30–45% dry matter in foods for dogs with cancer and 40–50% dry matter in foods for cats with cancer.[1]

Arginine is an essential amino acid that may have specific therapeutic value in pets with cancer. The minimum effective level of dietary arginine for animals with cancer is unknown; however, a positive correlation between plasma arginine concentrations and survival in dogs with lymphoma receiving chemotherapy suggests that it is appropriate to provide more than 2.5% arginine on a dry matter basis.[1,13] Arginine has also been shown to improve immune function in cancer patients, promote wound healing, and inhibit tumorigenesis.[1] Cats should receive foods with a similar level of arginine (i.e., >2%) until research discloses a more effective level. L-Arginine can be included in the diet by providing a supplement or a high level of good-quality protein.

Fat and Omega-3 Fatty Acids

Omega-3 fatty acids may have a preventive and therapeutic role in cancer therapy. There is epidemiologic evidence supporting the use of omega-3 fatty acids in human patients with cancer. Low cancer rates have been recognized in populations with high dietary intake of omega-3 fatty acids, which have been shown to reduce the risk of colorectal, prostate, and mammary cancer.[1,14] Omega-3 fatty acids increase the immunologic response

Table 39.2 Key nutritional factors for dogs and cats with cancer

	Protein	Soluble carbohydrate	Fat	Omega-3 fatty acids	Arginine	Crude fiber
Canine	30%–45%	<25%	25%–40%	>5%	>2.5%	>2.5%
Feline	40%–50%	<25%	25%–40%	>5%	>2.5%	>2.5%

against tumor cells, increase tumor susceptibility to oxidative stress, and decrease TNF-α production. In patients with cancer, a high level of omega-3 fatty acids has many clinical benefits, including reduced tumorigenesis, tumor growth, and metastasis as well as anticatabolic effects.[15–17]

In clinical trials of dogs with spontaneous cancer, high dietary levels of omega-3 fatty acids (specifically eicosapentaenoic acid [EPA] and docosahexaenoic acid [DHA]) and arginine were shown to benefit dogs with lymphoma, nasal carcinoma, hemangiosarcoma, and osteosarcoma.[13,14] In a double-blind, placebo-controlled clinical trial in which dogs underwent chemotherapy, the test food with high levels of omega-3 fatty acids and arginine was shown to reduce lactic acid consistently over a 12-week period compared with the control food.[14] Omega-3 fatty acids in conjunction with arginine were shown to influence clinical signs, increase survival time, provide longer remission time, and improve quality of life.[14]

Clinical Studies Using Omega-3 Fatty Acids in Patients with Cancer

The use of a high-fat, low-carbohydrate, arginine- and fish oil–supplemented food in normal, healthy dogs and in dogs undergoing chemotherapy for lymphoma or radiation therapy for nasal tumors have been evaluated in a number of clinical studies.[18] In normal dogs, food supplemented with a high level of fish oil increased serum concentrations of EPA and DHA within 1 week. These elevated concentrations persisted for several weeks after dietary supplementation was discontinued.[18]

Although clinical trials with functional foods have been performed for only a few types of cancer, the underlying metabolic abnormalities caused by cancer have been documented in dogs with many types of

tumors.[3,4,14] These findings suggest that similar clinical responses would be expected in animals with various cancers.

Overall, dietary supplementation with a high level of fish oil is safe for dogs. Potential adverse effects to be mindful of include poor wound healing, coagulopathies (platelet dysfunction), gastrointestinal upset (soft stools, diarrhea), pancreatitis, fishy breath odor, and nutrient interactions (e.g., the vitamin E requirement increases with the amount of polyunsaturated fatty acids, including omega-3 fatty acids, in the food).[14] Because of the potential for serious bleeding problems, cats with cancer should be given foods with a level of fish oil or omega-3 fatty acids lower than those recommended for dogs with cancer (Table 39.2).[14]

In general, using commercial therapeutic foods formulated to aid in nutritional management of dogs with cancer is preferable to supplementing typical pet foods with fish oil and arginine. The feeding of an appropriate therapeutic food is more economical and easier than administering multiple daily supplements. Clinical trials have shown that more than 90% of dogs accept and tolerate therapeutic foods.

Nutraceuticals

Antioxidant Vitamins

The use of antioxidants in cancer patients is somewhat controversial. Some veterinary professionals think that antioxidants improve the efficacy of cancer therapy, improve immune function, decrease toxicity to normal cells, and reverse metabolic changes contributing to cachexia. Others think that dietary antioxidants may protect cancer cells against damage from chemotherapy or radiation therapy.[13,14] It has been reported that many human cancer patients use vitamin supplements as complementary therapy, usually without the recommendation or knowledge of their physician.[19–22]

It is assumed that owners of pets with cancer may also commonly provide vitamin supplementation; however, this has not been studied.

The need for vitamin E in the diet is influenced by composition of the food. The vitamin E requirement increases with increasing levels of polyunsaturated fatty acids (including omega-3 fatty acids), oxidizing agents, and trace minerals and decreases with increasing levels of fat-soluble vitamins, sulfur-containing amino acids, and selenium. Manufacturers of many specialty-brand pet foods have increased levels of antioxidant vitamins such as vitamins E and C because they appear to improve immune function and reduce cell damage in normal animals. However, the role of antioxidant vitamins in animals with cancer is far more complex. Additional studies are needed to determine optimal antioxidant nutrient intake for pets with cancer. At the present time, if the animal is fed a complete and balanced commercial food, megadose vitamin therapy does not appear to be indicated. The levels of vitamin E and other antioxidant nutrients should be appropriate in regard to the levels of polyunsaturated fatty acids, trace minerals, and oxidants in the food.

Trace Minerals

Serum zinc, chromium, and iron concentrations are lower in dogs with lymphoma and osteosarcoma than in normal dogs.[23,24] The clinical significance of these abnormalities is unknown, especially given that serum levels may or may not correlate with tissue levels of trace minerals. Additional studies are warranted to determine the optimal trace mineral intake for cats and dogs with cancer. Currently, trace mineral supplementation does not seem to be indicated if the pet is fed a complete and balanced commercial food, but is very important if the owner plans to feeds home-prepared food.

Glutamine

Glutamine may have specific therapeutic value for pets with cancer. Glutamine is an essential precursor for nucleotide biosynthesis and an important oxidative fuel for enterocytes. Glutamine has recently been recognized as a conditionally essential amino acid in certain physiologic states, including stress. Cancer would be considered to elicit a stressful physiologic response. Glutamine has several important biochemical roles and is a preferred source of energy for cells with rapid turnover, such as lymphocytes, enterocytes, and cancer cells. Glutamine has been shown to stabilize weight loss, improve protein metabolism, improve immune response, and improve gut barrier function in rodent cancer models and in human clinical trials.[1] The optimal glutamine intake for cats and dogs with cancer has not yet been determined and additional studies are necessary. Glutamine is best supplied by high-quality, high-protein pet foods.

Tea Polyphenols

Tea polyphenols, found in the leaves of the tea plant *Camellia sinensis* protect against cancers induced by chemicals or ultraviolet radiation. Tea polyphenols have also been found to increase chemotherapy efficacy in animal cancer models.[14,25] Although green tea supplements are available, proper doseage has not been established for cats and dogs.

Vitamin A

Natural and synthetic vitamin A derivatives, also known as retinoids, are currently being studied for their effects on cancer. The functions of vitamin A include growth promotion, differentiation and maintenance of epithelial tissues, and maintenance of normal reproductive and visual functions. Retinoic acid affects differentiation and proliferation of epithelial cells by binding to and activating specific cell nuclear receptors that can modify rates of gene transcription. Human and veterinary studies suggest that retinoids, alone or with other agents, may be effective for treating certain types of malignancies. Retinoids promote cellular differentiation and may enhance the susceptibility of cancer cells to chemotherapy and radiation therapy.[1]

Pet owners are acutely aware of cancer in humans and thus relate their experiences with humans to their pets. Health care team members must remember to approach cats and dogs with cancer and their owners in a positive, compassionate, and well-informed fashion. Nutritional therapy and nutraceutical supplementation may influence remission time, survival time, and quality of life of veterinary patients with cancer. It is imperative that veterinary healthcare teams remember that nutritional management may help pets live longer and feel better and involving pet owners in their pets' care and treatment helps family members to feel a part of their pets' treatment.

References

1 Saker KE, Selting KA (2010) Cancer. In MS Hand, CD Thatcher, RL Remillard *et al.* (eds), *Small Animal Clinical Nutrition* (5th edn), pp. 587–607, Topeka, KS: Mark Morris Institute.

2 Fearon KC, Voss AC, Hustead DS (2006) Definition of cancer cachexia: effect of weight loss, reduced food intake, and systemic inflammation on functional status and prognosis. *Am J Clin Nutr* **83**:1345–50.

3 Ogilvie GK, Walters L, Salman MD *et al.* (1997) Alterations in carbohydrate metabolism in dogs with non-hematopoietic malignancies. *Am J Vet Res* **56**: 277–81.

4 Mazzaferro EM, Hackett TB, Stein TP *et al.* (2001) Metabolic alterations in dogs with osteosarcoma. *Am J Vet Res* **62**: 1234–9.

5 Costelli P, Baccino FM (2000) Cancer cachexia: from experimental models to patient management. *Curr Opin Clin Nutr Metab Care* **3**: 177–81.

6 Inui A (2002) Cancer anorexia-cachexia syndrome: current issues in research and management. *CA Cancer J Clin* **52**: 72–91.

7 Ogilvie GK, Vail DM, Wheeler SL (1988) Alterations in fat and protein metabolism in dogs with cancer [abstract]. *Proc Vet Cancer Soc* **31**.

8 Langhans W (2002) Peripheral mechanisms involved with catabolism. *Curr Opin Clin Nutr Metab Care* **5**: 419–26.

9 Ogilvie GK, Ford RD, Vail DM *et al.* (1994) Alterations in lipoprotein profiles in dogs with lymphoma. *J Vet Intern Med* **8**: 62–6.

10 Hansell DT, Davies JW, Shenkin A, Burns HJ (1986) The oxidation of body fuel stores in cancer patients. *Ann Surg* **204**: 637–42.

11 Ernst E (2001) Complementary therapies in palliative cancer care. *Cancer* **91**: 2181–5.

12 Bernstein BJ, Grasso T (2001) Prevalence of complementary and alternative medicine use in cancer patients. *Oncology (Hunting)* **15**: 1267–72.

13 Hemming L, Maher D (2005) Understanding cachexia and excessive weight loss in cancer. *Brit J Comm Nursing* **10**(**11**): 492–5.

14 Michel KE, Sorenmo K, Shofer FS (2004) Evaluation of body condition and weight loss in dogs presented to a veterinary oncology service. *JVIM* **18**: 692–5.

15 Delaney SJ (2006) Management of anorexia in dogs and cats. *Vet Clin Sm An Pract* **36**: 1243–9.

16 Burns, KM (2010) Therapeutic foods and nutraceuticals in cancer therapy. *Veterinary Technician*. April. Vetlearn.com. E1–E7.

17 Forrester SD, Roudebush P, Davenport DJ (2010) Supportive care of the cancer patient: nutritional management of the cancer patient. In CJ Henry, ML Higginbotham (eds), *Cancer Management in Small Animal Practice*, pp. 167–87, Maryland Heights, MO: Saunders Elsevier.

18 Roudebush P, Davenport DJ, Novotny BJ (2004) The use of nutraceuticals in cancer therapy. *Vet Clin North Am Small Anim Pract* **34**: 249–9.

19 Bougnoux P (1999) Omega-3 polyunsaturated fatty acids and cancer. *Curr Opin Clin Nutr Metab Care* **2**: 121–6.

20 Zhou J-R, Blackburn GL (1999) Dietary lipid modulation of immune response in tumorigenesis. In D Heber, GL Blackburn, VLW Go (eds), *Nutritional Oncology*, pp. 195–213, San Diego, CA: Academic Press.

21 Ross JA, Moses AGW, Fearon KCH (1999) The anti-catabolic effects of omega-3 fatty acids. *Curr Opin Clin Nutr Metab Care* **2**: 219–26.

22 Hansen RA, Ogilvie GK, Davenport DJ *et al.* (1998) Duration of effects of dietary fish oil supplementation on serum eicosapentaenoic acid and docosahexaenoic acid concentrations in dogs. *Am J Vet Res* **59**: 864–8.

23 Metz JM, Jones H, Devine P *et al.* (2000) Cancer patients use unconventional medical therapies far more frequently than standard history and physical examination suggest. *Cancer J* **7**: 149–54.

24 Kazmierski KJ, Ogilvie GK, Fettman MJ *et al.* (2001) Serum zinc, chromium and iron concentrations in dogs with lymphoma and osteosarcoma. *J Vet Intern Med* **15**: 585–8.

25 Sandler RS, Halabi S, Kaplan EB *et al.* (2001) Use of vitamins, minerals, and nutritional supplements by participants in a chemoprevention trial. *Cancer* **91**:1040–5.

40   Refeeding Syndrome

Refeeding syndrome (RS) refers to the metabolic alterations that occur after nutritional support is started in a severely malnourished, underweight, and/or starved patient. When a patient is in a starved state, the body maintains extracellular concentrations of electrolytes at the expense of intracellular concentrations. This may then result in inward restructuring when glucose and insulin are introduced to the patient with refeeding. The result of this shift is critical decreases in vital serum electrolyte concentrations which may be life threatening. When food is reintroduced to the patient, the blood glucose rises and the body releases insulin which pumps glucose and potassium intracellularly. Consequently, a profound hypokalemia may result. This can occur rather quickly in patients being fed parenterally, but may take days to appear when feeding enterally. The patient may also experience hypomagnesemia and hypophosphatemia. Hypophosphatemia has also been associated with hemolysis and may lead to additional cardiac and neurologic complications. Malnourished patients, especially those experiencing refeeding syndrome, may also have a thiamine deficiency, so it is imperative to monitor thiamine levels in malnourished patients.[1-3]

RS occurs in disease conditions such as starvation from feline hepatic lipidosis, overall malnutrition, and prolonged diuresis as ensues in uncontrolled diabetes renal failure. Again, the greatest risk is seen in patients that are severely malnourished and experiencing significant loss of lean body mass.[4] RS includes a variety of fluid and electrolyte abnormalities affecting multiple organ systems, including neurologic, cardiac, hematologic, neuromuscular, and pulmonary function which is especially prevalent in humans. In cats, RS affects are mainly seen in the hematologic and neurologic systems. In canines, the effects seen are typically in the hematologic, cardiac, and neurologic systems. It is believed that cats are more susceptible to refeeding syndrome as opposed to dogs,

because cats' hepatic glycogen stores are low and gluconeogenesis is accelerated within the first day of malnutrition. Veterinary technicians must be familiar with the risks that may lead to RS in both cats and dogs in addition to how to manage RS in all patients.

An in-depth history from the owner is critical when determining whether a patient is suffering from RS. If the patient has been hospitalized attentive nursing care and constant monitoring must be performed to watch for signs and laboratory evidence of RS. Oftentimes the owner will communicate the following signs upon history and physical examination of the patient: anorexia, weight loss, lethargy, weakness, nausea and/or vomiting, diarrhea, pigmenturia, restlessness, seizures, and coma.

The physiology of starvation helps to provide a clearer understanding of the development of clinical signs associated with refeeding a severely malnourished patient. Initially during the period of starvation (24–72 hours), the liver uses glycogen stores for energy and skeletal muscle to provide amino acids as a source for new glucose production (i.e., gluconeogenesis) for glucose-dependent tissues, such as the brain and red blood cells. After 72 hours of starvation, metabolic pathways shift and take energy from ketone production as a result of free fatty acid oxidation while sparing protein utilization from skeletal muscle. Also, the body's adaptive mechanisms include; an overall decrease in liver gluconeogenesis, a decline in basal metabolic rate, reduction in the secretion of insulin, and an increased use of free fatty acids by the brain as the primary energy source in place of glucose.[5,6]

In critically ill patients, endogenous protein catabolism is accelerated beyond the requirement of gluconeogenesis. The key to survival is whether the animal can recover from the underlying disease or injury. Amino acids are needed not just for gluconeogenesis, but also for the synthesis of new proteins

Nutrition and Disease Management for Veterinary Technicians and Nurses, Second Edition. Ann Wortinger, Kara M. Burns
© 2015 John Wiley & Sons, Inc. Published 2015 by John Wiley & Sons, Inc.
Companion Website: www.wiley.com/go/wortinger/nutrition

(e.g., clotting factors, immunoglobulins, granulation tissue). Consequently, endogenous proteins are reallocated from less essential tissues to tissues critical for survival, thus leading to the extreme catabolic response that is seen in the sickest patients. In stressed starvation, the hormones and peptides are released in response to tissue injury and inflammation, not simply due to a deficit of nutrient intake. Therefore the effects will not be simply reversed through feeding. Subsequently, while the goals of nutritional support should be to provide enough energy and protein to the patient to sustain the increased nutrient demands of critical illness and preserve the patient's endogenous tissues, the catabolic response will be, at best, blunted by the provision of nutrients in the face of ongoing disease.[7−9] Veterinary technicians must also remember that nutrients given in excess of the patient's needs will not be utilized in a critically ill patient, as they would in a healthy patient. Thus, overfed patients are at increased risk of developing hepatic lipidosis, hypercapnia, and a multitude of metabolic abnormalities.

The literature shows that metabolic disturbances of any type are less likely to occur if estimates of caloric needs are conservative. Current recommendations for feeding critically ill patients are to begin feeding equal to the patient's estimated resting energy expenditure. To cover all sizes of canines and felines the following calculation is recommended: RER = (kg × kg × kg, $\sqrt{}$, $\sqrt{}$) × 70. Make sure you do not use any stress/illness factors in your initial energy calculation. Particularly with critically ill patients, starting with an estimate of the patient's RER and making adjustments based on response is the safest course of action.

Electrolytes

Potassium
Hypokalemia is probably the most commonly detected electrolyte disturbance when providing nutritional support to a patient. Typically patients who are receiving nutritional support are also receiving intravenous fluids; thus the patients' serum sodium and potassium levels should be constantly monitored. Potassium is also affected by resumption of exogenous carbohydrate metabolism. With refeeding, glucose is absorbed, insulin is secreted and potassium is taken up by cells along with glucose. Veterinary technicians should look

for the following clinical signs that may accompany hypokalemia: glucose intolerance, muscle weakness, ileus, respiratory depression, cardiac arrhythmias, and ECG changes.

Phosphorus
Hypophosphatemia has been reported as a consequence of enteral nutrition in veterinary patients and of insulin administration in diabetic patients. Hypophosphatemia is actually an uncommon condition in dogs in cats. However, in refeeding syndrome, it is the most significant disturbance. Serum phosphorus levels are not as likely to be routinely monitored as serum potassium levels. Therefore it is important that the healthcare team recognizes "at-risk" patients so that they can be monitored more closely. The healthcare team should look for the following clinical signs associated with severe hypophosphatemia: hemolytic anemia, muscle weakness, acute ventilatory failure, and altered myocardial function. Liquid enteral diets may not contain maintenance quantities of phosphorus. This is not a problem for patients who are not phosphorus depleted but will be for those who become hypophosphatemic on feeding. Phosphorus can be supplemented in liquid diets by adding potassium phosphate. Dogs and cats that develop hypophosphatemia on enteral and parenteral feeding will require additional supplementation in their fluid therapy.

Magnesium
Magnesium abnormalities are being detected more often in critically ill dogs and cats, especially in patients suffering with prolonged starvation, diabetes mellitus, or renal disease. The clinical signs of hypomagnesemia include tetany and other neurological abnormalities, cardiac arrhythmias and ECG changes, and secondary effects on the homeostasis of other electrolytes. Magnesium is a co-factor in many enzyme systems including the ATPase associated with membrane-bound sodium-potassium pumps. It is the dysfunction in the sodium-potassium pump in the renal tubules that is believed to be the mechanism for the refractory hypokalemia that can be seen concurrent with hypomagnesemia. Hypocalcemia is another secondary electrolyte effect of hypomagnesemia. Magnesium is necessary for both parathyroid hormone (PTH) secretion and the actions of PTH on bone. Hypocalcemic patients will respond to parenteral calcium supplementation but will rapidly become hypocalcemic again once calcium infusion is ceased

unless serum magnesium levels are also corrected. Magnesium can be supplemented parenterally with magnesium sulfate in patients who have severe clinical signs and good urine output. Oral magnesium supplementation is not recommended in these patients as most oral magnesium preparations are cathartic and are poorly absorbed. Patients are able to better tolerate magnesium gluconate or amino acid chelates of magnesium.

Managing Refeeding Syndrome

When refeeding syndrome is suspected in a patient or to prevent refeeding syndrome in critically ill patients, begin feeding the patient *very* slowly. Also as discussed above, with refeeding syndrome patients, it is best to begin nourishment at a portion of the RER, with increasing amounts as tolerated, over the course of 3–5 days. Consideration should be given to starting nutrition at 25–30% of the calculated RER for the first 24 hours (small frequent meals) working up to 100% of the RER after 5 days. This should be done regardless of oral, other enteral, or parenteral feeding.[3,7,9,10]

Veterinary healthcare team members must monitor potential refeeding syndrome patients. Phosphate supplementation is justified in patients at risk for development of hypophosphatemia, patients with clinical signs resulting from hypophosphatemia, and patients with hypophosphatemia. When formulating enteral or parenteral nutrition solutions for patients with normal serum phosphorus levels, phosphates should be added to the solution to meet the patient's estimated daily requirements. The estimated daily phosphorus requirement is 200–400 mg in cats and 75 mg/kg in dogs. Patients with severe hypophosphatemia and patients exhibiting hemolytic anemia, IV potassium or sodium phosphate should be administered at 0.01–0.06 mmol/kg/hr until the patient is no longer severely hypophosphatemic or until serum phosphorus is >2 mg/dL.

If patients develop hypokalemia, potassium supplementation should begin. Potassium chloride or potassium phosphate may be added to parenteral fluid therapy dependent upon the level of hypokalemia. Patients with severe hypokalemia can be given a KCl IV infusion at 0.5 mEq/kg/hr for 6 hours. The KCl should be diluted in an equal volume of normal saline.

The overall potassium infusion should *not* exceed 0.5 mEq/kg/hr. The veterinary healthcare team must be cognizant of the contribution of potassium phosphate to the overall potassium supplementation especially if this solution is being used to correct hypophosphatemia.

In patients that develop hypomagnesemia supplementation of magnesium should be started by the healthcare team. Magnesium chloride or sulfate may be added to parenteral fluid therapy at 1 mEq/kg/day for the first 24 hours. If further magnesium supplementation is needed past the initial 24 hours, decrease the rate to 0.5–0.75 mEq/kg/day.

Remember to monitor the patients' thiamine level as thiamine supplementation is recommended in all malnourished patients. This is especially important when beginning to reintroduce nutrition to the patient. Cats and dogs should receive 10–100 mg/day SQ during the refeeding period.

The veterinary healthcare team should assess the patient's food intake or administration of nutritional support every day and often assessment multiple times a day is warranted. The patient's body weight and body condition score should be recorded in the medical record at least once a day. Dependent upon the amounts of fluids going into the patient, their weight may change numerous times throughout the day. Patients undergoing treatment with IV phosphates, serum phosphorus and serum calcium concentrations should be evaluated every 6–12 hours. Serum phosphate, glucose, potassium, and magnesium levels should be monitored at least once a day during the refeeding period (≥5 days) or more frequently for patients receiving potassium, magnesium, or insulin supplementation. PCV and HCT should be monitored for evidence of anemia, and serum should be monitored for evidence of hemolysis in animals with hypophosphatemia. Nursing care should also include monitoring patients frequently for signs of fluid overload and congestive heart failure.

Summary

RS is a serious condition that may develop in underweight, severely malnourished, or starved patients during nutrition repletion. RS involves significant electrolyte, fluid, and vitamin abnormalities that can lead to significant illness and possibly death. The veterinary healthcare team should be aware of RS, identify patients at risk of developing RS, how to manage RS should it develop in patients, and most importantly take steps to prevent RS. Patients who develop signs and symptoms of RS require aggressive electrolyte supplementation, vitamin supplementation, and supportive care, and nutrition support should be restarted, but with great caution.

References

1 Lippo N, Byers, CG (2008) Hypophosphatemia and Refeeding Syndrome. *Standards of Care: Emergency and Critical Care Medicine* **10** (4), May: 6–10.

2 Saker K, Remillard RL (2010) Critical care nutrition and enteral-assisted feeding. In MS Hand, CD Thatcher, RL Remillard *et al.* (eds), *Small Animal Clinical Nutrition* (5th edn), pp 439–76, Marceline, MO: Walsworth Publishing, Mark Morris Institute.

3 Larsen, JA (2012) Enteral nutrition and tube feeding. In A Fascetti, S Delaney (eds), *Applied Veterinary Clinical Nutrition*, pp. 328–52, Ames, IA: Wiley Blackwell.

4 Wortinger A (2007) Nutritional support. In *Nutrition for Veterinary Technicians and Nurses*, pp. 211–20, Ames, IA: Wiley-Blackwell.

5 Chandler ML, Guilford WG, Payne-James J. (2000) Use of peripheral parenteral nutritional support in dogs and cats. *J Am Vet Med Assoc* **216**: 669–73.

6 Proulx J (2000) Nutrition in critically ill Animals. In The Veterinary ICU Book, *pp*. 202–17, Jackson Hole, WY: Teton New Media.

7 Eirmann L, Michel K (2009) Enteral nutrition. In *Small Animal Critical Care Medicine*, pp. 53–8, St Louis, MO: Saunders.

8 Michel K (2011) Metabolic complications of nutritional support: prevention and troubleshooting. *Proceedings 17th IVECCS*, San Antonio, TX.

9 Chan DL, Freeman LM (2006) Nutrition in critical illness. *Veterinary Clinics of North America Small Animal Practice* **36** (6): 1225–41.

10 Delaney SJ, Fascetti AJ, Elliott DA (2006) Critical care nutrition of dogs. In P Pibot, V Biourge, D Elliot (eds), *Encyclopedia of Canine Clinical Nutrition*, pp. 426–51, Aniwa SAS, France: Royal Canin.

41 Cardiac Disease

Cardiovascular disease is a common disorder in dogs and cats, with 11% of canines and up to 20% of feline populations affected by cardiac disease.[1,2] Chronic valvular disease has been found to be the most common acquired heart disease in dogs with an overall incidence greater than 40%.[3] Chronic mitral valvular disease is the most common acquired cardiac abnormality in dogs, affecting more than one-third of patients over 10 years of age.[4] Approximately 30% of cases involve the tricuspid valve but disease of the tricuspid valve is usually less severe. Valvular disease is more prevalent in small breed dogs. Acquired valvular disease is rarely seen in cats. Taurine deficiency was discovered to be the principal cause of dilated cardiomyopathy in cats in 1987, and since this time the prevalence of this disease has decreased significantly.[3,4] Today, hypertrophic and restrictive cardiomyopathies are more prevalent causes of myocardial failure in cats.

Several types of myocardial disease not recognized 40 years ago now appear commonly in dogs. Large-breed dogs, especially males, are predisposed to dilated cardiomyopathy, and the Doberman pinscher breed seems to stand out as the pre-disposed breed. Hypertrophic cardiomyopathy in dogs is rarely seen. Arrhythmogenic right ventricular cardiomyopathy is common among boxer dogs.

Pulmonary vascular disease with secondary cor pulmonale is most often seen with *Dirofilaria immitis* infection (heartworm disease). This disease is more widespread in areas with higher mosquito and heartworm populations and is worsened when the dog does not receive appropriate preventive medication. Pulmonary hypertension appears to be more common than previously believed with diagnosis of pulmonary hypertension increasing due to heightened awareness. Pulmonary thromboembolism is most commonly associated with renal disease, hyperadrenocorticism, corticosteroid therapy, neoplasia, nephrotic syndrome,

pancreatitis, and immune-mediated hemolytic anemia. Primary systemic vascular disease is uncommon. Secondary aortic thromboembolism in cats may occur with any of the forms of cardiomyopathy and is the most frequently acquired feline vascular abnormality. Systemic hypertension in dogs and cats now appears to be more common than believed 40 years ago.

Dogs and cats with hypertension may present at any age, but typically hypertension is seen in middle-aged to geriatric patients. The mean age of dogs with hypertension is nine years and the mean age of cats is 15 years. The strength of the peripheral pulses does not help detect systemic hypertension. Retinal hemorrhages and detachments are common end-organ changes in patients with moderate to severe hypertension. These ocular signs are frequently the first signs seen associated with hypertensive disease. A fundic examination should be part of the routine evaluation of all dogs and cats. Other clinical signs of hypertension are most often related to the underlying disease that causes systemic hypertension. The effects of long-term or severe systemic hypertension may cause significant heart disease (e.g. left ventricular concentric hypertrophy), and hypertension may complicate the treatment of chronic mitral valvular disease in dogs by worsening valvular regurgitation. The healthcare team should screen dogs and cats with significant heart disease for the presence of systemic hypertension. The healthcare team should also search for underlying heart disease in patients with known hypertension, especially those exhibiting clinical signs that may be indicative of heart disease.

The most frequently encountered problems associated with cardiovascular disease that require nutritional modification are fluid retention states associated with chronic CHF, primary or secondary hypertension, obesity, cachexia and myocardial diseases related to a specific nutrient deficiency (taurine- and carnitine)

Nutrition and Disease Management for Veterinary Technicians and Nurses, Second Edition. Ann Wortinger, Kara M. Burns
© 2015 John Wiley & Sons, Inc. Published 2015 by John Wiley & Sons, Inc.
Companion Website: www.wiley.com/go/wortinger/nutrition

and electrolyte disorders that may predispose to cardiac dysrhythmias.

Effective treatment requires a multifaceted approach, of which nutritional managment is an important component. Foods designed for patients with cardiovascular disease should supply age-appropriate nutrition and specific nutrients that may help manage hypertension, decrease fluid retention and control the signs associated ascites, maintain heart muscle function, help slow the progression of concurrent kidney disease, and help counter the loss of nutrients in the urine of pets prescribed diuretics.

Heart failure is characterized by inadequate cardiac output and insufficient delivery of nutrients relative to tissue metabolic needs. Heart failure is a clinical syndrome which results from a variety of structural and functional disorders of the heart or great vessels. Clinical manifestations of heart failure are due to reduced cardiac output (weakness, exercise intolerance, syncope), pulmonary congestion (dyspnea, orthopnea, cough, abnormal breath sounds with crackles and wheezes), systemic fluid retention (jugular venous distention, hepatomegaly, ascites, pleural effusion) or a combination of these conditions. Obesity and chronic bronchitis often occur in dogs and cats with heart disease and cause clinical manifestations similar to those of heart failure, which can further complicate the diagnosis. Obesity can also exacerbate previously existing cardiac conditions.

Key Nutritional Factors

Sodium and Chloride
Sodium, chloride, and water retention are linked with CHF. Subsequently, the healthcare team should focus on these nutrients in patients with cardiovascular disease. A few hours after the ingestion of high levels of sodium, healthy dogs and cats easily excrete any excess in their urine. However, patients in early cardiac disease may lose this ability to excrete excess sodium. As heart disease worsens and CHF arises, the ability to excrete excess sodium is worsened. Historically, sodium retention was primarily implicated in the pathogenesis of CHF and some forms of hypertension. A number of studies have examined the interaction of sodium with other ions, including chloride. Chloride may also act as a direct renal vasoconstrictor. According the NRC

the minimum recommended allowance for sodium and chloride in foods for adult dogs is 0.08 and 0.12% dry matter (DM), respectively. In foods for adult cats it is 0.068 for sodium and 0.096% for chloride (DM).When dealing with patients with cardiovascular disease the sodium levels in foods designed to manage these patients should be limited to 0.08 to 0.25% DM for dogs and 0.07 to 0.3% DM for cats. Recommended chloride levels are typically 1.5 times sodium levels.

Avoiding excess sodium chloride in cat foods is more difficult than in dog foods as ingredients used to meet the higher protein requirement of cats also contain sodium and chloride and thus increase the sodium chloride content of cat food.

Taurine
Taurine is an important amino acid in dogs and cats with myocardial failure. The mechanism of heart failure in taurine-deficient cats and dogs is not well understood. Taurine may function in inactivation of free radicals, osmoregulation and calcium modulation. Taurine is also known for its direct effects on contractile proteins. Additionally, there may be other factors responsible for contributing to the development of myocardial failure in patients with taurine deficiency. Dilated cardiomyopathy and heart failure may result from an inciting or contributing factor combined with taurine deficiency. As we know, taurine is an essential amino acid in cats, therefore a minimum recommended allowance for taurine is necessary in cat foods. Taurine should be 0.04% DM. Taurine content of foods for cats with cardiovascular disease should contain at least 0.3% DM. Levels of taurine typically recommended for supplementation of feline cardiovascular patients (250–500 mg taurine/day) provide approximately twice that much.

Taurine is not an essential amino acid for dogs. Nevertheless, an association between dilated cardiomyopathy and plasma taurine deficiency and low myocardial taurine concentrations, has been observed. The association between taurine deficiency and dilated cardiomyopathy is strongest in American cocker spaniels and golden retrievers. An association between taurine deficiency and dilated cardiomyopathy has also been shown in Newfoundlands, Labrador retrievers, Dalmatians, English bulldogs, Portuguese water dogs and Irish wolfhounds. Even in canine dilated cardiomyopathy dogs with normal plasma and whole blood taurine levels, additional taurine may be warranted. Therefore foods for management of cardiovascular disease in dogs should contain added taurine. The level of taurine in foods for canine patients can be lower than for cats due to the fact that dogs can synthesize taurine. The recommendation for taurine in foods for canine cardiovascular disease patients is at least 0.1% DM. This is somewhat lower than would be supplied by the typical recommendation for taurine supplementation of foods for dogs with dilated cardiomyopathy (500–1000 mg taurine/day). Studies support the fact that in dogs and cats, taurine is considered safe.

L-Carnitine

Deficiency of L-carnitine in dogs has been linked to dilated cardiomyopathy in dogs. Cardiac muscle function benefits from carnitine because carnitine is a critical component of the mitochondrial membrane enzymes responsible for transporting activated fatty acids in the form of acyl-carnitine esters. These are transported across the mitochondrial membranes to the matrix. From here b-oxidation and high energy phosphate generation occur. Free L-carnitine serves as a mitochondrial detoxifying agent.

Currently, the recommendation for carnitine supplementation in dogs with dilated cardiomyopathy is 50–100-mg L-carnitine/kg body weight three times daily. It is widely accepted that even if the cause of cardiomyopathy in a heart disease patient is not due to carnitine deficiency, supplementing dogs with carnitine does not appear to do any harm and may in fact be beneficial. Foods for heart disease patients should provide at least 0.02% DM of carnitine.

Phosphorus

Patients with cardiac disease are often suffering from concurrent disease conditions. It is understood that phosphorus is a nutrient of concern in patients with concurrent chronic kidney disease and that kidney disease is one of the more prevalent diseases seen concurrently with cardiac disease. Therefore nutritional management should avoid excess phosphorus in patients with concurrent chronic kidney disease. The recommended amount of phosphorous in nutritional management of cardiac disease is 0.2–0.7% DM in dogs and 0.3–0.7% DM in cats.

Potassium and Magnesium

Another concern in cardiac disease patients is the metabolism of potassium and magnesium. Hypokalemia, hyperkalemia, and hypomagnesemia, all have the potential for complications when medication therapy is introduced in patients with cardiovascular disease. Veterinary technicians should be aware that potassium or magnesium homeostasis abnormalities can:
- cause cardiac dysrhythmias;
- decrease myocardial contractility;
- produce profound muscle weakness;
- potentiate adverse effects from cardiac glycosides and other cardiac drugs.

The amounts of potassium and magnesium recommended for adult maintenance in dogs and cats (0.4 and 0.52% DM potassium, respectively, and 0.06 and 0.04% DM magnesium) should be the minimum amounts included in nutritional management of CHF. If abnormalities in these electrolytes occur, the healthcare team should consider supplementation or switching to a different food.

Protein

Cardiac cachexia is a major concern in patients with cardiac disease. The protein requirements of patients with cardiac cachexia have not been investigated extensively to date. The metabolic changes associated with cachexia and their effect on overall nutrient requirements is only recently being investigated. Many patients with cachexia present with concomitant disease (i.e., chronic kidney disease), which also significantly affects nutrient requirements. Nutritionists do know that profound anorexia enhances protein-energy malnutrition in patients with cachexia. Subsequently, patients with cachexia or exhibiting signs potentially leading to cachexia should be encouraged to eat a complete and balanced food that contains adequate calories and adequate high-quality, highly digestible protein.

Omega-3 Fatty Acids

In cardiac cachexia, TNF and IL-1cytokines have been implicated as pathogenic mediators. Fish oil (known to be high in omega-3 (n-3) fatty acids) has been shown to alter cytokine production. Early investigations involving fish oil suggest that fish-oil-mediated alterations in cytokine production may help dogs with CHF. Consequently, it is believed that heart failure patients with cachexia may benefit from the alterations of cytokine production through omega-3 fatty acid supplementation.

It is believed that omega-3 fatty acids electrically stabilize heart cells through modulation of the fast voltage-dependent Na(+) currents and the L-type Ca(2+) channels which results in the heart cells becoming resistant to dysrhythmias. Clinical studies of fish oil as a source of long-chain omega-3 fatty acids have confirmed the reduction in frequency of ventricular arrhythmia in boxer dogs.

Omega- 3 fatty acids have been shown to have a significant effect on survival times when used in dogs diagnosed with DCM or chronic valvular disease. The effect of the omega-3 fatty acids may be attributed to: anti-inflammatory effects, cachexia prevention, improved appetite, or anti-arrhythmic effects. The veterinary healthcare team should also be aware of further effects of omega-3 fatty acids on the patient. The healthcare team must be mindful of the fact that omega-3 fatty acids have the potential to alter immune function. This alteration in immune function may contribute to the cardiovascular effects of omega-3 fatty acids. Also, omega-3 fatty acids reduce platelet aggregation resulting from the production of thromboxane B5. The reduction in platelet aggregation might be of benefit in cats with cardiac disease and at risk for thrombus formation. However, this effect is also important to be mindful of when using omega-3 fatty acids in animals with coagulopathies.

Additional studies and discussion are needed in the long term, but it is believed that dogs and cats with cardiac disease may benefit from omega-3 fatty acid supplementation. However, the healthcare team must consider a number of factors: (1) dose, (2) timing, and (3) omega-3 fatty acid form.

At this point in time, no optimal dose of omega-3 fatty acids has been established for humans, cats, or dogs. The current recommendation from nutritionists studying fatty acids and cardiac disease is a dose of 40 mg/kg EPA and 25 mg/kg DHA for both dogs and cats.

Timing also needs to be taken into consideration when supplementing omega-3 fatty acids. The healthcare team should remember and educate owners that the majority of omega-3 fatty acids benefits occur after peak plasma and tissue concentrations have been achieved. Although plasma concentrations may increase significantly in the first week of omega-3 fatty acid supplementation, typically 4–6 weeks are required to reach peak plasma concentrations.

EPA and DHA can be provided through the diet or as a dietary supplement. There are a few therapeutic pet foods with high levels of EPA and DHA, but the majority of foods manufactured today do not achieve the recommended level of EPA and DHA. The current recommended dose is 40 mg/kg EPA + 25 mg/kg DHA. Therefore a manufactured food would need to contain between 80 and 150 mg/100 kcal EPA + DHA. Other factors that would need to be taken into consideration would be the size of the pet and the amount of food consumed. If the pet is not prescribed one of the high fatty acid foods, a recommendation of fish oil supplementation would be necessitated. However, caution must be given when making a supplement recommendation, as fish oil supplements vary widely in the amount of EPA and DHA they contain. The healthcare team should be familiar with various brands of fish oil supplements and plan to make a recommendation based on a specific brand with which the concentration of EPA and DHA have been researched and confirmed.

Water

With all patients, veterinary technicians must remember to talk with clients about the importance of water for pets. Veterinary technicians need to remind clients that pets should be offered water free choice and it should be clean and fresh. Healthcare teams must also keep in mind that water quality varies considerably, even within the same community. We must be cognizant of the fact that water can be a significant source of sodium, chloride, and other minerals. Veterinary healthcare teams should be familiar with the mineral levels in their local water supply. Water samples can be submitted to state or other government laboratories for analysis. Also municipal water companies can be contacted to ask about mineral levels in local water supplies. Distilled water or water with less than 150 ppm sodium is recommended for patients with advanced heart disease and failure.

References

1 Buchanan JW (1999) Prevalence of cardiovascular disorders. In PR Fox, D Sisson, NS Moise (1999) *Textbook of Canine and Feline Cardiology* (2nd edn), pp. 457–70, Philadelphia, PA: Saunders.

2 Paige CF, Abbott JA, Elvinger F, Pyle RL (2009) Prevalence of cardiomyopathy in apparently healthy cats, *Journal of American Veterinary Medical Association* **234**: 1398–1403.

3 Rush JE (2009) Chronic valvular disease in dogs. In Bongura JD, Twedt DC (eds), *Kirk's Current Therapy XIV* (14th edn), St Louis, MO: Saunders Elsevier.

4 Roudebush P, Keene BW (2010) Cardiovascular disease. In M Hand C Thatcher, R Remillard *et al.* (eds), *Small Animal Clinical Nutrition* (5th edn), Topeka, KS: Mark Morris Institute.

Further reading

Freeman LM (2010) Beneficial effects of omega-3 fatty acids in cardiovascular disease, *Journal of Small Animal Practice* **51**, September, 462–70.

Lunn J, Theobald HE (2006) The health effects of dietary unsaturated fatty acids. *British Nutrition Foundation Nutrition Bulletin* **31**: 178–224.

Gross KL, Yamka RM, Khoo C *et al.* (2010) Macronutrients. In M Hand C Thatcher, R Remillard *et al.* (eds), *Small Animal Clinical Nutrition* (5th edn), Topeka, KS: Mark Morris Institute.

Freeman LM, Rush JE, Kehayias JJ, *et al.* (1998) Nutritional alterations and the effect of fish oil supplementation in dogs with heart failure. *Journal of Veterinary Internal Medicine* **12**: 440–8.

Slupe JL, Freeman LM, Rush JE (2008) Association of body weight and body condition with survival in dogs with heart failure, *Journal of Veterinary Internal Medicine* **22**: 561–5.

42　Musculoskeletal

Osteoarthritis (OA) is the most common form of arthritis recognized in humans and in all veterinary species. Typically OA is a slowly progressive condition and it is characterized by two main pathologic processes: degeneration of articular cartilage with a loss of both proteoglycan and collagen; and proliferation of new bone. In addition, there is a variable, low-grade inflammatory response within the synovial membrane.[1] Current estimates of the prevalence of arthritis in senior and geriatric dogs range from 20 to 25%. The prevalence of OA in adult cats is 33% with the prevalence in senior cats rising to 90%.[2] The objectives of treatment for OA are multifaceted; reduce pain and discomfort, decrease clinical signs, slow the progression of the disease, promote the repair of damaged tissue and improve the quality of life. It has been suggested that best results dogs with chronic pain due to OA include a combination of anti-inflammatory and analgesic medications, disease-modifying osteoarthritis agents (DMOAs), nutraceuticals, weight reduction, exercise programs, physical therapy and therapeutic foods. Applying an individualized combination of these management options to each patient will enhance quality of life which is the ultimate goal of therapy. This discussion will focus on the nutritional management of OA and the importance of the technician's role in managing OA.

Weight Reduction

Obesity is epidemic in companion animals. Numerous studies indicate that 25–40% of adult dogs are overweight or obese. Similar to the CDC estimate that approximately 33% of all adults suffer from arthritis, an estimated 20% of the adult canine population suffers from osteoarthritis (OA). One long-term study has documented that the prevalence of osteoarthritis is greater in overweight/obese dogs compared to ideal weight dogs (83% vs 50%).[3,4] Given these statistics, it is reasonable to assume a significant portion of arthritic dogs will be overweight/obese and vice versa. Managing these concurrent conditions presents many challenges.

Before a disease can be treated it must first be diagnosed. As disease entities, osteoarthritis and overweight/obesity present diagnostic challenges for very different reasons. Clinical signs of osteoarthritis are often not obvious on examination, particularly early in the disease process. Signs of overweight/obesity may be readily apparent, but often they are overlooked or dismissed as inconsequential. Diagnosis of osteoarthritis generally requires a combination of history, physical examination findings, and radiographic evidence of degenerative joint disease. This may seem straightforward, though historical clues which are crucial to diagnosis may not be readily apparent on routine veterinary examination. Often owners attribute many signs of OA to normal aging and consequently fail to report them unless prompted by the healthcare team.

Clinical signs of advanced arthritis include difficulty rising from rest, stiffness, or lameness. A thorough, disease specific history should be taken and may reveal evidence of subtle changes early in the course of OA such as reluctance to walk, run, climb stairs, jump, or play. Signs may be as discreet as lagging behind on walks. Owners are often unaware of the correlation between behavior changes and arthritis. Yelping or whimpering and even personality changes (i.e., withdrawal, aggressive behavior) may be indicative of the chronic pain of osteoarthritis. It is recommended to use an owner questionnaire with every potential OA patient to assist with early detection of osteoarthritis.

Recognizing signs of OA in cats is much more difficult. Cats often suffer in silence and the veterinary healthcare team must rely upon the owner's evaluation and a thorough history to discover potential signs and

Nutrition and Disease Management for Veterinary Technicians and Nurses, Second Edition. Ann Wortinger, Kara M. Burns
© 2015 John Wiley & Sons, Inc. Published 2015 by John Wiley & Sons, Inc.
Companion Website: www.wiley.com/go/wortinger/nutrition

symptoms of OA in cats. Oftentimes, the changes that may be noted by owners can be categorized into four groups: mobility, activity level, grooming, and temperament. Mobility changes include reluctance to jump; not jumping as high; and changes in toileting behavior due to inability to climb into the litter box. Activity level changes manifest in decreased playing and hunting and a change in sleep patterns. Grooming changes may be noticed when the cat may be more matted or unable to groom certain areas, and the claws may be overgrown because they cannot stretch out to "scratch/sharpen" claws. Changes in temperament are demonstrated by the cat hiding from owners or other pets in the house and seeming "grumpy."[4,5] Many of these signs are again attributed to "old age" in the cat by the owner. Thus it is important for the technician to take a thorough history and ask open-ended questions that may help uncover otherwise overlooked signs of OA in cats.

Diagnosing overweight/obesity is of the utmost importance and leads to diagnostic, curative, and preventive strategies that may be lost in the absence of a diagnosis. The first step to diagnosing overweight/obesity is consistent recording of both a body weight and body condition score. The body condition score (BCS) is a subjective assessment of an animal's body fat that takes into account the animal's frame size independent of its weight. In addition to body weight, BCS should always be documented at every exam. Body weight alone does not indicate how appropriate the weight is for an individual animal. A Labrador retriever weighing 30 kg may be underweight, optimal weight, or overweight. The BCS puts body weight in perspective for each individual patient. In both human and veterinary medicine timely identification of overweight/obesity by primary care providers remains the crucial initial step in their management.

Prevention

In dogs risk factors for developing osteoarthritis include age, large or giant breeds, genetics, developmental orthopedic disease, trauma and obesity. Risk factors for overweight/obesity in dogs include age, certain breeds, being neutered, consuming a semi-moist, homemade, or canned food as their major diet source and consumption of "other" foods (meat or other food products, commercial treats, or table scraps). The radiographic prevalence

of canine hip dysplasia, a leading cause of OA in dogs, has been reported to be as high as 70% in Golden Retrievers and Rottweilers.[6] Golden Retrievers, Rottweilers and Labrador Retrievers are over-represented in the population of overweight/obese dogs.

Dogs found to be overweight at nine to 12 months of age were 1.5 times more likely to become overweight adults.[7−10] Owners of dogs at risk for obesity and OA should be educated on the importance of lifelong weight management. The incidence and severity of OA secondary to canine hip dysplasia can be significantly influenced by environmental factors such as nutrition and lifestyle.[3,11] One long-term study has documented that the prevalence and severity of osteoarthritis is greater in dogs with body condition scores above normal compared to dogs maintained at an ideal body condition throughout life. Over the lifespan of these same dogs, the mean age at which 50% of the dogs required treatment for pain attributable to osteoarthritis was significantly earlier (10.3 years, p<0.01) in the overweight dogs as compared to the dogs with normal body condition scores (13.3 years). Obesity is also a risk factor for the most common traumatic cause of OA in dogs, ruptured cruciate ligaments. Overweight/obese dogs have a 2−3 times greater prevalence of ruptured cruciate ligaments compared to normal weight dogs. Understanding the correlation between maintaining their dog at a healthy weight and decreasing the risk of disease may be a powerful motivator for many owners.

In humans, the epidemic of obesity is largely attributed to changes in the availability, quantity, and composition of food and the decrease in the amount of physical activity needed for daily living. Physical activity levels of dogs often mirror their human companions. Owners should be encouraged to respond with play activities or praise rather than food rewards.

Nutritional Solutions

Weight Management

Historically, the stress of excess weight on the skeletal system has been thought to be the primary offender of the pathophysiology and progression of osteoarthritis. Yet, adipose tissue is no longer considered simply a storage site for energy; rather it is now recognized as a multifunctional organ. Adipose tissue plays an active role in a variety of homeostatic and pathologic processes.

Recent studies have documented that adipocytes secrete several hormones including leptin and adiponectin and produce a diverse range of proteins termed adipokines. Among the currently recognized adipokines is a growing list of mediators of inflammation: tumor necrosis factor-α, interleukin-6, interleukin-8 and interleukin-10.[12] These adipokines are found in human and canine adipocytes. Production of these proteins is increased in obesity, suggesting that obesity is a state of chronic low-grade inflammation. Low-grade inflammation may contribute to the pathophysiology of a number of diseases commonly associated with obesity including osteoarthritis. This might explain why relatively small reductions in body weight can result in significant improvement in clinical signs.

Nutrigenomics and Osteoarthritis

Nutritional supplementation of omega-3 fatty acids is a relatively new concept in the management of dogs with osteoarthritis. Recent studies provide high-quality data that show a food with high levels of total omega-3 fatty acids and eicosapentaenoic acid (EPA), can improve the clinical signs of canine osteoarthritis. The use of a therapeutic food (Hill's® Prescription Diet® j/d® Canine Mobility support) for the management of OA has been supported by four randomized, double-blinded, controlled clinical trials using client-owned dogs.[13–16] One 6-month study and two 3-month studies were conducted in US veterinary hospitals. Another 3-month prospective study was conducted in two veterinary teaching hospitals. In all, more than 500 dogs with OA were studied. Participating dogs were diagnosed with OA based on history, clinical signs, and radiographic evidence. Dogs were fed either a typical commercial dog food or a test mobility food, which has higher concentrations of total omega-3 fatty acids and EPA and lower omega-6: omega-3 fatty acid ratios. At baseline and throughout the studies, subjective and objective veterinary evaluations were performed. Owners were also asked to subjectively evaluate their dogs throughout the studies.

These studies provide high-quality evidence that illustrates the benefits of incorporating a food with high levels of omega-3 fatty acids, into the management of the pain of osteoarthritis in dogs. In normal canine cartilage, there is a balance between synthesis and degradation of cartilage matrix. In arthritic joints damage to chondrocytes incites a viscous circle which culminates

in the destruction of cartilage, inflammation and pain. The mechanisms responsible for the demonstrated clinical benefits of omega-3 fatty acids include controlling inflammation and reducing the expression and activity of cartilage degrading enzymes.

Cartilage degradation begins with loss of cartilage aggrecan and is followed by loss of cartilage collagens. This results in the loss of ability to resist compressive forces during movement of the joint. Eicosapentaenoic acid (EPA) is the only omega-3 fatty acid able to considerably decrease the loss of aggrecan in canine cartilagel. EPA inhibits the up regulation of aggrecanases by blocking the signal at the level of messenger RNA.[17,18]

Inflammation is a vital reaction and it also plays a fundamental role in the pathophysiology of osteoarthritis. The polyunsaturated fatty acids are critical components in the initiation and mediation of inflammation. Arachidonic acid (AA, 20:4n-6) and eicosapentaenoic acid (EPA, 20:5n-3) act as precursors for the synthesis of eicosanoids, a significant group of immunoregulatory molecules that function as local hormones and mediators of inflammation. The amounts and types of eicosanoids synthesized are determined by the availability of the fatty acid precursor and by the activities of the enzyme systems that synthesize them. In most conditions, the principal precursor for these compounds is AA, although EPA competes with AA for the same enzyme systems. The eicosanoids produced from AA are pro-inflammatory and when produced in excess amounts may result in pathologic conditions. In contrast, eicosanoids derived from EPA promote minimal to no inflammatory activity.[19]

Ingestion of foods containing omega-3 fatty acids results in a decrease in membrane AA levels because omega-3 fatty acids replace AA in the substrate pool. This produces an accompanying decrease in the capacity to synthesize eicosanoids from AA. Studies have documented that inflammatory eicosanoids produced from AA are depressed when dogs consume foods with high levels of omega-3 fatty acids. In addition to their role in modulating the production of inflammatory eicosanoids, omega-3 fatty acids have a direct role in the resolution of inflammation. Resolution of inflammation is a progressive, active process involving a switch in the production of lipid-derived mediators over time. Pro-inflammatory products of omega- 6 fatty acids metabolim (PGE2, PGE12, LTB4) are thought to initiate this sequence. Arachidonic acid-derived mediators foster the extravasation of inflammatory cells. With time and in the presence of sufficient levels of omega-3 fatty acids, a class shift occurs towards production of pro-resolving omega-3 derived mediators (resolvins, protectins). These mediators serve as endogenous stop signals by preventing inflammatory cell recruitment, stopping "cell entry" and promoting resolution by removing inflammatory cells from the site. The identification of these two new families of omega-3 derived chemical mediators (resolvins and protectins) may clarify the mechanisms that underlie the many reported benefits of dietary omega-3 PUFAs. Absence of sufficient dietary levels of omega-3 fatty acids may contribute to "resolution failure" and perpetuation of chronic inflammation.

In cats with OA two therapeutic foods are available for management of OA in the US. Hill's® Prescription Diet® Feline j/d™ is available in the US as well as Europe. The active ingredients include high levels of n-3 polyunsaturated fatty acids (DHA), natural sources of glucosamine and chondroitin, methionine and manganese. Just as in dogs, high levels of n-3 PUFAs control inflammation in cats. However, in cats DHA rather than EPA inhibits the aggrecanase enzymes responsible for cartilage degradation.[4,20] Natural sources of glucosamine and chondroitin increase proteoglycan production by chondrocytes and inhibit inflammatory mediators. Methionine and manganese enhance chondrocyte viability, provide building blocks and act as a sulfur donor for the production of proteoglycans. Royal Canin Veterinary Diet® Mobility Support JS® Feline is available in the US and Canada. The chief ingredient is green lipped muscle, which contains anti-inflammatory constituents aimed at improving joint health; other active ingredients are DHA, EPA, glycosaminoglycans, such as chondroitin sulfate, which are components of cartilage; an amino acid glutamine, which is a precursor of glycosaminoglycans as well as minerals important to maintaining healthy cartilage (i.e., zinc, copper and manganese). The efficacy of therapeutic nutrition (Prescription Diet® Feline j/d®) is supported by three studies.[4,21–23] The efficacy of therapeutic nutrition (Royal Canin Veterinary Diet® Mobility Support JS® Feline) is supported by one published study.[24]

As studies suggest therapeutic nutrition provides an effective and safe way to manage both dogs and cats with osteoarthritis. Foods with high levels of n-3 fatty acids have the dual value of controlling inflammation and pain while slowing progression of the disease by reducing cartilage degradation. Efficacy of therapeutic nutrition for osteoarthritis is supported by multiple clinical trials in arthritic pets.

Developmental Orthopedic Disease

The goal of a feeding plan for pediatric pets is to create a healthy adult. The specific objectives of a good feeding plan are to achieve healthy growth, optimize trainability and immune function and minimize obesity and developmental orthopedic disease. Growth is a complex process involving interactions between genetics, nutrition, and other environmental influences. Nutrition plays a role in the health and development of growing pets and directly affects the immune system body composition, growth rate, and skeletal development.

Developmental orthopedic diseases (DOD) are a diverse group of musculoskeletal disorders that occur in growing puppies and may be related to nutrition. Canine hip dysplasia (CHD) and osteochondrosis are the most common musculoskeletal problems with a nutrition related etiology. Specific nutritional factors that are thought to increase the risk of DOD in young dogs include: (1) free choice feeding (excess energy consumption), (2) feeding high energy foods (rapid growth) and (3) excessive intake of calcium from food, treats and or supplements (dietary imbalance).[25–27] OA secondary to DOD can be minimized by educating young dog owners to offer appropriate nutrition during the critical growth phase. All puppies whose adult weight is estimated to be ≥50 lbs should be fed a growth food specifically formulated for large breed dogs. As discussed earlier, maintaining an ideal body condition score throughout life will decrease trauma to joints and the development of OA.

Patient Assessment

Pediatric patients should be assessed for risk factors before weaning to allow implementation of recommendations for appropriate nutrition. A thorough history and physical evaluation are necessary. Special attention should be paid to large- and giant breed puppies, breeds, and gender (including intact and neutered) at risk for obesity. In addition, growth rates and body condition scores (BCS) provide valuable information about nutritional risks. Growth rates of young dogs are affected by the nutrient density of the food and the amount of food fed. It is important that puppies be fed to grow at an optimal rate for bone development and body condition rather than at a maximal rate. Growing animals reach a similar adult weight and size whether growth rate is rapid or slow. Feeding for maximum growth puts puppies at increased risk for skeletal deformities and has been found to decrease longevity in other species.[25] In Labrador retrievers, even moderate overfeeding resulted in overweight adults and decreased longevity. The most practical indicator of whether or not a puppy's and kitten's growth rate is healthy is its BCS. Healthcare team members should be comfortable body condition scoring all patients; and with growing patients should reassess at least every two weeks to allow for adjustments in amounts fed and, thus, growth rates. Owners can and should be taught to assess body condition and are likely to become more aware of the appearance of a healthy growing puppy and kitten. Regularly assessing body condition provides immediate feedback about optimal nutrition.

Key Nutritional Factors

The requirements for all nutrients are increased during growth compared with requirements for adult dogs. Most nutrients supplied in excess of that needed for growth cause little to no harm. However, excess energy and calcium are of special concern; these concerns include energy for puppies of small and medium breeds (for obesity prevention) and energy and calcium for puppies of large and giant breeds (for skeletal health). Also, essential fatty acids can affect neural development and trainability of puppies.

Energy
Energy requirements for growing puppies consist of energy needed for maintenance and growth. During the first weeks after weaning body weight is relatively small and the growth rate is high; puppies use about 50% of their total energy intake for maintenance and 50% for growth. Gradually, the growth curves reach a plateau, as puppies become young adults. The proportion of energy needed for maintenance increases progressively, whereas the part for growth decreases. Energy needed for growth decreases to about 8 to 10% of the total energy requirement when puppies reach 80% or more

of adult body weight. A puppy's daily energy requirement (DER) should be about $3 \times$ its resting energy requirement (RER) until it reaches about 50% of its adult body weight.[26] Thereafter, energy intake should be about $2.5 \times$ RER and can be reduced progressively to $2 \times$ RER. When approximately 80% of adult size is reached, 1.8 to $2 \times$ RER is usually sufficient.

$$RER\ (kcal/day) = 70 \times BW(kg)^{0.75}$$

$$RER\ (kcal/day) = (BW_{kg} \times BW_{kg} \times BW_{kg},\ \sqrt{},\ \sqrt{}) \times 70$$

These factors are general recommendations or starting points to estimate energy needs. Body condition scoring should be used to adjust these energy estimates to individual puppies.

Prevention of obesity is essential and should start at weaning. After puppies and kittens become overweight, it is challenging to return to, and maintain, normal weight. Too much food intake during growth may contribute to skeletal disorders in large- and giant-breed puppies. If the pet is overweight and/or obese and this is carried into adulthood, the risk for several important diseases is increased. These include hypertension, heart disease, diabetes mellitus, dyslipidemias, osteoarthritis, heat and exercise intolerance and decreased immune function. Studies show that moderate energy and food restriction during the postweaning growth period reduces the prevalence of hip dysplasia in large-breed (Labrador retriever) puppies and increases longevity in rats without hindering adult size.[25,26] However, the pet may not receive enough energy and nutrients to support optimal growth if fed a food with a very low energy density and low digestibility. This may lead to consumption of large quantities of the food, which can overload the gastrointestinal (GI) tract resulting in vomiting and diarrhea. Healthcare team members should initiate monitoring of energy and food intake and body condition at an early age to help keep the pet at a healthy weight throughout life.

Protein
Protein requirements of growing dogs differ from the requirements of adult dogs. During puppyhood, protein requirements are highest at weaning and decrease progressively until adulthood. Puppies 14 weeks and older, should receive at least the minimum recommended allowance for crude protein which is 17.5% DM. The recommended protein range in foods intended for

growth in all puppies (small, medium and large breed) is 22–32% DM. Most dry commercial foods marketed for puppy growth provide protein levels within this range.[26]

Protein levels above the upper end of this range have not been shown to be detrimental but are well above the level in bitch's milk. Protein requirements of growing dogs differ from those of adults. An important difference is that arginine is an essential amino acid for puppies, whereas it is only conditionally essential for adult dogs. Foods formulated for adult dogs *should not* be fed to puppies.[25] Although protein levels may be adequate, energy levels and other nutrients may not be balanced for growth.

Fat

Dietary fat serves three primary functions:
1 a source of essential fatty acids;
2 a carrier for fat-soluble vitamins;
3 a concentrated source of energy.

Growing dogs have an estimated daily requirement for essential fatty acids (linoleic acid) of about 250 mg/kg body weight, which can be provided by a food containing between 5% and 10% DM fat. Studies indicate that docosahexaenoic acid (DHA) is essential for normal neural, retinal and auditory development in puppies. Inclusion of fish oil as a source of DHA in puppy foods improves trainability and should be considered essential for growth. The minimum recommended allowance for DHA plus eicosapentaenoic acid (EPA) is 0.05% DM; EPA should not exceed 60% of the total. Thus, DHA needs to be at least 40% of the total DHA plus EPA, or 0.02% DM.[26]

When feeding young pets we must remember that fat contributes greatly to the energy density of a food and excessive energy intake can cause overweight/obesity and developmental orthopedic disease. The minimum recommended allowance of dietary fat for growth (8.5% DM) is much less than that needed for nursing, but more than is needed for adult maintenance (5.5% DM). In order to deliver a DM energy density between 3.5 to 4.5 kcal/g; 10 to 25% DM fat is necessary. This range of dietary fat is recommended from postweaning to adulthood.[26]

Calcium and Phosphorus

Although growing dogs need more calcium and phosphorus than adult dogs, the healthcare team must remember and educate owners that the minimum requirements are relatively low. Puppies have been successfully raised when fed foods containing 0.37–0.6% DM calcium and 0.33% DM phosphorus.[26]

Foods for large- and giant-breed puppies should contain 0.7–1.2% DM calcium (0.6–1.1% phosphorus). Foods with a calcium content of 1.1% DM provide more calcium to puppies just after weaning than if bitch's milk is fed exclusively. Small- to medium-sized breeds are less sensitive to slightly overfeeding or underfeeding calcium; thus the level of calcium in foods for these puppies can range from 0.7% to 1.7% DM (0.6–1.3% phosphorus) without risk. The phosphorus intake is less critical than the calcium intake, provided the minimum requirements of 0.35% DM are met and the calcium–phosphorus ratio is between 1:1 and 1.8:1. For large- and giant-breed dogs, the calcium/phosphorus ratio should be between 1:1 and 1.5:1.[26]

Digestibility

Puppies that are fed foods low in energy density and digestibility will need to eat larger amounts of food to achieve growth. This will increase the risk of flatulence, vomiting, diarrhea, and the development of a "pot-bellied" appearance. As a result, foods recommended for puppies should be more digestible than typical adult foods. An indirect indicator of digestibility is energy density. Foods with a higher energy density are likely to be more digestible.[25,26]

Carbohydrates

While no specific level of digestible (soluble) carbohydrates exists for growing puppies, it is recommended that the level of digestible (soluble) carbohydrates around 20% (DM) may optimize health.

Successful treatment and prevention of musculoskeletal disease conditions require a comprehensive approach which includes preventive measures and a multimodal management program. Clinical signs of musculoskeletal diseases are often not obvious on examination, especially early in the disease process. Although signs of overweight/obesity are readily apparent they are often overlooked or dismissed as inconsequential. Documenting a diagnosis of overweight/obesity is critical to the management of these disease conditions. Diagnosing overweight/obesity requires consistent recording of both a body weight and body condition score. Early diagnosis of OA and DOD enables early intervention which in turn often improves the long-term outcome for the patient. Consistent use of a thorough, disease specific history may raise awareness of subtle changes early in the course of OA and DOD. Successful management of OA/DOD and obesity requires nutritional intervention.

References

1 Anandacoomarasamy A, Caterson I, Sambrook P *et al.* (2008) The impact of obesity on the musculoskeletal system, *Int J Obes (Lond)* **32**: 211–22.

2 Lascelles BD, Robertson SA (2010) *J Feline Med Surg* **12**: 200–12.

3 Kealy RD, Lawler DF, Ballam JM *et al.* (2000) Evaluation of the effect of limited food consumption on radiographic evidence of osteoarthritis in dogs, *JAVMA* **217**: 1678–80.

4 Burns, KM (2011) Are your patients suffering in silence? Managing osteoarthritis in pets. *NAVTA Journal*, Convention Issue, 16–22.

5 Bennett D, Morton C (2009) A study of owner observed behavioural and lifestyle changes in cats with musculoskeletal disease before and after analgesic therapy. *J Feline Med Surg* **11(12)**: 997–1004.

6 Paster ER, LaFond E, Biery DN, *et al.* (2005) Estimates of prevalence of hip dysplasia in Golden Retrievers and Rottweilers and the influence of bias on published prevalence figures, *JAVMA* **226(3)**: 387–92.

7 Eby J, Colditz G (2008) Obesity/overweight: prevention and weight management. In S Quah, K Heggenhougen (eds), *International Encyclopedia of Public Health*, pp. 602–9, St Louis: Elsevier.

8 Kienzle E, Bergler R, Mandernach A (1998) A comparison of the feeding behavior and the human-animal relationship in owners of normal and obese dogs, *J Nutr* **128**: 2779S–2782S.

9 Anandacoomarasamy A, Fransen M, March L (2009) Obesity and the musculoskeletal system, *Curr Opin Rheumatol* **21**: 71–7.

10 Christensen R, Bartels EM, Astrup A, Bliddal H (2007) Effect of weight reduction in obese patients diagnosed with knee osteoarthritis: a systematic review and meta-analysis, *Ann Rheum Dis* **66**: 433–9.

11 Impellizeri JA, Tetrick MA, Muir P (2000) Effect of weight reduction on clinical signs of lameness in dogs with hip osteoarthritis. *JAVMA* **216**: 1089–91.

12 Towell TL, Burns KM (2011) Multimodal management of osteoarthritis. *NAVC Proceedings*.

13 Roush JK Dodd CE, Fritsch DA, *et al.* (2010) Multicenter practice assessment of the effects of omega-3 fatty acids on osteoarthritis in dogs, *JAVMA* **236 (1)**: 59–66.

14 Fritsch D, Allen TA, Dodd CE *et al.* (2010) Dose-titration effects of fish oil in osteoarthritic dogs, *J Vet Intern Med* **24**: 1020–6.

15 Roush JK Cross AR, Renberg WC, *et al.* (2010) Evaluation of the effects of dietary supplementation with fish oil Omega-3 Fatty Acids on weight bearing in dogs with osteoarthritis, 3-month feeding study, *JAVMA* **236(1)**: 67–73.

16 Fritsch DA, Allen TA, Dodd CE *et al.* (2010) A multi-center study of the effect of dietary supplemetation with fish oil omega-3 fatty acids on carprofen dosage in dogs with osteoarthritis, *JAVMA* **236**: 535–9.

17 Caterson B, Flannery CR, Hughes CE *et al.* (2000) Mechanisms involved in cartilage proteoglycan catabolism. *Matrix Biology* **19**: 333–44.

18 Caterson G (2004) Omega-3 fatty acids-incorporation in canine chondrocyte membranes. Unpublished data. Cardiff University, Wales.

19 Wander RC Hall JA, Gradin JL, *et al.* (1997) The ratio of dietary (n-6) to (n-3) fatty acids influences immune system function, eicosanoid metabolism, lipid peroxidation and vitamin E status in aged dogs, *J Nutr* **127**: 1198–1205.

20 Innes J, Gabriel N, Vaughan-Thomas A, *et al.* (2008) *Proceedings Hill's Global Mobility Symposium*, 22–6.

21 Sparkes A, Debraekeleer J, Hahn KA (2010) An open-label, prospective study evaluating the response to feeding a veterinary therapeutic diet in cats with degenerative joint disease. *J Vet Intern Med* **24**: 771.

22 Fritsch D, Allen TA, Sparkes A *et al.* (2010) Improvement of clinical signs of osteoarthritis in cats by dietary intervention. *J Vet Intern Med* **24**: 771–2.

23 Frantz NZ, Hahn K, MacLeay J *et al.* (2010) Effect of a test food on whole blood gene expression in cats with appendicular degenerative joint disease. *J Vet Intern Med* **24**: 771.

24 Lascelles BDX, DePuy V, Thomson A *et al.* (2010) Evaluation of a therapeutic diet for feline degenerative joint disease. *J Vet Intern Med* **24**: 487–95.

25 Burns KM (2014) Pediatric nutrition: Optimal care for life! *NAVC Proceedings*.

26 Richardson DC, Zentek J, Hazewinkel HAW *et al.* (2010) Developmental orthopedic disease in dogs. In M Hand, CD Thatcher, R Remillard R (eds), *Small Animal Clinical Nutrition* (5th edn), pp. 667–93, Topeka, KS: Mark Morris Institute.

27 Wortinger A (2007) *Nutrition for Veterinary Technicians and Nurses*, pp. 159–67, Ames, IO: Blackwell.

SECTION 5
Feeding Management of Other Species

43 Avian

One area of veterinary medicine that affects every pet that comes into the hospital including companion birds is nutrition. Every bird that presents to the hospital should have a nutritional assessment every time they present. Many of the problems for which birds present to veterinary hospitals are nutrition related. Psittacine and passerine species have unique nutritional requirements and if owners are not familiar with the proper care and feeding of the particular species owned, the bird is at risk for disease or malnutrition.[1,2] Each avian species has differing nutritional demands and it is important to review the needs of the particular breed of bird with the owner.

Nutritional deficiencies and excesses may result in immune dysfunction, increased susceptibility to infectious diseases, and metabolic and biochemical derangements. Clinically veterinary teams may see the following result: nutritional secondary hyperparathyroidism, thyroid hyperplasia (dysplasia), hemochromatosis, and the potential for many other issues. Healthcare teams must familiarize themselves with the reasons for the development of nutritionally induced illnesses occurring in companion psittacine and passerine birds. Until recently, specific nutritional requirements for these birds were unidentified. Consequently veterinary team members would compare the well-known nutrient needs of poultry to other avian species. Today the profession is aware of nutritional differences between poultry and other avian species and has commercially prepared foods specific to the individual physiologic and nutrient needs of the companion bird species. Another reason for nutrition induced problems is the perception that allseed diets, especially those comprised on only one seed type (e.g., millet or sunflower) as well as diets made up of fruits, vegetables, and other human foods, are complete and provide all the nutrients birds need. This is a misperception, as the majority of seeds available commercially are deficient in specific nutrients (e.g., specific amino acids, vitamins, and trace minerals, and macrominerals such as calcium and sodium). Therefore, owners must be educated that seeds are not and should not be the main diet for most species of companion birds.

Additionally, it is suggested that the most common cause of dietary-induced diseases in companion birds occurs when fruits and vegetables are added to commercially prepared foods or supplemented seed mixtures. The most readily available fruits and vegetables are comprised mainly of water, carbohydrates, and fiber and are deficient in protein, vitamins, and minerals – especially when compared to the nutrient recommendations for psittacine and passerine birds.[3] As a result, fruits and vegetables mainly dilute vital nutrients present in nutritionally balanced commercially prepared foods. Because of the high moisture content most birds prefer fruits and vegetables as opposed to dry extruded or pelleted foods and seed mixtures. Birds will often select food items based on water content, texture, color or taste, instead of nutrient content.[3] This selection process can lead to imbalanced nutrient intake and is another reason companion birds develop nutritional deficiencies. Again this leads to another myth – that birds are able to balance their diets. The end result oftentimes is that a bird may become habituated to or fixated on a particular food item (e.g., sunflower, safflower, millet seeds, grapes, oranges, etc.) and refuse to eat other food items which provide a complete and balanced array of nutrients.

As with other species presenting to the veterinary hospital one of the most important steps is to obtain a detailed history from the owner (Table 43.1). We have discussed the fact that nutrition and husbandry-related problems are very common findings and can lead to various medical conditions. The patient history should include a list of foods offered daily. In addition, clients should be encouraged to provide a sample of

Nutrition and Disease Management for Veterinary Technicians and Nurses, Second Edition. Ann Wortinger, Kara M. Burns
© 2015 John Wiley & Sons, Inc. Published 2015 by John Wiley & Sons, Inc.
Companion Website: www.wiley.com/go/wortinger/nutrition

Table 43.1 Avian history questionnaire

- Signalment – gender, age, species
- Chief complaint – reason for bringing bird to hospital
- From where did you acquire the bird? Breeder? Prior owners?
- Living environment –
  - Type of cage
  - What is cage lined with; newspapers, shavings, etc.?
  - Perches – number and type
  - Toys in cage – what kind and what are they made from? How are they attached to cage?
  - Where in house is bird kept?
  - Any cleaners or other household supplies used near the bird cage?
  - Is the bird allowed out of cage? Flight? Supervised? Interactive playthings?
  - How often is bird handled?
- Diet
  - What is bird being fed?
  - How often is bird fed?
  - How is the birds' appetite?
  - How much is fed?
  - What types of bowls are used?
  - Where is the water bowl?
  - What is the source of the birds' water?
  - How often is water changed?
  - Any supplements added to food or water?
  - Is food commercially prepared or homemade?
  - How is food stored?
- Cage mates
  - Are there other birds in the cage? If so, what species?
  - Are there other birds in the house? If so, what species?
- Behavior
  - Overall attitude?
  - Does the bird vocalize?
  - Any changes to vocalizations?
  - Past behavior related problems?
- Medical History
  - Any illness prior?
  - Has bird ever been prescribed medications? What was the reason? What was the medication?
  - Any illness in other birds in house, or other pets in house?
  - Has this bird been to a veterinary hospital prior?

any commercially prepared foods they feed. A good idea is to ask the owners to take a picture of the birds' home environment, including all items that are offered to their bird to eat and/or drink. If the typical food fed is a commercially prepared food, observe the label for nutrient information or guarantees. The key nutrients of concern are protein and calcium. Many foods commonly fed to companion birds are composed primarily of carbohydrates and fat. When reviewing the label of an acceptable commercially prepared food the guaranteed amount of protein should be at least 12%. Additionally, the healthcare team should be able to determine the source of calcium included in the food by the ingredients listed on the label. It is important to note that seeds ordinarily contain more phosphorus than calcium (Table 43.1).

If the food label does not contain nutrient information or is just a list of ingredients such as seeds or dried fruit, it is recommended to not use this particular food long term. It is essential for all birds that their foods be appropriately balanced with carbohydrates, proteins, fats, vitamins, minerals and water. Good nutrition is important for companion birds to insure:

- the health of the bird;
- proper growth and maturation;
- defense against disease;
- reproductive health.

Three methods of providing nutrients and achieving these objectives are: (1) commercially prepared foods, (2) seeds and seed mixtures, and (3) homemade mixed foods.

The benefits of using commercially prepared, nutritionally complete foods are similar in birds as in other companion animals. Ninety percent or more of the nutrients for companion dogs and cats in North America can be supplied through commercially prepared foods and has been determined to contribute markedly to the health of these animals. The same is true of companion birds. Nutrient balance and owner convenience are benefits which commercially prepared foods offer. Most manufacturers follow established nutrient recommendations[3] (Table 43.2) to formulate foods for companion birds. Extruded or pelleted diets are recommended as they tend to supply all the nutrients in a pellet. Pelleted diets help prevent the variation of nutrients. Well-meaning owners may feed imbalanced seeds or human foods. Also some birds may consume various quantities of imbalanced foods fed separately.

Healthcare team members should encourage owners to bring the bird food package in with their bird and compare the nutrient levels of the food to those recommended in Table 43.2. By reviewing the package of the

Table 43.2 Nutrition recommendations for avian foods[3]

Nutrient	Psittacine Minimum	Maximum	Minimum	Passerine Maximum
Gross energy (kcal/kg)**	3200	4200	3500	4500
Total protein (%)	12.0	–	14.0	–
Linoleic acid (%)	1.0	–	1.0	–
Amino acids				
Lysine (%)	0.65	–	0.75	–
Methionine (%)	0.30	–	0.35	–
Methionine + cystine (%)	0.50	–	0.58	–
Arginine (%)	0.65	–	0.75	–
Threonine (%)	0.40	–	0.46	–
Vitamins (fat soluble)				
Vitamin A activity (total) IU/kg	8000	–	8000	–
Vitamin D3 (IU/kg)	500	2000	1000	2500
Vitamin E (ppm)	50	–	50	–
Vitamin K (ppm)	1.0	–	1.0	–
Vitamins (water soluble)				
Thiamin (ppm)	4.0	–	4.0	–
Riboflavin (ppm)	6.0	–	6.0	–
Niacin (ppm)	50.0	–	50.0	–
Pyridoxine (ppm)	6.0	–	6.0	–
Pantothenic acid (ppm)	20.0	–	20.0	–
Biotin (ppm)	0.25	–	0.25	–
Folic acid (ppm)	1.50	–	1.50	–
Vitamin B12 (ppm)	0.01	–	0.01	–
Choline (ppm)	1500	–	1500	–
Minerals				
Calcium (%)	0.30	1.20	0.50	1.20
Phosphorus (%)	0.30	–	0.50	–
Calcium–phosphorus ratio	1.0–1.0	2.0–1.0	1.0–1.0	2.0–1.0
Potassium (%)	0.40	–	0.40	–
Sodium (%)	0.12	–	0.12	–
Chloride (%)	0.12	–	0.12	–
Magnesium (ppm)	600	–	600	–
Trace minerals				
Manganese (ppm) 6	5.0	–	65.0	–
Iron (ppm)	80.0	–	80.0	–
Zinc (ppm)	50.0	–	50.0	–
Selenium (ppm)	0.10	–	0.10	–

Source: Kollias GV, Kollias HW (2010) Feeding passerine and psittacine birds. In MS Hand, CD Thatcher, RL Remillard et al. (eds), Small Animal Clinical Nutrition (5th edn), pp. 1255–69, Marceline, MO: Walsworth Publishing, Mark Morris Institute.

bird food, this will help to decide if there are any incongruities in the nutrient profile.

As mentioned earlier, it is suggested that a formulated diet be provided to best achieve the balance of nutrients required for companion birds. These formulated foods come in a variety of forms with the most popular being:[4]

1 pellets;

2 extruded diets with a pellet appearance;

3 whole grains and/or seeds with added pelleted material.

A seed-based food with a vitamin/mineral mix coating on the outside of the seed is another option. However, typically the seed is not hulled. When the bird dehulls the coated seed, necessary vitamins and minerals are removed thus creating a nutritional imbalance putting the bird's health at risk.

Two processes are used when pelleted diets are manufactured – bound and extruded. Bound pellet manufacturing involves the grinding of grains such as corn, soybean, and oat groats (oat berries). Following the grinding process vitamins, minerals, and other components are added to produce a balanced food (per the manufacturer's recommendation). The grinding process produces a consistent pellet which makes it difficult for birds to pick out their favorite part of the diet. With bound pellets in general, the food material is not cooked and the diet will have a longer fiber chain length. Bound pelleted diets may not be as palatable as the extruded diet.[4,5]

Extruded pellets utilize finely ground grains which are mixed with vitamins, minerals, etc. until a balanced formulation is reached. This pellet mixture is then forced through an extruder, under pressure and high temperatures. The mixture will take on the shape of the "die" in the extrusion process. This allows for extruded pellets to be made into different shapes and colors.[5]

Extruded pelleted diets come in a variety of sizes and should be selected based on the species and size of bird. Owners must be instructed to monitor their bird to prevent picking out certain colored pellets and ignoring others. Owners should not choose colors or shapes because their bird "likes these" as this can be expensive and wasteful. Companion birds are healthier when they are psychologically stimulated and this can occur by presenting multi colored pellets in an assortment of shapes (Figure 43.1).

Historically, providing diets for birds has included seed-based diets. Although pelleted diets have allowed bird owners to provide a better balanced diet without vitamin and mineral supplementation, not every bird will eat them.[6] Also as discussed earlier, each species has different nutritional requirements. For example, certain passerine species (e.g., canary and finch) require seed in their base diet. However, for the psittacine species (e.g., budgerigar, cockatiel, lovebird, etc.) seed is not the recommended diet and a balanced pelleted food is advised as the appropriate base diet. Overall, many seed diets are high in fat and lower in other essential nutrients and therefore should be considered a treat. As with any species, treats should be offered in small quantities or the bird will be at risk for malnutrition – most likely obesity.

Transition from a seed diet to a pellet is believed to be difficult. However, this is not the case even in older birds. Healthcare team members must educate owners on what to look for when transitioning a bird from seed to pellets. Owners should insure that their pet is ingesting the food not simply crushing the pellet in the hopes of finding a kernel inside. Two signs that indicate that the bird is actually eating the pellets are seen in the production of fecal material and a color change of the fecal material associated with the pellet color being ingested.[5]

To aid owners in transitioning their birds from seed to pellet, formed seed products have been manufactured (i.e., Nutriberries® Lafeber Co., Cornell, IL) (Figure 43.2). These products are comprised of whole grains and seeds which are mixed with additional components and are affixed together. This is similar to

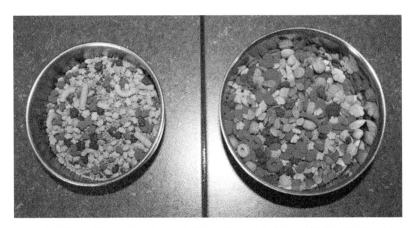

Figure 43.1 Smaller pellets: Left (cockatiels) and the larger; right (small parrots). (Copyright Kara M. Burns.)

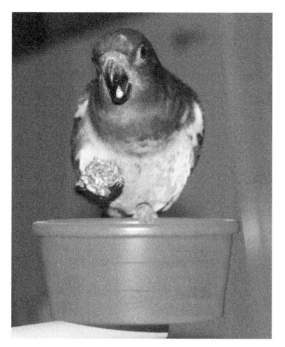

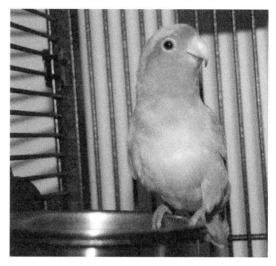

Figure 43.3   Lovebird with water bowl. (Copyright Kara M. Burns.)

Figure 43.2 Meyer's parrot with Seed Ball/Nutriberries® Lafeber Co., Cornell, IL. (Copyright Kara M. Burns.)

pellets but this product is not ground. The bird must pick off the seed to eat.

Owners can also learn to transition their birds from seed to pellets through the slow introduction of increased pellets in the seed mixture over a period of time. The transition is recommended to take 7–14 days with the final diet consisting of 100% pellets.

Avian Key Nutritional Factors

Water

Water is the most critical nutrient, and all birds should have access to fresh, clean water at all times (Figure 43.3). Water should be changed on a daily basis and the healthcare team is responsible for reviewing this important piece of husbandry with owners. Water is important for birds as it acts as a food carrier and aids in digestion. As we have seen in other species of companion animals, some foods are higher in water than others. Some avian species are more physiologically proficient at extracting water from their foods. Birds should never go for more than a few hours without

access to fresh clean water. More than 50% of a bird's body weight is made up of water and in young birds; the percentage may be even higher. Water intake plays an important role in avian thermoregulation. It is important to note that reproducing females may require more water for egg production and for heat regulation while incubating eggs. Water should be provided in bowls or dishes that the bird can reach easily. They should not be located in a place that collects feces, feathers, food, etc. Healthcare team members should educate owners to attach water bowls to the wall of enclosures, near or above food bowls. Water bowls should not be placed directly under the favorite perching area to cut down on excrement in the water. Separate bowls should be provided specifically for bathing.

Birds typically accept municipal tap water, but it is recommended that well water be boiled before allowing the bird to drink freely. If owners are hesitant to boil water, the healthcare team should recommend providing bottled water to their birds. This recommendation is made due to the fact that well water can be contaminated easily by bacteria colonies in the pipes leading to the faucet.[7]

Protein and Amino Acids

Protein requirements differ among species. The minimum recommended protein allowance for maintenance in psittacine companion birds is 12% and in the passerine species it is 14%.[3,8]

As with all foods, the quality of the protein is dependent up on bioavailability and essential amino acid content. Bird food formulations must avoid excess and deficiency of proteins and amino acids. For the majority of companion birds the following amino acids are considered essential: arginine, isoleucine, lysine, methionine, phenylalanine, valine, tryptophan, and threonine. Budgies also require glycine.[8] Too much protein in the diet of birds has been associated with renal disease, behavioral changes (biting, feather picking, nervousness, rejection of food), and regurgitation. Poor weight gain, poor feathering, stress lines on feathers, plumage color changes, and poor reproductive performance are clinical signs associated with protein and amino acid deficiencies.[8]

Fats and Essential Fatty Acids

Fats are a more concentrated source of energy in a diet. Essential fatty acids (linoleic and arachidonic) are required in birds for the following: the formation of membranes and cell organelles, hormone precursors, and the basis for psittacofulvins (i.e. feather pigments found in psittacine species). The typical recommended linoleic allowance for psittacine and passerine companion bird diets is approximately 1%.[3] It is important for healthcare team members to note that in birds, lipogenesis takes place primarily in the liver. Pet birds fed high energy diets may develop illness associated with hepatic lipidosis. This is heightened if exercise is restricted in the bird.

As with other companion animals and humans, too much fat in the diet of a bird may result in obesity, hepatic lipidosis, congestive heart failure, diarrhea, and oily feather texture. Increased fat levels may also interfere with the absorption of other nutrients such as calcium. Low amounts of fat in the diet may lead to weight loss, reduced disease resistance, and overall poor growth, especially when coupled with restriction of other energy producing nutrients.[3,7,9]

Carbohydrates

Carbohydrates are another energy source which in birds can be converted into fat in the liver and vice versa. Glucagon is the major component of carbohydrate metabolism in birds. The result of inadequate carbohydrates in the diet is the utilization of glucogenic amino acids to manufacture carbohydrates. The process involves amino acids being shifted away from growth and production and instead utilized in glucose synthesis.[9] Carbohydrates are the only source of energy utilizable by the nervous system; therefore neurological abnormalities may indicate deficiency in a diet that is otherwise adequate in kilojoule content.[7,9]

Calcium

Calcium is an important dietary element for companion and caged birds. Calcium is essential for bone and eggshell formation. Calcium is also necessary for blood coagulation and nerve and muscle function. Remember to review the list of ingredients on the bird food label, as this will help determine if a source of calcium is included in the food. Seeds commonly contain more phosphorus than calcium. Thus, an added calcium source such as calcium carbonate, dicalcium phosphate, bone meal, ground limestone or ground oyster shells helps balance the calcium-phosphorus ratio of bird foods.

It is recommended that all birds' nutritional regimen be reviewed to insure proper amount of calcium is being fed. This is especially true for birds fed a seed diet. Calcium supplementation can be provided in the form of a cuttlebone, mineral block, crushed oyster shell, or baked crushed eggshell. Birds will eat the calcium if provided and when needed to meet physiologic demands. Cuttlebones should be placed in the cage with the soft side facing the bird. Cuttlebones are strictly a calcium source and are not beak sharpening devices.[5] It should also be noted that high phosphorus in the diet can negate adequate amounts of calcium in the diet. High phosphorous levels will interfere with calcium absorption from the intestinal tract. The calcium to phosphorus ratio for psittacine and passerine companion birds should be range from 1:1 to 2:1.[5,9] This is another reason to provide a nutritionally balanced diet as seeds, fruit, vegetables, meat are extremely calcium deficient but do have higher amounts of phosphorous. For example corn has a 1:37 ratio and muscle meat has a 1:20 ratio.[5]

Vitamins and Minerals

Vitamin requirements for companion birds are similar to those of companion mammals. The major exception is that the active form of vitamin D required by birds is vitamin D3 (cholecalciferol) as opposed to vitamin

D2 (ergocholeciferol). Vitamin C is important in specific fruit-eating species, but for the majority of passerine and psittacine species a complete and balanced diet will provide the necessary amounts of vitamin C. However, vitamin C supplementation has been suggested to assist debilitated birds as the ability to create vitamin C is reduced and the patients' requirements are greater.[7,9]

If the bird is prescribed antibiotics, the healthcare team should monitor the patient closely as vitamin deficiencies may result from the antibiotics interfering with normal intestinal microflora. Intestinal infections (e.g. giardiasis) may block vitamin absorption from the intestine (e.g. vitamin E, vitamin A). Hypervitaminosis has become an increasing problem, as clients may over-supplement formulated food or multivitamin preparations, thereby causing renal failure due to hypervitaminosis D. Hypervitaminosis A can also result in disease, especially in nectarivorous (those birds that eat the sugar rich nectar of flowering plants or the jouices of frutis) birds.[5,7,9]

Fruits and Vegetables

Fruits and vegetables are typically presented as supplementation to the pet birds' commercial diet. Fruits are made up of mainly sugars and water and thus should not be offered in excess. Fruit is a necessary part of the diet for some psittacine species such as eclectus and lories, but these are exceptions. Fruit should not be fed more than a couple of times in a seven-day period.

Companion birds receive greater nutritional benefit from vegetables as opposed to fruits. As much as possible, fresh or cooked dark green, red, and orange vegetables should be offered on a daily basis. One vegetable that should *not* be offered is comfrey. Comfrey is a green leaf herb especially popular in canary aviaries, which may to lead to liver damage. Proper husbandry suggests the healthcare team educate owners to place fruit and vegetables in a separate container and leave in cage no longer than 30 minutes. Time restriction will help decrease the likelihood of microorganism growth.[5]

References

1 Rupley AE (1997) *Manual of Avian Practice*. Philadelphia, PA: Saunders.
2 Burns KM, Renda-Francis L (2014) Birds and reptiles. In *Textbook for the Veterinary Assistant*. Ames, IA: Wiley Blackwell.
3 Kollias GV, Kollias HW (2010) Feeding passerine and psittacine birds. In MS Hand, CD Thatcher, RL Remillard *et al.* (eds), *Small Animal Clinical Nutrition* (5th edn), pp. 1255–69, Marceline, MO: Walsworth Publishing, Mark Morris Institute.
4 Orosz SE (2007) Formulated diets in avian nutrition. September 2007. http://lafebervet.com/avian-medicine-2/avian-nutrition (last accessed 12/03/2014).
5 Tully T (2009) Birds. In M Mitchell, T Tully, *Manual of Exotic Pet Practice*, pp. 250–98, St Louis MO: Saunders Elsevier.
6 Hess L (2009) The nutritional content of pet bird diets. October. http://lafebervet.com/avian-medicine-2/avian-nutrition (last accessed 12/03/2014).
7 Macwhirter P (2009) Basic anatomy, physiology, and nutrition. In T Tully, GM Dorrestein, AK Jones (eds), *Handbook of Avian Medicine* (2nd edn), pp. 25–55, St Louis MO: Saunders Elsevier.
8 Brue RN (1994) Nutrition. In B Ritchie, G Harrison, L Harrison (eds), *Avian Medicine: Principles and Application*, pp. 70–85, Lake Worth, FL: Wingers.
9 McDonald D (2006) Nutritional considerations: Section I: Nutrition and dietary supplementation. In GJ Harrison, TL Lightfoot (eds), *Clinical Avian Medicine*, Volume 1, pp. 85–107, Palm Beach, FL: Spix Publishing.

44   Small Pet Mammals

Small mammals are extremely popular pets that are brought to veterinary hospitals for advice about proper care, including nutritional management and treatment of medical disorders. As with the other species we have discussed in this book, each species of small mammal presents its own unique nutritional challenges. Nutritional management of ferrets, rabbits, guinea pigs, and other small mammals should be dependent upon lifestage, level of physical activity, and state of health. Pet parents of small mammals will need information about proper feeding to meet the needs of maintenance, growth, reproduction, or stress. Disorders may result in these mammals due to an improper diet or poor husbandry.

Nutritional management begins with assessment of the pet, the animal's food, and the method of feeding. From this assessment the healthcare team can begin to formulate a feeding plan. The nutritional assessment is similar to that performed in other species. It begins with a detailed history of the animal, a nutritional history, husbandry practices, and the animal's environment. A systematic physical examination should be performed and the BCS and pets' weight recorded. The five-point BCS system appears to be most useful in assessing the BCS in small mammals. BCS is a qualitative assessment of body fat and muscle. BCS should be performed at every visit and documented in the medical record. With small mammals' husbandry, diet, and/or disease may lead to loss of body fat and is suggestive of starvation. Excessive loss of muscle is indicative of advanced starvation, forced inactivity, or altered metabolic states.

Ferrets

Ferrets are popular pets because of their low maintenance needs, their relatively small size, and their fun inquisitive nature. Ferrets are strict carnivores that have a very short, simple gastrointestinal (GI) tract. Ferrets' GI tract lacks a cecum and ileocolic valve. Because of their shorter GI tract, ferrets' GI transit time is rapid – approximately 3–6 hours. Highly digestible foods containing large amounts of protein and fat should be offered. Also the nutritional make-up should include minimal digestible (soluble) carbohydrate and fiber.[1,2]

Ferrets are obligate carnivores, and as with other carnivorous species young ferrets imprint on food by smell and develop strong food preferences by the time they are a few months old. Consequently, ferrets should be exposed to a variety of food tastes, textures, smells. Also providing exposure to various protein sources as juveniles will assist in diet flexibility as an adult. This can be extremely helpful when ferrets experience medical conditions that may require restricted or altered diets at an older age.[3]

Foods with higher animal fat for energy, higher amounts of good-quality meat (not plant) protein, and minimal carbohydrate and fiber are recommended for ferrets. Whole-prey diets are appropriate, but owners typically do not want to feed a whole prey diet. In the United States dry kibble is commonly the diet fed to ferrets. Usually, dry foods are recommended for ferrets because they are more energy efficient, cost less, and are easier to store and feed than moist foods or whole prey diets. Healthcare team members should familiarize themselves with the ingredients listed on the package and be prepared to educate owners. The crude protein should be 30–35% DMB and composed primarily of high-quality meat sources and the fat content should be 15–20% DMB. Growing kits need 35% protein DMB and 20% fat DMB, and lactating females require 20% DMB fat and twice the calories of the nonpregnant ferret.[2]

Ferrets find commercial grocery store cat foods very palatable due to the coating on the kibble. This coating

Nutrition and Disease Management for Veterinary Technicians and Nurses, Second Edition. Ann Wortinger, Kara M. Burns
© 2015 John Wiley & Sons, Inc. Published 2015 by John Wiley & Sons, Inc.
Companion Website: www.wiley.com/go/wortinger/nutrition

is made from animal fat and digest. However, these foods may not be nutritionally adequate for the various lifestages. Minimally stressed ferrets may live on these foods for years, but nutritional deficiencies may occur especially in breeding animals.[2] Pelleted ferret food is the preferred diet, although premium dry kitten food is generally acceptable for meeting the ferret's nutritional requirements for growth and reproduction. Moist/Canned food as the major part of the diet should be avoided as ferrets most likely are not able to consume enough protein and fat on a dry matter basis (DMB).[1]

The specific amino acid requirements for ferrets are not known, but the assumption is that the requirements are similar to those of cats. It should be noted that strict carnivores need high biologic value proteins. Therefore, nutritional protein for ferrets should come from animal-based ingredients.

As discussed, ferrets do well when eating commercial foods containing 15–20% DMB fat.[2,3] Ferrets are assumed to require linoleic and arachidonic acids in their diets. Linoleic acid is abundant in vegetable oils. Arachidonic acids are found in animal-based ingredients. Fatty acid requirements should be met by providing meat-based commercial cat or mink foods.

It is believed that ferrets do not have dietary requirement for carbohydrates, including fiber, as is seen in other obligate carnivores. Glucose is provided by hepatic gluconeogenesis, using amino acids. Dietary fiber is considered to be a factor in weight control and reduction. It is also considered to play a role in certain specific GI disorders. The short digestive tract of ferrets dictates hydrolysis of most dietary fuels, with little or no hindgut fermentation of fiber. The intestinal tract of ferrets is relatively deficient in brush-border enzymes, therefore creating an inability to absorb calories from carbohydrates.[1,2] As a rule, foods with additional fiber should not be fed to healthy or lactating ferrets or young kits. Additional fiber may be considered in ferrets with fiber responsive disorders.

It is highly recommended to offer a ferret a variety of food items throughout life. This may include a minimum of weekly whole-prey foods, daily high-quality ferret kibble, and small amounts of high-quality canned cat food or other meat-based treats fed two to three times a week. This variety would be mentally enriching for the ferret. Ferrets are intelligent animals and will need environmental enrichment to keep them stimulated.

This feeding strategy would also increase the variety of the ferret's diet preferences.

Fasting a ferret for longer than 3 hours should not be recommended due to their short GI tract and the short GI transit time. In the United States, many ferrets over 2 years of age are likely to develop insulinoma. Fasting a ferret with an insulinoma for more than 3 hours could result in a serious hypoglycemic condition.[1,3,4]

Clean, fresh water should always be available. The best method for watering ferrets is with a sipper bottle or a heavy crock-type bowl. Ferrets are fun-loving animals and they especially love to play in the water, so the healthcare team must educate owners to provide bowls that are not easy to tip over.

Rabbits

Rabbits are popular pets because they are small, relatively easy to care for, fastidious, quiet mannered, and can be litter-box trained. Two pair of upper incisor teeth differentiates lagomorphs from rodents. The smaller, second upper incisors (peg teeth) are found behind the first. These peg teeth lack a cutting edge. Rabbit teeth are hypsodont. Malocclusion and overgrowth commonly occur with the incisor teeth as these can grow 10–12 cm a year during the course of the rabbits' life. Rabbit teeth are developed for a high-fiber, herbivorous diet.[1,5] Rabbits are herbivorous hindgut fermenters and have a GI system similar to horses.[6] The rabbits' GI tract consists of a noncompartmentalized stomach and a large cecum. The simple stomach has thin walls and indistinctly separated glandular and nonglandular areas. It is important to note with owners that rabbits are unable to vomit due to a well-developed cardiac sphincter.

Nutritional management of a rabbit should provide sufficient fiber to support normal GI motility as well as to ensure sufficient amounts and types of digestible nutrients are available to the cecal microflora for fermentation. Rabbits also need enrichment and thus, the diet should stimulate normal foraging behavior throughout the day (Figure 44.1).

Rabbits derive amino acids directly from the foods they ingest, as well as from cecotrophs. Essential amino acids in the rabbit include arginine, glycine, histidine, isoleucine, leucine, lysine, methionine, phenylalanine, threonine, tryptophan, and valine. Grasses tend to

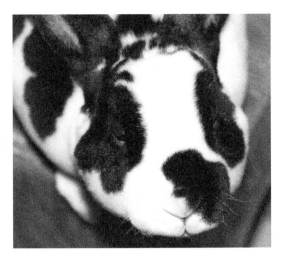

Figure 44.1 Rex Rabbit (exhibiting Broken Rex color pattern). (Reproduced with permission from Susan A. Holland. LVT, VTS (Anesthesia, Surgery))

contain limited amounts of methionine and isoleucine; however they are abundant in arginine, glutamine, and lysine. Synthetic amino acids are regularly added to commercial mixes for rabbits as these cereals are often low in methionine and lysine. Conversely legumes are high in lysine and may be used to balance low lysine levels in cereal-based diets. Rabbits have the ability to digest forage-based protein because of the increase in protein digestibility that occurs as a result of cecotrophy. An appropriate protein level for pet rabbits is 12–16% DMB. For lactating does, the level may increase to 18–19% protein DMB.

Although simple sugars and starches can be used for energy, excessive levels of these should not be fed. Lagomorphs have a rapid gut transit time resulting in starch and simple sugars not being completely digested in the small intestine. These are then directed into the cecum, where they may be used for fermentation by the cecal microorganisms. Carbohydrate overload in the cecum predisposes to enterotoxemia, especially in young animals. Low-energy grains such as oats are recommended for the rabbits' diet as opposed to corn or wheat. Care should be taken to not process the grains too finely.

Fiber is an essential nutrient for the maintenance of GI health. Fiber also helps to promote normal dental attrition and encourages normal foraging behavior, thus decreasing the potential for behavioral issues. The digestion of fiber in rabbits overall is poor; however, indigestible fiber is essential for stimulating gut motility and

helping to control gut transit time. Manufacturing processes play a role in the digestibility of commercial rabbit foods. For example, the finer the grinding, the longer the gut transit and cecal retention times which lead to greater potential for cecal dysbiosis.[5,7]

In the dietary management of rabbits balance must be established between providing enough indigestible fiber to maintain normal motility, cell regeneration, secretion, absorption, and excretion; while simultaneously providing enough digestible fiber for sufficient bacterial fermentation in the gut. The total dietary fiber levels recommended for pet rabbits is 20–25% DMB. Healthcare team members should educate owners to provide an ad libitum source of indigestible fiber (e.g., grass and/or hay). Also owners should insure the amounts of other dietary components are limited. This will insure that the rabbit actually eats the primary fiber source. Commercial foods used as a portion of the diet should preferably have a crude fiber content of >18% DMB, with indigestible fiber at >12.5% DMB.

Fat provides another source of energy and increases palatability. Fat also decreases dustiness and crumbling of commercially manufactured pellets. As with other species, rabbits are prone to obesity. Rabbits are also at risk for hepatic lipidosis. Consequently high-fat diets must be avoided. The recommended level of fat for rabbits is 2.5–4% DMB.

In the nutritional management of rabbits, vitamins A, D and E are important and should be part of the dietary make-up. Gut bacteria synthesize B vitamins in sufficient quantities. So, adding B vitamins to commercial foods may be unnecessary. Vitamin K synthesis in the gut is not as efficient. Therefore vitamin K is often added to the commercial formulation by the rabbit food manufacturer. Vitamins A and E are readily destroyed by oxidation, so it is imperative that food preparation and storage methods prevent losses from excess light or heat. The recommendation is to store rabbit feed at 15°C (60°F) and feed within 90 days of milling.[8] If the food is comprised of more than 30% alfalfa meal there should be sufficient vitamin A in the form of the precursor b-carotene. However, if the alfalfa is over a year post harvest, vitamin A deficiency can occur. Vitamin recommendations for pet rabbits include:[1,9]

• 7000 to 18,000 IU vitamin A/kg food;
• 40–70 mg vitamin E/kg food;
• 2 mg vitamin K/kg food.

Calcium regulation and vitamin D's role differs in rabbits than in other species. The presence of vitamin D is not required for the intestinal absorption of calcium. Vitamin D is important for the metabolism of phosphorus. Vitamin D deficiencies can lead to hypophosphatemia and osteomalacia[1,5,9]. Husbandry education should include cage placement as sunlight is necessary for endogenous synthesis of vitamin D in rabbits. Commercially prepared rabbit pellets are supplemented with vitamin D. For pet rabbits, a level of 800 to 1200 IU/kg is recommended.[1,9]

Guinea Pigs

Guinea pigs are herbivores with simple stomachs. The teeth of guinea pigs are open-rooted and erupt continuously. Unlike other rodents which typically have yellow incisors, a distinguishing factor of guinea pigs is white incisors. The guinea pig digestive tract is long and has a gastric emptying time of roughly two hours. The total GI transit time ranges from 8 to 20 hours. The normal flora found in the GI tract includes mainly lactobacillus and occasionally Streptococcus spp., yeast, and soil bacteria. The majority of the digestive process happens in the cecum. The cecum of a guinea pig is a thin-walled sac divided into several lateral pouches by smooth muscle bands (taenia coli). The cecum is normally found on the central and left side of the abdomen and may contain as much as 65% of the GI contents.[1,10] Guinea pigs exhibit coprophagous behavior, a fact which is important to educate owners (Figures 44.2 and 44.3).

Guinea pigs do not like change. Guinea pigs develop dietary preferences early in life, and do not adjust readily to changes in type, appearance, or presentation of their food or water. Guinea pig owners are encouraged to expose their pets to small amounts of different foods and vegetables while they are young. This will help the guinea pig accept variety in their feedstuffs. This reluctance to change can be a dangerous characteristic of guinea pigs; thus it is important to educate owners to be cognizant of this fact and to gradually transition guinea pigs if introducing something new in the diet. Client education will hopefully prevent a self-imposed fast by a pet guinea pig that is fed new food.

A crude protein level of 18–20% DMB is sufficient for growth and lactation. The recommended minimum level of crude fiber is 10% DMB.

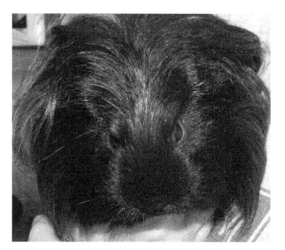

Figure 44.2 Silkie breed of Cavy. (Reproduced with permission from Susan A. Holland. LVT, VTS (Anesthesia, Surgery).)

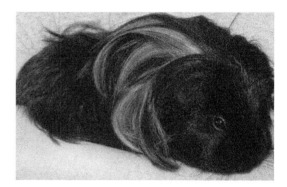

Figure 44.3 Silkie breed of Cavy – young adult.

Guinea pigs require a dietary source of vitamin C (ascorbic acid) because they lack the enzyme involved in synthesizing glucose to ascorbic acid. This enzyme is l-gulonolactone oxidase. Nonbreeding adult guinea pigs require 10 mg/kg daily of ascorbic acid with higher levels needed for growing and pregnant animals; 30 mg/kg daily is recommended during pregnancy.

The recommended diet for pet guinea pigs consists of guinea pig pellets and grass hay, supplemented with fresh vegetables.[11] Good-quality grass hay should be available at all times. A variety of leafy greens can be offered in handfuls, as guinea pigs like greens. Remember to advise owners to wash and prepare fresh foods. Also it is important to advise owners that fresh foods should not be left in the cage and should be removed after a few hours if not eaten. Fruits, rolled oats, and dry cereals should be offered only in very small quantities, if at all, as treats.[1,10,11] Any additions or changes to the diet should be made gradually.

Commercially prepared guinea pig foods typically contain 18–20% DMB crude protein and 10–16% DMB fiber. Pellets are fortified with ascorbic acid; but almost half of the initial vitamin C content may be oxidized and lost 90 days after the diet has been mixed and stored at 22°C. Many commercially prepared guinea pig diets are now available with stabilized vitamin C and these diets should be stored in a cool, dry area (<70°F (22°C)). Foods can be refrigerated or frozen but should be protected from condensation and increased storage temperature and humidity in vegetables and fruits or in the drinking water. Foods with higher levels of ascorbic acid are:

* red and green peppers;
* broccoli;
* tomatoes;
* kiwi fruit;
* oranges.

Many types of leafy greens (kale, parsley, beet greens, chicory, spinach) are high in vitamin C, but many contain high levels of calcium or oxalates; these should be offered in only small amounts. Vitamin C can be added to the water at 1 g/L. In an open container, water with added vitamin C loses more than 50% of its vitamin C content in 24 hours. Water must be changed daily to ensure adequate activity of the vitamin.

Other Small Mammals

Hamsters, gerbils, mice, and rats naturally hoard food items. Therefore it is difficult to determine truly how much food is actually being ingested. Education of owners must include information on the natural hoarding tendencies of rodents. Although owners need to be aware when the food dish of these small mammals is empty; consistently filling the bowl may result in obese small mammals.

Most rodents are omnivorous, often eating grasses, seeds, grain, and occasionally invertebrates in the wild.[12,13] Dietary requirements of species in laboratory settings are well established. However, for pet small mammals, needs are best met with a formulated diet supplemented with small amounts of fresh foods and seeds for variety and interest. Seed mixtures are popular choices for small mammals; however, seed mixtures regularly lead to selective feeding. A nutritional imbalance can result from small mammals eating high-calorie seeds (sunflower) while ignoring the formulated pellets. Many rodents have a short life span so determining a nutritional deficiency is rare. The most common form of malnutrition in rats is obesity. Studies show an increase in length of life as well as a decrease in certain disease conditions in rats fed a calorie-restricted diet.[14] Gerbils exhibit sensitivity to high fat, high cholesterol diets resulting in changes in the gerbils' levels of blood cholesterol.

Protein requirements for rodents range from 14% to 17% DMB in hamsters, from 14% to 16% DMB in rats and mice, and up to 22% DMB in gerbils.[12,13] Nutritional management of hamsters, rats, mice, and gerbils should insure these ranges are followed. Nutritional management of reproducing small mammals should contain higher levels of protein.

As with other species water is extremely important and should be discussed with small mammal owners. Fresh, clean water should be provided. Typically water bottles are used as these help prevent bedding from getting wet and are often preferred by small mammals. However, with time water bottles may become clogged or start to leak. It is best for the healthcare team to educate owners to change water and test water bottles every day.

References

1 James W, Carpenter JW, Wolf KN, Kolmstetter C (2010) Feeding small pet mammals. In MS Hand, CD Thatcher, RL Remillard *et al.* (eds), *Small Animal Clinical Nutrition* (5th edn), pp. 1215–36, Marceline, MO: Walsworth Publishing, Mark Morris Institute.

2 Bell JA (1999) Ferret nutrition. *Vet Clin North Am Exot Anim Pract* **2**: 169–92.

3 Powers LV, Brown SA (2012) Basic anatomy, physiology, and husbandry. In K Quesenberry, J Carpenter (eds), *Ferrets, Rabbits, and Rodents* (3rd edn), pp. 340–53, St Louis, MO: Saunders.

4 Wolf TM (2008) Ferrets. In M Mitchell, T Tully (eds), *Manual of Exotic Pet Practice*, pp. 346–75, St Louis, MO; W.B. Saunders.

5 Campbell-Ward ML (2012) Gastrointestinal physiology and nutrition. In K Quesenberry, J Carpenter (eds), *Ferrets, Rabbits, and Rodents* (3rd edn), pp. 232–44, St Louis, MO; Saunders.

6 Cheeke PR (1994) Nutrition and nutritional diseases. In PJ Manning, DH Ringler, CE Newcomer (eds), *The Biology of the Laboratory Rabbit* (2nd edn), pp. 321–35, New York: Academic Press.

7 Pinheiro V, Guedes CM, Outor-Monteiro D *et al.* (2009) Effects of fibre level and dietary mannanoligosaccharides on digestibility, caecal volatile fatty acids and performances of growing rabbits. *Anim Feed Sci Tech* **148**: 288–300.

8 Brooks DL (2004) Nutrition and gastrointestinal physiology. In KE Quesenberry, JW Carpenter (eds), *Ferrets, Rabbits and Rodents: Clinical Medicine and Surgery* (2nd edn), pp. 155–60, St Louis, MO: W.B. Saunders,

9 Harcourt-Brown FM (2002) *Textbook of Rabbit Medicine*, Edinburgh: Butterworth-Heinemann.

10 Quesenberry KE, Donnelly TM, Mans C (2012) Biology, husbandry, and clinical techniques of guinea pigs and chinchillas. In K Quesenberry, J Carpenter (eds), *Ferrets, Rabbits, and Rodents* (3rd edn), pp. 280–94, St Louis, MO; Saunders.

11 Riggs SM (2008) Guinea pigs. In M Mitchell, T Tully (eds), *Manual of Exotic Pet Practice*, pp. 457–74, St Louis, MO; W.B. Saunders.

12 Lennox AM, Bauck L (2012) Basic anatomy, physiology, husbandry, and clinical techniques. In K Quesenberry, J Carpenter (eds), *Ferrets, Rabbits, and Rodents* (3rd edn), pp. 340–53, St Louis, MO; Saunders.

13 Keeble E (2009). Rodents: biology and husbandry. In E Keeble, A Meredith (eds), *BSAVA Manual of Rodents and Ferrets*, pp. 1–17, Gloucester, UK: British Small Animal Veterinary Association.

14 Masoro EJ (2009) Caloric restriction-induced life extension of rats and mice: A critique of proposed mechanisms. *Biochim Biophys Acta* **1790**(**10**): 1040–8.

45 Equine

Feeding the precise amount and finding the correct balance of nutrients is important to the overall health and well-being of horses. Today, horses are domesticated and considered companion animals. Companion horses today consume a variety of feeds ranging in physical form, from forage with a high content of moisture to cereals with a high amount of starch; and from hay in the form of physically long fibrous stems to salt licks and water. Horses are nonruminant herbivores that naturally spend 60 to 75% of their day grazing. Typically they ingest approximately 2% of their body weight (dry matter basis) per day while grazing (Figure 45.1).[1–7]

Domesticating horses has resulted in adaptations in feed, feeding times, and feeding methods – similar to domesticated cats and dogs – where the horse is "meal fed" and materials such as starchy cereals, protein concentrates, and dried forages have been introduced. Companion horses are confined more of the time in stalls or smaller pastures, are typically fed only 1–2 times per day, and spend less time of the day (approximately 40%) eating.

The diets formulated for horses contain on average 5% fat and 7–12% protein, with carbohydrate being the major source of energy (~80%). This is a result of the evolution of horses to eating grass and other forages. Grasses and hays provide a strong foundation for the feeding of horses. Protein is essential to the maintenance and replacement of tissues but is sometimes considered to be an expensive source of energy; however, dietary protein and fat can contribute to meeting the physiological energy demands of the horse. Protein converts the carbon chain of amino acids to intermediary acids and some of the carbon chains to glucose. Fat can aid in meeting energy demands following its hydrolysis to glycerol and fatty acids. Subsequently, the glycerol can be converted to glucose and the fatty acid chain can be broken down by a stepwise process called ß oxidation in

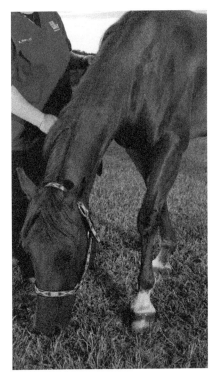

Figure 45.1 American quarter horse grazing.

the mitochondria which yields adenosine triphosphate (ATP) and acetate or acetyl coenzyme A and requiring tissue oxygen.[1–7]

Carbohydrate digestion and fermentation yield mostly glucose and acetic, propionic, and butyric volatile fatty acids. The portal venous system collects these nutrients and a proportion of them are removed from the blood as they pass through the liver. Both propionate and glucose contribute to glycogen (liver starch) reserves and acetate and butyrate bolster the fat pool and comprise primary energy sources for many tissues.

Nutrition and Disease Management for Veterinary Technicians and Nurses, Second Edition. Ann Wortinger, Kara M. Burns
© 2015 John Wiley & Sons, Inc. Published 2015 by John Wiley & Sons, Inc.
Companion Website: www.wiley.com/go/wortinger/nutrition

Nutritional Physiology

Multiple compartments make up the digestive tract of the horse and therefore, the nutritional physiology of cats and dogs differs significantly from that of the horse. Each compartment has its own function in terms of utilizing ingested feed. The oral cavity is responsible for physically processing foods into smaller particles (~1.6 mm). This allows for passage through the esophagus and increases the surface area for the small intestine enzymatic action. The oral cavity also breaks down structural carbohydrate for bacterial fermentation in the large intestine. Horses chew an average of 60,000 times per day. It is only during chewing that the salivation process is activated. Given the increased chewing in the equine species, a horse will average 5–10 liters per day of saliva, which in turn acts as a lubricant for passage into the esophagus.[3−5]

The stomach is responsible for ~8% of the total capacity of the equine GI tract. The stomach's retention time can range from 2 to 18 hours. The fundus and the pylorus are the two main regions making up the stomach. The pyloric region secretes 10–30 liters of gastric juice per day. The small intestine of the horse measures 50–70 feet long and has a volume of 40–50 liters. The transit time of the small intestine averages 2–8 hours. Toward the anterior end of the small intestine, pancreatic juice aids in the digestion of lipids, protein, and nonstructural carbohydrates. Microvilli line the small intestine thus increasing the surface area of the gut. As mentioned earlier, digestion in the small intestine is dependent upon oral processing and types of feed (e.g., forage is less digested than processed feed). The large intestine has the ability to hold large volume (100 liters) and has a very slow transit time of approximately 50 hours.[1] The large intestine is responsible for the fermentation of structural carbohydrates to volatile fatty acids which are responsible for 50% of the metabolizable energy. Additionally, the large intestine absorbs roughly 80 liters of water per day. B vitamins are produced by the bacteria absorbed in the large intestine. Nonprotein nitrogen is not utilized well in the large intestine.

Key Nutritional Factors for Horses

Water, energy, protein, minerals, and vitamins are the main nutrients with which veterinary healthcare teams should be concerned. Water is the most important nutrient in any mammalian species. Fresh, abundant water should be available at all times. Horses drink an average of 25 liters of water per day. In conditions of extreme heat or stress the number of liters a horse will drink per day increases to 100. In addition, healthcare team members should remind owners that the more grain their horse ingests the more water intake the horse will need.

Energy is measured in terms of digestible energy (DE) and fed in kilocalories. The amount of DE horses need, will be dependent upon various factors; physiologic state, activity level, environment, and the size of the individual horse. The majority of energy utilized by the horse is from carbohydrates that are ingested through the horses' natural feed. The amount of kcal/kg in various carbohydrate feeds is shown as follows:

Feed kcal/kg	
Oats	3000
Alfalfa (early bloom)	2100
Bermuda grass hay	1800
Corn cobs	1250

As with other species fat in the diet provides the horse with high density energy. Nevertheless, fat should not exceed 20% of the total equine diet or 30% of concentrate. Surpassing these levels puts the horse at risk for loose stools and most likely will result in decreased palatability.

The amount of protein in the diet is generally expressed as "crude protein (CP)" and is communicated as % dry matter (DM). Again the amount of protein needed by an individual horse is dependent upon many factors including physiologic state, type of diet, age, quality of diet, etc. The protein quality increases the closer the proportions of each of the various indispensable amino acids in the dietary protein conform to the proportions in the mixture required by the tissues.[3−5]

Calcium and phosphorous are considered together because of their interdependent role as the main elements of the crystal apatite, which provides the building blocks for the skeletal system. The physiologic state of the horse will aid in predicting the calcium requirement of the individual horse. The average adult horse weighing approximately 500 kg will need ~20 g of calcium and 14 g of phosphorous per day. It is important to balance the ratio of calcium to phosphorous with a mature horse needing a ratio of 1.1:1 to 6:1. The ratio for a growing horse is recommended to be 1.1:1 to 3:1.

Sodium is the principal determinant of the osmolarity of extracellular fluid and as a result, the volume of that fluid. Chloride concentration in the extracellular fluid is directly related to that of sodium. Rarely do companion animals have an excess or deficiency of sodium or chloride; however, these are both conditions of which to be watchful. Daily sodium requirements are recommended to be approximately 0.18–0.36% DM. If the requirements for sodium are met, a chloride deficiency is rare. Good sources of sodium and chloride can be found in grains with premixture and salt blocks.

Potassium is the main intracellular cation. Deficiencies in equines are rare; excess potassium is not a common problem. However, excess potassium can lead to hyperkalaemic periodic paralysis, a syndrome of intermittent weakness in horses accompanied by elevated serum potassium concentration. This syndrome appears to be confined to descendants of the American Quarter Horse. Forages are approximately 1–4% potassium. Cereals are relatively poor sources of potassium.

A trace element needed to aid in antioxidant defense in horses is known as selenium. Selenium forms an integral part of the GSH-Px molecule and catalyses peroxide detoxification in body tissues at which time reduced glutathione (GSH) is oxidized. It is closely involved with the activity of α-tocopherol (vitamin E), which protects polyunsaturated fatty acids from peridoxication. The requirement is 1–2 mg/day for a 500 kg horse or 0.1–2 ppm. Selenium deficiencies produce pale, weak muscles in foals and a yellowing of the depot fat, known as "White Muscle Disease." It is imperative that pregnant mares receive adequate amounts of selenium in their diet. Selenium is highly toxic to animals, with the minimum toxic dose through continuous intake is 2–5 mg/kg feed. Too much selenium results in skin, coat, and hoof abnormalities.[3–5]

Grazing horses derive their vitamin A from the carotenoid pigments present in herbage. The principal one is β-carotene with 1 mg of β-carotene equating to approximately 400 IU of vitamin A. Horses that graze for 4–6 weeks build up a 3–6 month supply of vitamin A in the liver.

Carotene levels (mg/kg DM) amounts

Pasture grass/alfalfa	300–600
Good hay	20–40
Poor hay	4–5

Requirements for vitamin A during certain lifestages are as follows:
- Mature horses require 30 IU/kg body weight.
- Gestation/lactation stage requires 60 IU/kg body weight.
- Growth stage requires ~50 IU/kg body weight.

Vitamin E functions as a cellular antioxidant in conjunction with vitamin A and is required for normal immune function. Fresh green forage and the germ of cereal grains are rich sources of vitamin E. Adult horses require 80–100 IU/kg DM. Although deficiencies are rare, two neurological disorders of horses have been recognized to involve α-tocopherol status: equine degenerative myeloencephalopathy and equine motor neuron disease. These diseases typically are seen in horses that do not have access to pastures, with the consumption of poor quality hay, and in horses with low concentrations of circulating levels of α-tocopherol.

Types of Feed

There are three types of feed that are commonly used in the feeding of horses; roughages, concentrates, and complete feeds. Roughages include grasses and forage legumes cut for hay. Most common species of grass are suitable, but the preferred are the more popular and productive grasses such as rye grasses, fescues, timothy, and cocksfoot. Other grasses found in permanent pastures are acceptable as well and include; meadow grasses, brome, bent grass, and foxtails. Legumes utilized are: red, white, alsike, and crimson clovers and trefoils; lucerne; and sainfoin. Roughages are relatively low in energy and have >18% crude fiber. Roughages are considered to be the foundation to an equine feeding program. Quality hay can provide energy for the maintenance requirements of the horse. Legumes and nonlegume grasses that are well managed and fertilized (proteinaceous roughages) provide >10% CP as opposed to carbonaceous grasses (those that are

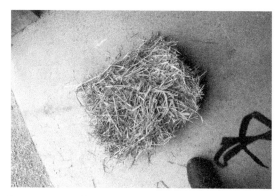

Figure 45.2 Roughage that meets quality criteria. (Reprinted with permission from L Lien, S Loly, S Ferguson (eds), *Large Animal Medicine for Veterinary Technicians* (2014). John Wiley & Sons, Inc.)

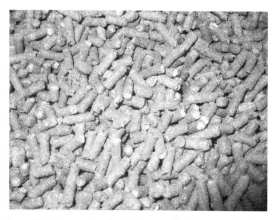

Figure 45.3 A complete feed. (Reprinted with permission from L Lien, S Loly, S Ferguson (eds), *Large Animal Medicine for Veterinary Technicians* (2014). John Wiley & Sons, Inc.)

not well maintained or fertilized) provide <10% CP. It is important that the healthcare team educate clients on the features of satisfactory roughage including the following:

- mold free;
- tactile softness and flexibility;
- leafy with fine stems (2/3E, ¾ protein);
- pleasing, fragrant aroma;
- bright green with no brown or yellow.

It is also important to educate owners that additional handling of roughages can result in loss of:

- ¼ of the leaves;
- ¼ to 1/3 energy and protein;
- 90% of β-carotene.

(See Figure 45.2.)

Concentrates are typically a cereal grain that may or may not have supplemented protein, minerals, and vitamins. Concentrates are high in energy (typically 50% greater than forage), and are less than 18% crude fiber. Oftentimes, concentrates are used as a supplement if forage is insufficient in nutrients – especially energy and protein. Concentrates are needed more often in certain lifestages such as gestation (especially later in the gestation period), lactation, growth, and in work horses. As a rule it is best to not exceed 50:50 (wt:wt) concentrate to roughage. Anything new should be introduced and transitioned slowly. It is important for healthcare team members and owners alike to remember that concentrates are energy dense, especially compared to roughages; therefore, excess concentrate may lead to

laminitis, rhabdomyolysis, developmental orthopedic disease, and obesity.

Complete feeds are typically a mixture of roughage and concentrate – usually an 80% roughage to 20% concentrate mixture. Complete feeds are manufactured by completely grinding the food and formulating it into a pellet, thus making it easier (all in one) for the owner at the same time as potential increase cost for the convenience. Because the complete feed is pelleted or wafered, care must be given to the potential risks associated with inadequate particle size, including; colic, choking risk, wood chewing, coprophagy, to name a few (Figure 45.3).

Healthcare team members must discuss the need for fresh, clean water to be available at all times when discussing nutritional management of horses with clients. Energy for maintenance can be met completely with quality hay. However, owners may supplement with concentrate if necessary. It is imperative that the horse is not supplemented in excess of 50% by weight with concentrate. Adequate amounts of vitamins A & E are supplied through good quality green roughage. Nutrition is the foundation for good health and affects every horse; thus nutrition should be discussed with every visit.

Pediatric Equine Nutrition and Care

The objective of a feeding plan for foals and young horses is to create a healthy animal which will lead to a healthy adult horse. The specific objectives of a feeding plan for a young horse are to achieve healthy growth, optimize trainability and immune function, and minimize obesity and developmental orthopedic disease. Growth is a complex process involving interactions between genetics, nutrition, and other environmental influences. Nutrition plays a role in the health and development of growing horses and directly affects the immune system body composition, growth rate, and skeletal development.

Foals should be assessed for risk factors before weaning to allow implementation of recommendations for appropriate nutrition. A thorough history and physical evaluation are necessary. Additionally, body condition scores (BCS) provide valuable information about nutritional risks. Growth rates of young horses are affected by the energy density of the food and the amount of food fed. It is important that horses be fed to grow at an optimal rate for physiologic development and body condition rather than at a maximal rate.[8]

Nutritional requirements and dietary composition of the foal change markedly from the time they are transitioned from neonate to weanling. The foal is transitioning from a continuous supply of nutrients from the dam in utero to sporadic absorption of ingested nutrients post birth. Concurrently, the neonate's metabolism no longer is dependent upon the maternal glucose concentration to maintain normal glucose levels, and the pancreas initiates the regulation of glucose homeostasis. This alteration in energy metabolism is dramatic and does not always occur smoothly, leading to limited energy reserves (glycogen and fat) in the neonatal foal. Even in the "normal" neonatal foal hypoglycemia occurs frequently and veterinary healthcare teams must be aware of this fact. In the sick foal, severe hypoglycemia will result if the foal is deprived of energy for even a short period of time.[1,9,10]

The neonatal foal has a high metabolic rate and thus frequent ingestion of high volumes of milk to meet its energy requirements for maintenance and growth are needed. During the first week to months of foals' life, calorie needs are as follows:

- First week ~150 kcal/kg/day
- Three weeks ~120 kcal/kg/day
- One to two months ~80 to 100 kcal/kg/day

Healthy foals less than seven days old will nurse approximately 7 times per hour for approximately 1–2 minutes a time. After 7 days, there is a decrease in the number of times a foal will nurse, but conversely there is an increase in the duration of time nursing. The mare's milk averages about 64% sugar (as lactose), 22% protein, and 13% fat. Thus the main energy source of energy for the foal is glucose.[9–12]

After the first 24 hours, foals will start to eat small amounts of hay, grass, and grain along with the mare's feces. It is understood that the feces provide the initial microbial flora needed by the foal to aid in the digestion of the hay, grass, and grain. Until several weeks of age, the roughage and grain are not well digested by the foal. It is at this time that transitioning from weaning (milk based diet) to a forage based diet is gradually occurring. The milk amount produced by the mare peaks after approximately 2 months of lactation and then the amount of milk produced begins to decline. Shortly thereafter the foal will be weaned from the mare and rely on solid feed for an increasing proportion of its nutritional requirements. Maturation of hindgut function is complete around 3 or 4 months of age.

Energy Requirement

The energy requirement of growing horses is determined through calculating the total energy required for maintenance in addition to the energy required for growth or gain. The daily energy requirement (DER) is dependent upon a number of factors; the environment, the foal's age, the desired average daily gain (ADG), and individual characteristics with the specific foal. The individual characteristics healthcare team members must take into account when calculating the daily energy requirement include metabolic and health characteristics. The optimal growth rate for horses has yet to have been determined; therefore it is difficult to determine the exact energy requirement. If horses grow too quickly and too much weight is added skeletal integrity and longevity may be adversely affected. On the other hand, inadequate energy intake will result in poor and slower growth rates and young horses will look unhealthy. Most nutritionists and equine specialists will follow the formula recommended by the National Research Council (NRC). This formula calculates the daily energy requirement of growing horses in the following manner:

DE (Mcal/day) = (56.5x − 0.145) × BW

$$+ (1.99 + 1.21x - 0.021 \times 2) \times ADG$$

(x is age in months; ADG is average daily gain;

BW is body weight in kilograms)

The majority of horse owners will feed to achieve ADG of 1.1–1.4 kg/day and with some owners aiming slightly higher. Veterinary healthcare teams and owners must be aware of what feed is being fed, how much is being fed, other feedstuffs that are being added to the diet, etc., as well as the energy concentration for total diets consumed. The team must perform a nutritional assessment prior to beginning a feeding plan and on every subsequent patient visit (whether farm visit or hospital visit). The average energy concentration for the total amount of feed (on an as-fed basis) given to a growing horse can range from 2.5 Mcal/kg with diets consisting of 70% concentrate to 30% hay ratio to 0.72 Mcal/kg for certain pasture fed growing horses. Young horses have been found to gain enough energy from pasture feeding to sustain adequate growth. Many factors must be taken into consideration whether the horse is pasture fed or concentrate and roughage fed. These factors would include the forage type and quality (if pasture fed), training level of the young horse, environmental conditions, body condition, and health of the growing horse. Again, the feed or pasture will also need to be evaluated for protein level, protein quality, vitamin and mineral level, etc. Any and all of these factors will influence the desired rate of growth in young horses. Restrictions in protein have a direct correlation to restrictions in the growth rate of a young horse.

Crude protein requirements for the growing horse can be calculated using the following equation:

CP requirement = (BW × 1.44g CP/kg BW)

$$+((ADG \times 0.20)/E)/0.79$$

The E in the equation represents the efficiency of the use of dietary protein. Estimates from the NRC for the efficiency of use of dietary protein in the young horse are as follows:

- ~50% for 4–6 month old horses;
- ~45% for 7–8 month old horses;
- ~40% for 9–10 month old horses;
- ~35% for 11 month old horses;
- ~30% for 12 month and older horses.

It is important also to remember the quality of protein, as defined by amino acid composition, also plays a huge role in the growing horse; and poor quality protein sources can have significant effects on growing horses. Also, inadequate amounts of dietary energy will be consumed if the feed is too low in either digestible energy or protein, even though plenty of feed may be available. Thus growth rate in the young horse will decrease if inadequate intake of dietary energy or protein occurs. A slower growth rate has the potential to mask other nutritional deficiencies, and if slowed significantly may reduce the body size of the horse at maturation. At a fast growth rate, a deficiency in minerals may result. If a deficiency of calcium, phosphorous, zinc, or copper occurs, developmental orthopedic disease may result. Conversely, if the young horse has too high dietary protein and energy intake, a rapid growth rate may occur, increasing the risk of developmental orthopedic disease and obesity.[9–12]

When feeding the young horse from nursing to maturity, fresh, clean water should be available at all times. Oftentimes busy veterinary healthcare team members forget to mention the importance of this key nutrient.

The weight of growing horses should be obtained by owners as often as possible (bi-weekly is recommended). This can be accomplished through the use of a weight tape if scales are not available. Also the healthcare team and the owner should record body weight and food intake. A BCS should be obtained at least every two weeks. This level of attention to BCS is important to the development of a healthy growing horse. Also, routinely assessing body condition delivers immediate feedback about optimal nutritional. This will prepare the owner to continue these observations throughout the life of the horse. Routine BCS will monitor horses throughout their lifespan, and should result in fewer skeletal diseases, overweight or obesity, and many other related problems. Veterinary healthcare team members should reassess growing horses during farm calls and work in conjunction with the owners observations to detect the potential or occurrence of under- or overnutrition. Reexamination should include body weight and body condition scoring, nutritional assessment, and determination of correct feed amount calculations.

References

1 Burns KM (2014) Nutrition. In L Lien, S Loly, S Ferguson (eds), *Large Animal Internal Medicine for Veterinary Technicians*, pp. 107–44, Ames, IA: Wiley Blackwell.

2 Davies Z (2009) *Introduction to Horse Nutrition*, Ames, IA: Wiley-Blackwell.

3 Frape D (2010) *Equine Nutrition and Feeding* (4rd edn), Ames, IA: Wiley-Blackwell.

4 Geor R (2009) *Equine Nutrition, Veterinary Clinics of North America: Equine Practice*, St Louis, MO: Elsevier/Saunders.

5 Pilliner S (2009) *Horse Nutrition and Feeding* (2nd edn), Ames, IA: Wiley-Blackwell.

6 Reed S, Bayly WM, Sellon DC, *et al.* (2009) *Equine Internal Medicine*. St Louis, MO: Elsevier/Saunders.

7 Reeder D, Miller S, Wilfong D, *et al.* (2009) *AAEVT's Equine Manual for Veterinary Technicians*, Ames, IA: Wiley-Blackwell.

8 Burns KM (2011) Equine nutrition. *Canadian Veterinary Technician*. Fall, **3**(**4**).

9 Lewis LD (1996) Growing horse feeding and care. In *Feeding and Care of the Horse* (2nd edn), pp. 264–76, Media, PA: Williams & Wilkins.

10 Lewis LD (1995) Growing horse feeding and care. In *Equine Clinical Nutrition: Feeding and Care*, pp. 334–52, Baltimore: Williams & Wilkins.

11 Geor RJ (2010) Aspects of clinical nutrition. In SM Reed, WM Bayly, DC Sellon (eds), *Equine Internal Medicine* (3rd edn), pp. 205–32, St Louis, MO: Saunders Elsevier.

12 Gordon MB, Young JK, Davison KE, Raub RH (2009) Equine nutrition. In D Reeder, S Miller, D Wilfong, *et al.* (eds), *Equine Manual for Veterinary Technicians*, pp. 11–46, Ames, IA: Wiley-Blackwell.

Index

Locators in *italic* refer to figures and tables

A

AAFCO. *see* American Association of Feed Control Officials
AAHA (American Animal Health Association), 71
acidemia, 173–4
ad lib feeding regimens, dogs and cats, *94*, 95–6, *96*
adaptations, cats, 140–3. *see also* evolution
adaptive thermogenesis, 44
additives and preservatives, 80–4, *82*, *83*
   nutrition myths, 145–6
   preservation methods, *80*
   see also antioxidants
adenosine triphosphate (ATP), 3, 29, 134
adipose tissue, 180. *see also* obesity
adult maintenance
   cats, *46*, *119*, 124–7, *126*
   dogs, *46*, 105, 114, 116, *117*, 121–3, *122*, *123*
   feeding trials, 66
   homemade diets, 85
   pet food labels, 63
adverse food reactions, 193, *193*, 194, 195, 196
African wild cat (*Felis silvestris libyca*), 76, 141
aging dog and cats, *128*, 128–32, *131*, 212
Agronomy Guide, Penn State, 147
alkalemia, 173–4
allergies, 193, *193*, 194, 195, 196
alpha-linoleic acid, 17–18, *18*, 72, 108, *229*
alpha-S1 casein, cow's milk, 188
alpha-tocopherol, 81, 146. *see also* vitamin E
American Animal Health Association (AAHA), 71
American Association of Feed Control Officials (AAFCO)
   adult maintenance in cats, 124
   adult maintenance in dogs, 121
   feeding trials, 4, *5*, 145
   growth in dogs, 113–14
   meat by-products, 144
   pet food labels, 59, 63
   regulation of commercial pet foods, 56–8, 76
American quarter horse, *240*
American Veterinary Medical Association (AVMA), 6
amino acids, essential and nonessential, 20, *20*. *see also*
   proteins/amino acids
ammonia toxicity, cats, 142
anabolic reactions, 3
anatomic adaptations, cats, 140
antimicrobial additives and preservatives, 82, *83*
antioxidants, 80–2, *82*, *83*, 83
   cancer patients, 205–6

geriatric dog and cats, 129, 131
   horses, 242
   nutrition myths, 145–6
   performance in dogs, 136
arachidonic acid, 17–18, *18*, 72, 87
arginine, 141, 142, 204, 205, *205*, *229*
ascorbic acid (vitamin C), 24, 31, 81, *82*, 146
assessment, veterinary
   developmental orthopedic diseases, 220–1
   homemade diets, 88–9
   nutritional management of illness, 150–1
   obesity, 180–1, *182*
assisted feeding, *161*, *164*, *165*
   complications, 162–5
   enteral feeding tubes, 157–61, *158*, *159*
Association of American Feed Control Officials. *see* American
   Association of Feed Control Officials
athletes, canine. *see* performance in dogs
ATP (adenosine triphosphate), 3, 29, 134
automated timed feeder, *98*. *see also* time-controlled-feeding
avian species (birds), 227–33, *228*, *229*, *230*, *231*
AVMA (American Veterinary Medical Association), 6

B

B-complex vitamins, 24, 27–31, 143, *229*
Bacillus cereus, 82
bacterial contamination in food, 77. *see also* infection
balanced food, 63
   definition, 59
   feeding regimens, 94
   moist pet foods, 74
   pregnancy and lactation in dogs, 103
   raw food diets, 76–7
BARF (biologically appropriate raw food), 74, 78. *see also* raw food
basal energy requirement (BER), 43
Baylisascaris proconis, 78
BCS. *see* body condition scoring
behaviors, feeding
   begging behavior, 95, 96, 97, 98
   cats, 139
Bennett, F. H., 55
beta-carotene. *see* carotenoids
BHA (butylated hydroxyanisole), 81, *82*, 146
BHT (butylated hydroxytoluene), 81, *82*, 146
bile salts, 40
bioflavonoids, 32
biologic value, corn, 147–8
biologically appropriate raw food. *see* BARF

Nutrition and Disease Management for Veterinary Technicians and Nurses, Second Edition. Ann Wortinger, Kara M. Burns
© 2015 John Wiley & Sons, Inc. Published 2015 by John Wiley & Sons, Inc.
Companion Website: www.wiley.com/go/wortinger/nutrition